CANCER
Principles & Practice of Oncology:

Handbook of Clinical Cancer Genetics

Ellen T. Matloff, MS

Research Scientist, Department of Genetics
Director, Cancer Genetic Counseling
Yale Cancer Center
New Haven, Connecticut

Wolters Kluwer | Lippincott Williams & Wilkins
Health

Philadelphia • Baltimore • New York • London
Buenos Aires • Hong Kong • Sydney • Tokyo

Senior Executive Editor: Jonathan W. Pine, Jr.
Senior Product Manager: Emilie Moyer
Vendor Manager: Alicia Jackson
Marketing Manager: Alexander Burns
Senior Designer: Stephen Druding
Production Service: Aptara Corp.

Chapters 2–15 of this book were originally published in *The Cancer Journal: The Journal of Principles and Practice of Oncology* Volume 18, Number 4, July/August 2012, edited by Vincent T. DeVita, Jr., Theodore S. Lawrence, and Steven A. Rosenberg, and published by Lippincott Williams & Wilkins.
Chapter 1 was originally published in *DeVita, Hellman, and Rosenberg's Cancer: Principles and Practice of Oncology,* 9th edition, edited by Vincent T. DeVita, Jr., Theodore S. Lawrence, and Steven A. Rosenberg, and published by Lippincott Williams & Wilkins, copyright 2011.

Printed in China

Library of Congress Cataloging-in-Publication Data available upon request

ISBN 978-1-4511-9098-4

Care has been taken to confirm the accuracy of the information presented and to describe generally accepted practices. However, the authors, editors, and publisher are not responsible for errors or omissions or for any consequences from application of the information in this book and make no warranty, expressed or implied, with respect to the currency, completeness, or accuracy of the contents of the publication. Application of the information in a particular situation remains the professional responsibility of the practitioner.

The authors, editors, and publisher have exerted every effort to ensure that drug selection and dosage set forth in this text are in accordance with current recommendations and practice at the time of publication. However, in view of ongoing research, changes in government regulations, and the constant flow of information relating to drug therapy and drug reactions, the reader is urged to check the package insert for each drug for any change in indications and dosage and for added warnings and precautions. This is particularly important when the recommended agent is a new or infrequently employed drug.

Some drugs and medical devices presented in the publication have Food and Drug Administration (FDA) clearance for limited use in restricted research settings. It is the responsibility of the health care provider to ascertain the FDA status of each drug or device planned for use in their clinical practice.

To purchase additional copies of this book, call our customer service department at (800) 638-3030 or fax orders to (301) 223-2320. International customers should call (301) 223-2300.

Visit Lippincott Williams & Wilkins on the Internet: at LWW.com. Lippincott Williams & Wilkins customer service representatives are available from 8:30 am to 6 pm, EST.

10 9 8 7 6 5 4 3 2 1

Contents

Preface

We stand at an interesting crossroads in the field of cancer genetic counseling and testing. Less than two decades ago, clinical testing for hereditary cancer syndromes was a rare event reserved for infrequently observed syndromes that a clinician might see once or twice in a lifetime. A small handful of specialized laboratories performed such testing and it was not unusual to send a sample to another country for processing as the options were limited and expertise sparse.

All of that changed early in 1996 when clinical testing became available for mutations within *BRCA1* and *BRCA2*. Those of us on the front lines were besieged with phone calls from patients wanting the test, reporters enquiring what we would do with the information, and medical colleagues questioning if and how these data would be useful. I remember lecturing to a small group of research clinicians at my institution soon after *BRCA* testing became available and discussing the option of prophylactic mastectomy and oophorectomy for women who tested *BRCA* positive. I found myself dodging angry accusations of "mutilating" women's bodies based on "genetic fortune telling," and opening Pandora's box, psychologically and emotionally ruining women who would then be uninsurable and societal castaways. Let's just say that cancer genetic testing was not welcomed with open arms by everyone.

The truth is that we didn't know how testing would unfold. Those of us providing counseling and testing had no information on how real-life patients outside of carefully proctored research protocols would handle this information. Would they be forever depressed? Would their anxiety levels make it impossible for them to function? Could this possibly make patients suicidal? We didn't know and we were worried. But, once testing hit the marketplace, there was no holding back the surge.

We were also concerned about insurability. Would patients who tested positive lose their health insurance coverage and, therefore, the ability to have the careful surveillance and expensive risk reduction surgeries we were recommending? If employers learned this information, would patients be passed up for promotions or even lose their jobs for fear that they would cost their companies too much money?

And, speaking of the surveillance and risk reduction surgeries we were offering, would they even work? I had multiple "academic conversations" with physicians at my institution who questioned whether prophylactic oophorectomy would adequately reduce the risk of ovarian cancer in *BRCA* carriers. Perhaps mutation carriers would then be at high risk to develop primary cancers in other locations? Although we thought that unlikely (and luckily, we were right), we had no long-term data to support this, or any, of our hypotheses.

Much has changed since 1996. We now have data demonstrating that there are no serious long-term psychological and emotional sequelae associated with genetic testing. Our fears regarding health insurance discrimination have not played out, perhaps in part to aggressive and supportive legislation via HIPAA and GINA protecting patients from genetic discrimination. Also, the employment and social repercussions have not been reported as major issues.

The surveillance and risk reduction surgeries we recommended, albeit far from perfect, have proven to be extremely effective in reducing cancer risk in carriers. While we have fewer data regarding chemoprevention in these populations, we are optimistic that these drugs may also reduce risk in these high risk families.

Interestingly, the issues that have generated the greatest dangers in the field of genetic counseling and testing are those we did not anticipate. Namely, how gene patents would create corporate monopolies and thwart competition, research and data-sharing in the field, and how this would impact pricing, access, and marketing of genetic testing. As you will read in Brierley et al.'s chapter, in part because of aggressive marketing of patented testing to clinicians without expertise in genetic counseling, there have been serious, adverse clinical outcomes for patients and their well-meaning physicians who ordered genetic testing in lieu of adequate counseling by a certified provider. And, as you will read in the thorough "Disease site" chapters, genetic testing encompasses many more genes than simply *BRCA* and Lynch syndrome genes. Risk assessment for these syndromes is not as simple as punching a few details into a risk calculator or taking just a family history of cancer; there are varied cancerous and noncancerous findings that impact the chance that a syndrome is present and influence what test should be ordered.

At this critical crossroads in our field, we see that targeted testing for one or two disease genes at a time may soon be coming to an end. Panels of disease genes and whole-exome sequencing, as you will read in O'Daniel and Lee's chapter, may soon become less expensive and much more informative than single-gene testing. The amount and complexity of data these new tests will yield is staggering. The amount of ambiguity in test results may increase by hundred-fold, making genetic counseling and result interpretation substantially more challenging—even for those of us who are experts in this field. And yet, ironically, complex genetic testing is now being marketed directly to consumers. (*See* Bellcross's chapter).

And so, the journey picks up speed and continues. Many thanks to my colleagues, some of the brightest minds in this field, who have donated their time and expertise to write the elegant and thorough chapters you will now have the opportunity to read.

Ellen T. Matloff, MS

Contributors

Jennifer E. Axilbund, MS, CGC
Cancer Risk Assessment Program
The Johns Hopkins Hospital
Baltimore, Maryland

Cecelia A. Bellcross, PhD, MS, CGC
Assistant Professor
Director, Genetic Counseling Training
  Program
Department of Human Genetics
Emory University School of Medicine
Atlanta, Georgia

Erica Blouch, MS, CGC
Center for Cancer Risk Assessment
Massachusetts General Hospital
Boston, Massachusetts

Karina L. Brierley, MS, CGC
Senior Genetic Counselor
Yale Cancer Center
New Haven, Connecticut

Gayun Chan-Smutko, MS, CGC
Massachusetts General Hospital Cancer Center
Boston, Massachusetts

Anu Chittenden, CGC
Genetic Counselor
Dana-Farber Cancer Institute
Boston, Massachusetts

Nicolette M. Chun, MS, LCGC
Clinical Assistant Professor of Pediatrics/
  Genetics
Stanford Cancer Genetics Clinic
Stanford, California

Whitney Cogswell, MS, CGC
Medical Center of Central Georgia
Macon, Georgia

Molly S. Daniels, MS, CGC
University of Texas, MD Anderson Cancer
  Center
Houston, Texas

James M. Ford, MD
Associate Professor of Medicine and
  Genetics
Stanford University School of Medicine
Division of Oncology
Stanford University School of Medicine
Stanford, California

Michele J. Gabree, MS
Certified Genetic Counselor
Center for Cancer Risk Assessment
Massachusetts General Hospital
Boston, Massachusetts

Jeanne P. Homer, MS, CGC
Hoag Hospital
Newport Beach, California

Kory W. Jasperson, MS, CGC
Huntsman Cancer Institute
Salt Lake City, Utah

Kristy Lee, MS
Certified Genetic Counselor
University of North Carolina Cancer &
  Adult Program
Chapel Hill, North Carolina

Ellen T. Matloff, MS
Research Scientist, Department of
  Genetics
Director, Cancer Genetic Counseling
Yale Cancer Center
New Haven, Connecticut

Dana Meaney-Delman, MS, CGC
Department of Obstetrics and
  Gynecology
Emory University School of Medicine
Atlanta, Georgia

Rebecca Nagy, MS, CGC
Clinical Cancer Genetics Program
The Ohio State University
Columbus, Ohio

Anna Newlin, MS, CGC
Center for Medical Genetics
NorthShore University HealthSystem
Evanston, Illinois

Julianne M. O'Daniel, MS
Illumina, Inc.
San Diego, California

Tricia Z. Page, MS, CGC
Director, Genetic Counseling Services
Instructor
Emory University
Decatur, Georgia

Debbie Pencarinha
Kingsport Hematology and Oncology
Wellmont Cancer Center
Kingsport, Tennessee

Robert Pilarski, MS, CGC, MSW, LSW
Clinical Cancer Genetics Program
The Ohio State University
Columbus, Ohio

Meredith Seidel, MS, CGC
Center for Cancer Risk Assessment
Massachusetts General Hospital
Boston, Massachusetts

Leigha Senter, MS, CGC
Assistant Professor
Human Genetics
The Ohio State University
Columbus, Ohio

Kristen Mahoney Shannon, MS, CGC
Program Manager/Senior Genetic
   Counselor
Center for Cancer Risk Assessment
Massachusetts General Hospital Cancer
   Center
Boston, Massachusetts

Christine L. Stanislaw, MS, CGC
Division of Medical Genetics
Emory University
Decatur, Georgia

Shelly Weiss, MS, CGC
Certified Genetic Counselor
Evanston, Illinois

Scott M. Weissman, MS, LGC
Licensed Genetic Counselor
Center for Medical Genetics
Evanston, Illinois

Elizabeth A. Wiley, MS
Department of Oncology
The Johns Hopkins University School of
   Medicine
Baltimore, Maryland

1

Cancer Genetic Counseling

Ellen T. Matloff and Danielle C. Bonadies

I n the past 15 years, clinically based genetic testing has evolved from an uncommon analysis ordered for the rare hereditary cancer family to a widely available tool ordered on a routine basis to assist in surgical decision making, chemoprevention, and surveillance of the patient with cancer, as well as management of the entire family. The evolution of this field has created a need for accurate cancer genetic counseling and risk assessment. Extensive coverage of this topic by the media and widespread advertising by commercial testing laboratories have further fueled the demand for counseling and testing.

Cancer genetic counseling is a communication process between a health care professional and an individual concerning cancer occurrence and risk in his or her family.[1] The process, which may include the entire family through a blend of genetic, medical, and psychosocial assessment and intervention, has been described as a bridge between the fields of traditional oncology and genetic counseling.[1]

The goals of this process include providing the client with an assessment of individual cancer risk, while offering the emotional support needed to understand and cope with this information. It also involves deciphering whether the cancers in a family are likely to be caused by a mutation in a cancer gene and, if so, *which one*. There are >30 hereditary cancer syndromes, many of which can be caused by mutations in different genes. Therefore, testing for these syndromes can be complicated. Advertisements by genetic testing companies bill genetic testing as a simple process that can be carried out by health care professionals with no training in this area; however, there are many genes involved in cancer, the interpretation of the test results is often complicated, the risk of result misinterpretation is great and associated with potential liability, and the emotional and psychological ramifications for the patient and family can be powerful. A few hours of training by a company generating a profit from the sale of these tests does not adequately prepare providers to offer their own genetic counseling and testing services.[2] Furthermore, the delegation of genetic testing responsibilities to office staff is alarming[3] and likely presents a huge liability for these ordering physicians, their practices, and their institutions. *Providers should proceed with caution before taking on the role of primary genetic counselor for their patients.*

1

Counseling about hereditary cancers differs from "traditional" genetic counseling in several ways. Clients seeking cancer genetic counseling are rarely concerned with reproductive decisions that are often the primary focus in traditional genetic counseling, but are instead seeking information about their own and other relatives' chances of developing cancer.[1] In addition, the risks given are not absolute but change over time as the family and personal history changes and the patient ages. The risk reduction options available are often radical (e.g., chemoprevention or prophylactic surgery), and are not appropriate for every patient at every age. The surveillance and management plan must be tailored to the patient's age, childbearing status, menopausal status, risk category, ease of screening, and personal preferences, and will likely change over time with the patient. The ultimate goal of cancer genetic counseling is to help the patient reach the decision best suited to her personal situation, needs, and circumstances.

There are now a significant number of referral centers across the country specializing in cancer genetic counseling and the numbers are growing. However, some experts insist that the only way to keep up with the overwhelming demand for counseling will be to educate more physicians and nurses in cancer genetics. The feasibility of adding another specialized and time-consuming task to the clinical burden of these professionals is questionable, particularly with average patient encounters of 19.5 and 21.6 minutes for general practitioners and gynecologists, respectively.[4,5] A more practical goal may be to better educate primary care providers in the area of generalized risk assessment so that they can screen their patient populations for individuals at

TABLE 1.1	How to Find a Genetic Counselor for your Patient

Gene tests

www.ncbi.nlm.nih.gov/sites/GeneTests/clinic—(206) 616–4089

gtclinic@u.washington.edu

A listing of US and international genetics clinics providing evaluation and genetic counseling

Informed medical decisions

www.informeddna.com–(800) 975–4819

Nationwide network of independent genetic counselors that use telephone and internet technology to bring genetic counseling to patients and providers. Covered by many insurance companies.

National society of genetic counselors

www.nsgc.org—click "Find a Counselor" button—(312) 321–6834

For a listing of genetic counselors in your area who specialize in cancer.

NCI cancer genetics services directory

www.cancer.gov/cancertopics/genetics/directory—(800) 4-CANCER

A free service designed to locate providers of cancer risk counseling and testing services.

high risk for hereditary cancer and refer them on to comprehensive counseling and testing programs. Access to genetic counseling is no longer an issue because there are now internet-, phone-, and satellite-based telemedicine services available (Table 1.1), and several major health insurance companies now cover these services.[6–8]

WHO IS A CANDIDATE FOR CANCER GENETIC COUNSELING?

Only 5% to 10% of most cancers are due to single mutations within autosomal dominant inherited cancer susceptibility genes.[9] The key for clinicians is to determine which patients are at greatest risk to carry a hereditary mutation. There are seven critical risk factors in hereditary cancer (Table 1.2). The first is early age of cancer onset. This risk factor, *even in the absence of a family history*, has been shown to be associated with an increased frequency of germline mutations in many types of cancers.[10] The second risk factor is the presence of the same cancer in multiple affected relatives on the same side of the pedigree. These cancers do not need to be of similar histologic type in order to be caused by a single mutation. The third risk factor is the clustering of cancers known to be caused by a single gene mutation in one family (e.g., breast/ovarian/pancreatic cancer or colon/ovarian/uterine cancers). The fourth risk factor is

TABLE 1.2	Risk Factors that Warrant Genetic Counseling for Hereditary Cancer Syndromes

1. Early age of onset (e.g., <50 years for breast, colon, and uterine cancer)
2. Multiple family members on the same side of the pedigree with the same cancer
3. Clustering of cancers in the family known to be caused by a single gene mutation (e.g., breast/ovarian/pancreatic; colon/uterine/ovarian; colon cancer/polyps/desmoid tumors/osteomas)
4. Multiple primary cancers in one individual (e.g., breast/ovarian cancer; colon/uterine; synchronous/metachronous colon cancers; >15 gastrointestinal polyps; >5 hamartomatous or juvenile polyps)
5. Ethnicity (e.g., Jewish ancestry for breast/ovarian cancer syndrome)
6. Unusual presentation of cancer/tumor (e.g., breast cancer in a male; medullary thyroid cancer; retinoblastoma; even one sebaceous carcinoma or adenoma)
7. Pathology[a] (e.g., triple-negative (ER/PR/*Her2*) breast cancer <60; medullary breast cancers are over-represented in women with hereditary breast and ovarian cancer; a colon tumor with an abnormal microsatellite instability (MSI) or immunohistochemistry (IHC) result increases the risk for a hereditary colon cancer syndrome)

[a]An evolving area of risk assessment

the occurrence of multiple primary cancers in one individual. This includes multiple primary breast or colon cancers as well as a single individual with separate cancers known to be caused by a single gene mutation (e.g., breast and ovarian cancer in a single individual). Ethnicity also plays a role in determining who is at greatest risk to carry a hereditary cancer mutation. Individuals of Jewish ancestry are at increased risk to carry three specific *BRCA1/2* mutations.[11] The presence of a cancer that presents unusually, in this case breast cancer in a male, represents a sixth risk factor and is important even when it is the only risk factor present. Finally, the last risk factor is pathology. This risk factor is listed in Table 1.1 in italics because it is a new and evolving entity. It appears that certain types of cancer are overrepresented in hereditary cancer families. For example, medullary breast cancer appears to be overrepresented in *BRCA1* families.[12] Triple-negative breast cancers (ER−, PR−, *Her2*−) are also overrepresented in *BRCA1* families,[13] and the National Comprehensive Cancer Network (NCCN) has recently updated their *BRCA* testing guidelines to include individuals diagnosed with a triple-negative breast cancer <age 60.[14] However, breast cancer patients without these pathologic findings are *not* necessarily at lower risk to carry a mutation. In contrast, patients with a borderline or mucinous ovarian carcinoma appear to be at lower risk to carry a *BRCA1* or *BRCA2* mutation[15] and may instead carry a mutation in a different gene. It is already well established that medullary thyroid carcinoma (MTC), sebaceous adenoma or carcinoma, adrenocortical carcinoma before the age of 25, and multiple adenomatous, hamartomatous, or juvenile colon polyps are indicative of other rare hereditary cancer syndromes.[16,17] These risk factors should be viewed in the context of the entire family history, and must be weighed in proportion to the number of individuals who have not developed cancer. Risk assessment is often limited in families that are small or have few female relatives; in such families, a single risk factor may carry more weight.

A less common, but extremely important, finding is the presence of unusual physical findings or birth defects that are known to be associated with rare hereditary cancer syndromes. Examples include benign skin findings, autism, large head circumference[18,19] and thyroid disorders in Cowden syndrome, ontogenic keratocysts in Gorlin syndrome,[20] and desmoid tumors or dental abnormalities in familial adenomatous polyposis (FAP).[21] These and other findings should prompt further investigation of the patient's family history and consideration of a referral to genetic counseling.

In this chapter, the breast/ovarian cancer counseling session with a female patient will serve as a paradigm by which all other sessions may follow broadly. However, as testing evolves from targeted testing of 1 or 2 genes to multigene panels, genetic counseling and test interpretation will become more complex.

COMPONENTS OF THE CANCER GENETIC COUNSELING SESSION
Precounseling Information

Before coming in for genetic counseling, the counselee should be given some basic information about the process. This information, which can be imparted by telephone or in the form of written material, should outline what the counselee can expect at each session, and what information he/she should collect before the first visit. The counselee can then begin to collect medical and family history information and pathology reports that will be essential for the genetic counseling session.

Family History

An accurate family history is undoubtedly one of the most essential components of the cancer genetic counseling session. Optimally, a family history should include at least three generations; however, patients do not always have this information. For each individual affected with cancer, it is important to document the exact diagnosis, age at diagnosis, treatment strategies, and environmental exposures (i.e., occupational exposures, cigarettes, other agents).[21] The current age of the individual, laterality, and occurrence of any other cancers must also be documented. Cancer diagnoses should be confirmed with pathology reports whenever possible. A study by Love et al.[22] revealed that individuals accurately reported the primary site of cancer only 83% of the time in their first-degree relatives with cancer, and 67% and 60% of the time in second- and third-degree relatives, respectively. It is common for patients to report a uterine cancer as an ovarian cancer, or a colon polyp as an invasive colorectal cancer. These differences, although seemingly subtle to the patient, can make a tremendous difference in risk assessment. Individuals should be asked if there are any consanguineous (inbred) relationships in the family, if any relatives were born with birth defects or mental retardation, and whether other genetic diseases run in the family (e.g., Fanconi Anemia or Cowden syndrome), as these pieces of information could prove important in reaching a diagnosis.

The most common misconception in family history taking is that somehow a maternal family history of breast, ovarian, or uterine cancer is more significant than a paternal history. Conversely, many still believe that a paternal history of prostate cancer is more significant than a maternal history. Few cancer genes discovered thus far are located on the sex chromosomes, and therefore both maternal and paternal history are significant and must be explored thoroughly. It has also become necessary to elicit the spouse's personal and family history of cancer. This has bearing on the cancer status of common children, but may also determine if children are at increased risk for a serious recessive genetic disease such as Fanconi anemia.[23] Children who inherit two copies of a *BRCA2* mutation (one from each parent) are now known to have this serious disorder characterized by defective DNA repair and high rates of birth defects, aplastic anemia, leukemia, and solid tumors.[23] Patients should be encouraged to report changes in their family history over time (e.g., new cancer diagnoses, genetic testing results in relatives), as this may change their risk assessment and counseling.

A detailed family history should also include genetic diseases, birth defects, mental retardation, multiple miscarriages, and infant deaths. A history of certain recessive genetic diseases (e.g., ataxia telangiectasia, Fanconi anemia) can indicate that healthy family members who carry just one copy of the genetic mutation may be at increased risk to develop cancer.[23,24] Other genetic disorders, such as hereditary hemorrhagic telangiectasia, can be associated with a hereditary cancer syndrome caused by a mutation in the same gene; in this case juvenile polyposis.[25]

Dysmorphology Screening

Congenital anomalies, benign tumors, and unusual dermatologic features occur in a large number of hereditary cancer predisposition syndromes. Examples include osteomas of the jaw in FAP, palmar pits in Gorlin syndrome, and papillomas of the lips and mucous membranes in Cowden syndrome. Obtaining an accurate past medical history of benign lesions and birth defects, and screening for such dysmorphology can greatly impact diagnosis, counseling, and testing. For example, BRCA1/2 testing is inappropriate in a patient with breast cancer who has a family history of thyroid cancer and the orocutaneous manifestations of Cowden syndrome.

Risk Assessment

Risk assessment is one of the most complicated components of the genetic counseling session. It is crucial to remember that risk assessment changes over time as the person ages and as the health status of their family members change. Risk assessment can be broken down into three separate components:

(1) What is the chance that the counselee will develop the cancer observed in his/her family (or a genetically related cancer such as ovarian cancer due to a family history of breast cancer)?
(2) What is the chance that the cancers in this family are caused by a single gene mutation?
(3) What is the chance that we can identify the gene mutation in this family with our current knowledge and laboratory techniques?

Cancer clustering in a family may be due to genetic and/or environmental factors, or may be coincidental because some cancers are very common in the general population.[26] While inherited factors may be the primary cause of cancers in some families, in others, cancer may develop because an inherited factor increases the individual's susceptibility to environmental carcinogens. It is also possible that members of the same family may be exposed to similar environmental exposures, due to shared geography or patterns in behavior and diet, that may increase the risk of cancer.[27] Therefore, it is important to distinguish the difference between a familial pattern of cancer (due to environmental factors or chance) and a hereditary pattern of cancer (due to a shared genetic mutation). Emerging research is also evaluating the role and clinical utility of more common low-penetrance susceptibility genes and single-nucleotide polymorphisms (SNPs) that may account for a proportion of familial cancers.[28]

Several models are available to calculate the chance that a woman will develop breast cancer including the Gail and Claus models.[29,30] Computer-based models are also available to help determine the chance that a BRCA mutation will be found in a family.[31] At first glance, many of these models appear simple and easy to use and it may be tempting to rely on these models, exclusively, to assess cancer risk. However, each model has its strengths and weaknesses, and the counselor needs to understand the limitations well and know which are validated, which are considered problematic, when a model will not work on a particular patient, or when another genetic syndrome should be considered. For example, none of the existing models are able to factor in other risks that may be essential in hereditary risk calculation (e.g., a sister who was diagnosed with breast cancer after radiation treatment for Hodgkin's disease).

DNA Testing

DNA testing is now available for a variety of hereditary cancer syndromes. However, despite misrepresentation by the media, testing is feasible for only a small percentage of individuals with cancer. DNA testing offers the important advantage of presenting clients with *actual risks* instead of the empiric risks derived from risk calculation models. DNA testing can be very expensive (full sequencing of the *BRCA1/2* genes currently costs >$3,300). All patients being offered *BRCA* testing should also be offered *BRCA* rearrangement testing (BART) which looks for large structural rearrangements within these genes.[14] It is the clinician's responsibility to discuss and order this test separately (an additional $700). Importantly, testing should begin in an affected family member, whenever possible. Most insurance companies now cover cancer genetic testing in families where the test is medically indicated.

The results of DNA testing are generally provided in person in a result disclosure session. It is recommended that patients bring a close friend or relative with them to this session who can provide them with emotional support and who can help them listen to and process the information provided.

One of the most crucial aspects of DNA testing is accurate result interpretation. One study found that test results for the hereditary colon cancer syndrome FAP were misinterpreted more than 30% of the time by those ordering the testing.[32] More recent data have shown that many medical providers have difficulty interpreting even basic pedigrees and genetic test results.[33–35] In a survey of over 2,000 physicians, only 13% of internists, 21% of Ob/Gyns, and 40% of oncologists correctly answered four basic knowledge questions about genetic aspects of breast cancer and *BRCA* testing. This deficiency in knowledge did not necessarily deter them from discussing or ordering testing.[5] Misinterpretation of results is now the greatest risk of genetic testing and is very common.[36] Interpretation is becoming increasingly complicated as more tests become available. For example, one study demonstrated that approximately 12% of high-risk families who test negative by standard *BRCA1* and *BRCA2* testing are found to carry a deletion or duplication in one of these genes, or a mutation in another gene.[37] This is particularly concerning in an era in which testing companies are canvassing physicians' offices and are encouraging them to perform their own counseling and testing. The potential impact of test results on the patient and his/her family is great, and therefore, accurate interpretation of the results is paramount. Professional groups have recognized this and have adopted standards encouraging clinicians to refer patients to genetics experts to ensure proper ordering and interpretation of genetic tests. The US Preventive Services Task Force recommends that women whose family history is suggestive of a *BRCA* mutation be referred for genetic counseling before being offered genetic testing.[38] The American College of Surgeons Commission on Cancer standards include "cancer risk assessment, genetic counseling, and testing services provided to patients either on site or by referral, by a qualified genetics professional."[2]

Results can fall into a few broad categories. It is important to note that a "negative" test result can actually be interpreted in three different ways, detailed in (2), (3), and (4) below:

(1) *Deleterious mutation "positive"*: When a deleterious mutation in a cancer gene is discovered, the cancer risks for the patient and her family are relatively straightforward. The risks associated with most genes are not precise and should be presented to patients as a risk range.[39,40] When a true mutation is found, it is critical to test both parents—whenever possible—to determine from which side of the family the mutation is originating, even when the answer appears obvious.

(2) *True negative*: An individual does not carry the deleterious mutation found in her family which ideally has been proven to segregate with the cancer family history. In this case, the patient's cancer risks are usually reduced to the population risks.

(3) *Negative*: A mutation was not detected and the cancers in the family are not likely to be hereditary based on the personal and family history assessment. For example, a patient is diagnosed with breast cancer at age 38 and comes from a large family with no other cancer diagnoses and relatives who died at old ages of other causes.

(4) *Uninformative*: A mutation cannot be found in affected family members of a family in which the cancer pattern appears to be hereditary; there is likely an undetectable mutation within the gene, or the family carries a mutation in a different gene. If, for example, the patient developed breast cancer at age 38 has a father with breast cancer and paternal aunt who developed breast and ovarian cancers before age 50, a negative test result would be almost meaningless. It would simply mean that the family has a mutation that could not be identified with our current testing methods or a mutation in another cancer gene. The entire family would be followed as high risk.

(5) *Variant of uncertain significance*: A genetic change is identified whose significance is unknown. It is possible that this change is deleterious or completely benign. It may be helpful to test other *affected* family members to see if the mutation segregates with disease in the family. If it does not segregate, the variant is less likely to be significant. If it does, the variant is more likely to be significant. Other tools, including a splice site predictor, in conjunction with data on species conservation and amino acid difference scores can also be helpful in determining the likelihood that a variant is significant. It is rarely helpful (and can be detrimental) to test *unaffected* family members for such variants.

In order to pinpoint the mutation in a family, an affected individual most likely to carry the mutation should be tested first, whenever possible. This is most often a person affected with the cancer in question at the earliest age. Test subjects should be selected with care, as it is possible for a person to develop sporadic cancer in a hereditary cancer family. For example, in an early-onset breast cancer family it would not be ideal to first test a woman diagnosed with breast cancer at age 65, as she may represent a sporadic case.

If a mutation is detected in an affected relative, other family members can be tested for the same mutation with a great degree of accuracy. Family members who do not carry the mutation found in their family are deemed "true negative." Those who are found to carry the mutation in their family will have more definitive information about their risks to develop cancer. This information can be crucial in assisting patients in decision making regarding surveillance and risk reduction.

If a mutation is not identified in the affected relative it usually means that either the cancers in the family (a) are not hereditary or (b) are caused by an undetectable mutation or a mutation in a different gene. A careful review of the family history and the risk factors will help to decipher whether interpretation (a) or (b) is more likely. Additional genetic testing may need to be ordered at this point. In cases in which the cancers appear hereditary and no mutation is found, DNA banking should be offered to the proband for a time in the future when improved testing may become available. A letter indicating exactly who in the family has access to the DNA should accompany the banked sample.

The penetrance of mutations in cancer susceptibility genes is also difficult to interpret. Initial estimates derived from high-risk families provided very high cancer risks for *BRCA1* and *BRCA2* mutation carriers.[41] More recent studies done on populations that were not selected for family history have revealed lower penetrances.[42] Since exact penetrance rates cannot be determined for individual families at this time, and because precise genotype/phenotype correlations remain unclear, it is prudent to provide patients with a range of cancer risk, and to explain that their risk probably falls somewhere within this spectrum.

Female carriers of *BRCA1* and *BRCA2* mutations have a 50% to 85% lifetime risk to develop breast cancer and between a 15% and 60% lifetime risk to develop ovarian cancer.[11,40,41] It is important to note that the classification "ovarian cancer" also includes cancer of the fallopian tubes and primary peritoneal carcinoma.[42,43] *BRCA2* carriers also have an increased lifetime risk of male breast cancer, pancreatic cancer, and possibly melanoma.[44,45] Carriers of Lynch syndrome mutations (also known as hereditary nonpolyposis colorectal cancer [HNPCC]) have a 65% to 85% lifetime risk to develop colon cancer, and female carriers have at least a 40% to 60% lifetime risk of uterine cancer, and as great as a 10% to 12% risk of ovarian cancer.[46,47] Individuals with Lynch syndrome have an increased risk for a variety of other types of cancers, including head and neck, other gastrointestinal, urinary tract, and hematologic malignancies.

Options for Surveillance and Risk Reduction

The cancer risk counseling session is a forum to provide counselees with information, support, options, and hope. Mutation carriers can be offered: earlier and more aggressive surveillance, chemoprevention, and/or prophylactic surgery. Detailed management options for BRCA carriers are discussed in this chapter; however, management options for some of the other major cancer syndromes are listed in the site-specific chapters.

Surveillance recommendations are evolving with newer techniques and additional data.

At this time, it is recommended that individuals at increased risk for breast cancer, particularly those who carry a BRCA mutation have annual mammograms beginning at age 25, with a clinical breast examination by a breast specialist, a yearly breast MRI with a clinical breast examination by a breast specialist, and a yearly clinical breast examination by a gynecologist.[48,49] It is suggested that the mammogram and MRI be spaced out around the calendar year so that some intervention is planned every 6 months. Recent data suggest that MRI may be safer and more effective in BRCA carriers <40 years and may someday replace mammograms in this population.[50]

BRCA carriers may take tamoxifen or Evista in hopes of reducing their risks of developing breast cancer. Both of these medications are selective estrogen receptor modulators (SERMs) that have been proven effective in women at risk due to a positive family history of breast cancer.[51,52] There are limited data on the effectiveness of prophylactic SERMs in BRCA carriers[53–55]; however, there are some data to suggest that BRCA carriers taking tamoxifen as treatment for a breast cancer reduce their risk of a contralateral breast cancer.[56] In addition, the majority of BRCA2 carriers who develop breast cancer develop an estrogen-positive form of the disease,[57] and it is hoped that this population will respond especially well to chemoprevention. Further studies in this area are necessary before drawing conclusions about the efficacy of SERMs in this population. Prophylactic bilateral mastectomy appears to reduce the risk of breast cancer by >90% in women at high risk for the disease.[58] Before genetic testing was available, it was not uncommon for entire generations of cancer families to have at-risk tissues removed without knowing if they were *personally* at increased risk for their familial cancer. Fifty percent of unaffected individuals in hereditary cancer families will *not* carry the inherited predisposition gene, and can be spared prophylactic surgery or invasive high-risk surveillance regimens. Therefore, it is clearly not appropriate to offer prophylactic surgery until a patient is referred for genetic counseling and, if possible, testing.[59]

Women who carry BRCA1/2 mutations are also at increased risk to develop second contralateral and ipsilateral primaries of the breast.[60] These data bring into question the option of breast-conserving surgery in women at high risk to develop a second primary within the same breast. For this reason, BRCA1/2 carrier status can have a profound impact on surgical decision making[61] and many patients have genetic counseling and testing immediately after diagnosis and before surgery or radiation therapy. Those patients who test positive and opt for prophylactic mastectomy can often be spared radiation and the resulting side effects that can complicate reconstruction. Approximately 30% to 60% of previously irradiated patients who later opt for mastectomy with reconstruction report significant complications or unfavorable cosmetic results.[61,62]

Women who carry *BRCA1/2* mutations are also at increased risk to develop ovarian, fallopian tube, and primary peritoneal cancer, even if no one in their family has developed these cancers. Surveillance for ovarian cancer is complex, with the recommended interventions being annual transvaginal ultrasounds and CA-125 levels beginning between the ages of 25 and 35 years.[63] The effectiveness of such surveillance in detecting ovarian cancers at early, more treatable stages has not been proven in any population. Some data have indicated that oral contraceptives reduce the risk of ovarian cancer in women carrying *BRCA* mutations.[64] Recent data indicate that the impact of this intervention on increasing breast cancer risk, if any, is low.[55,65] Given the difficulties in screening and treatment of ovarian cancer, risk/benefit analysis likely favors the use of oral contraceptives in young carriers of *BRCA1/2* mutations[27] who are not yet ready to have their ovaries removed. Prophylactic bilateral salpingo-oophorectomy (BSO) is currently the most effective means to reduce the risk of ovarian cancer and is recommended to *BRCA1/2* carriers by the age of 35 to 40 or when childbearing is complete.[66] Specific operative and pathologic protocols have been developed for this prophylactic surgery.[67] In *BRCA1/2* carriers whose pathology comes back normal, this surgery is highly effective in reducing the subsequent risk of ovarian cancer.[68] A decision analysis comparing various surveillance and risk-reducing options available to *BRCA* carriers has shown an increase in life expectancy if BSO is pursued by age 40.[69] A relatively small percentage of women who have this procedure may develop primary peritoneal carcinoma.[42,70] There has been some debate about whether *BRCA1/2* carriers should also opt for total abdominal hysterectomy (TAH) due to the fact that small stumps of the fallopian tubes remain after BSO alone. The question of whether or not *BRCA* carriers are at increased risk for uterine serous papillary carcinoma (USPC) has also been raised.[71–73] If a relationship does exist between *BRCA* mutations and uterine cancer, the risk appears to be low and not elevated over that of the general population.[74] Removing the uterus may make it possible for a *BRCA* carrier to take unopposed estrogen or tamoxifen in the future without risk of uterine cancer, but this surgery is associated with a longer recovery time and has more side effects than does BSO alone. Each patient should be counseled about the pros and cons of each procedure.

A secondary, but important, reason for female *BRCA* carriers to consider prophylactic oophorectomy is that it also significantly reduces the risk of a subsequent breast cancer, particularly if they have this surgery before menopause.[75,76] The reduction in breast cancer risk remains even if a healthy premenopausal carrier elects to take low-dose hormone replacement therapy (HRT) after this surgery.[77] Early data suggest that tamoxifen in addition to premenopausal oophorectomy in *BRCA* carriers may have little additional benefit in terms of breast cancer risk reduction.[78] Research is needed in balancing quality-of-life issues secondary to estrogen deprivation with cancer risk reduction in these young female *BRCA1/2* carriers.

Genetic counseling and testing are also available for many other cancer syndromes, including Lynch syndrome, von Hippel–Lindau, multiple endocrine neoplasias, and FAP. Surveillance and risk reduction for patients who are known mutation carriers for such conditions may decrease the associated morbidity and mortality of these syndromes.

Follow-up

A follow-up letter to the patient is a concrete means of documenting the information conveyed in the sessions so that the patient and his/her family members can review it over time. This letter should be sent to the patient and health care professionals to whom the patient has granted access to this information. A follow-up phone call and/or counseling session may also be helpful, particularly in the case of a positive test result. Some programs provide patients with an annual or biannual newsletter updating them on new information in the field of cancer genetics or patient support groups. It is now recommended that patients return for follow-up counseling sessions months, or even years, after their initial consult to discuss advances in genetic testing and changes in surveillance and risk reduction options. This can be beneficial for individuals who have been found to carry a hereditary predisposition, for those in whom a syndrome/mutation is suspected but yet unidentified and for those who are ready to move forward with genetic testing. Follow-up counseling is also recommended for patients whose life circumstances have changed (e.g., preconception, after childbearing is complete), are preparing for prophylactic surgery, or are ready to discuss the family genetics with their children.

ISSUES IN CANCER GENETIC COUNSELING
Psychosocial Issues

The psychosocial impact of cancer genetic counseling cannot be underestimated. Just the process of scheduling a cancer risk counseling session may be quite difficult for some individuals with a family history who are not only frightened about their own cancer risk, but are reliving painful experiences associated with the cancer of their loved ones.[9] Counselees may be faced with an onslaught of emotions, including anger, fear of developing cancer, fear of disfigurement and dying, grief, lack of control, negative body image, and a sense of isolation.[21] Some counselees are wrestling with the fear that insurance companies, employers, family members, and even future partners will react negatively to their cancer risks. For many it is a double-edged sword as they balance their fears and apprehensions about dredging up these issues with the possibility of obtaining reassuring news and much needed information.

A person's perceived cancer risk is often dependent on many "nonmedical" variables. They may estimate that their risk is higher if they look like an affected individual, or share some of their personality traits.[21] Their perceived risks will vary depending on if their relatives were cancer survivors, or died painful deaths from the disease. Many people wonder not "if" they are going to get cancer, but "when."

The counseling session is an opportunity for individuals to express why they believe they have developed cancer, or why their family members have cancer. Some explanations may revolve around family folklore, and it is important to listen to and address these explanations rather than dismiss them.[21] In doing this, the counselor will allow the clients to alleviate their greatest fears, and to give more credibility to the "medical" theory. Understanding a patient's perceived cancer risk is important, in that fear may *decrease* surveillance and preventive health care behaviors.[79] For patients and families who are moving forward with DNA testing, a referral to a mental health care professional is often very helpful. Genetic testing has an impact not only on the patient, but also on his/her children, siblings, parents, and extended relatives. This can be overwhelming for an individual and the family, and should be discussed in detail before testing.

To date, studies conducted in the setting of pre- and postgenetic counseling have revealed that, at least in the short term, most patients do not experience adverse psychological outcomes after receiving their test results.[80,81] In fact, preliminary data have revealed that individuals in families with known mutations who seek testing seem to fare better psychologically at 6 months than those who avoid testing.[80] Among individuals who learn they are *BRCA* mutation carriers, anxiety and distress levels appear to increase slightly after receiving their test results but returned to pretest levels in several weeks.[82] While these data are reassuring, it is important to recognize that genetic testing is an individual decision and will not be right for every patient or every family.

Presymptomatic Testing in Children

Presymptomatic testing in children has been widely discussed, and most concur that it is appropriate only when the onset of the condition regularly occurs in childhood or there are useful interventions that can be applied.[83] For example, genetic testing for mutations in the *BRCA* genes and other adult-onset diseases is generally limited to individuals who are >18 years of age. The American College of Medical Genetics states that if the "medical or psychosocial benefits of a genetic test will not accrue until adulthood…genetic testing generally should be deferred."[84] In contrast, DNA-based diagnosis of children and young adults at risk for hereditary MTC is appropriate and has improved the management of these patients.[85] DNA-based testing for MTC is virtually 100% accurate and allows at-risk family members to make informed decisions about prophylactic thyroidectomy. FAP is a disorder that occurs in childhood, and in which mortality can be reduced if detection is presymptomatic.[86] Testing is clearly indicated in these instances.

Questions have been raised about parents' right to demand testing for adult-onset diseases. Parents may have a constitutionally protected right to demand that unwilling physicians order this test, but there is little risk for liability for damages unless the child suffers physical harm as a direct result of this refusal.[83] The child's right *not* to be tested must be considered. Whenever childhood testing is not medically indicated it is preferable that testing decisions are postponed until the children are adults and can decide for themselves whether or not to be tested.

Confidentiality

The level of confidentiality surrounding cancer genetic testing is paramount due to concerns of genetic discrimination. Some programs opt to keep shadow files, keep their databases off-line, limit patient information in e-mails, and take precautions to protect confidentially when leaving voice mail messages for patients. Genetic counseling summary letters are often sent directly to patients and are copied to the referring physicians only with the explicit permission of the patient. These measures are taken because confidentiality and genetic discrimination are a grave concern for many of the patients seen in the cancer genetic counseling clinic.[87] Careful consideration should be given to the confidentiality of family history information, pedigrees, genetic test results, pathology reports, and the carrier status of other family members, as many hospitals and medical centers transition to electronic medical record systems. The goal of electronic records is to share information about the patient with his/her entire health care team. However, genetics is a unique specialty that involves the whole family. Patient's charts often contain HIPAA (Health Insurance Portability and Accountability Act)-protected health information and genetic test results for many other family members. This information may not be appropriate to enter into an electronic record. In addition, the hand-drawn pedigrees that genetics professionals rely on are difficult to translate into an electronic medical record. The unique issues of genetics services need to be considered when designing electronic medical record standards.

Confidentiality of test results *within* a family can also be of issue, as genetic counseling and testing often reveal the risk status of family members other than the patient. Under confidentiality codes, the patient needs to grant permission before at-risk family members can be contacted. It has been questioned whether or not a family member could sue a health care professional for negligence if they were identified at high risk yet not informed.[88] Most recommendations have stated that the burden of confidentiality lies between the provider and the patient. However, more recent recommendations state that confidentiality *should* be violated if the potential harm of not notifying other family members outweighs the harm of breaking a confidence to the patient.[89] There is no patent solution for this difficult dilemma, and situations must be considered on a case-by-case basis with the assistance of the in-house legal department and ethics committee.

Patients should be counseled about the benefits to other family members of knowing testing results, but, at the present time, the decision is ultimately the patient's. Extended family members who are notified, with the patient's consent, may not always be grateful to receive this information, and may feel that their privacy has been invaded by being contacted.

Insurance and Discrimination Issues

When genetic testing for cancer predisposition first became widely available, the fear of health insurance discrimination—by both patients and providers—was one of the most common concerns.[87,90] It appears that the risks of health insurance discrimination were overstated and that almost no discrimination by health insurers has been reported.[91] The HIPAA of 1996 banned the use of genetic information as a pre-existing condition.[92,93] In May 2008, Congress passed the Genetic Information Nondiscrimination Act (GINA) (HR 493) that provides broad protection of an individual's genetic information against health insurance and employment discrimination.[94] In addition, the 2010 Heath Care Reform (HR 4872) prohibits group health plans from denying insurance based on pre-existing conditions and from increasing premiums based on health status.[95] Health care providers can now more confidently reassure their patients that genetic counseling and testing will not put them at risk of losing group or individual health insurance.

More and more patients are choosing to submit their genetic counseling and/or testing charges to their health insurance companies. In the past few years, more insurance companies have agreed to pay for counseling and/or testing,[96] perhaps in light of decision analyses that show these services and subsequent prophylactic surgeries to be cost-effective.[97] The risk of life or disability insurance discrimination, however, is more realistic. Patients should be counseled about such risks before they pursue genetic testing.

Future Directions

The field of cancer genetic counseling and testing has grown tremendously over the past 15 years. Although cancer genetic counseling has traditionally been targeted at individuals with strong personal or family histories of cancer, this focus has broadened. Genetic counseling and testing is now offered to patients diagnosed with early-onset breast and colon cancer as a critical tool to guide surgical and radiation decision making, as the risk of new primaries is greater in individuals who carry germline mutations.[59,60]

Clinicians should be aware that technology to perform gene panels, whole exome and whole genome sequencing, has exploded onto the marketplace. Gene panels simultaneously analyze groups of genes that contribute to increased risk for breast, colon, ovarian, uterine, and other cancers while whole exome and genome sequencing deliver enormous amounts of data related to the entire exome/genome. These tests can identify mutations associated with rare and common disorders that may be overlooked by targeted, single gene testing; however, each have risks and benefits that should be weighed carefully. The cost of this technology continues to decrease and now costs, roughly, just a few hundred dollars more than full testing for *BRCA1* and *BRCA2*. Testing by whole exome and whole genome sequencing presents unique advantages and challenges that are further detailed in the chapter entitled "Whole-Genome and Whole-Exome Sequencing in Hereditary Cancer."

A remarkable limitation of this technology in the field of cancer genetics is specific gene patents that prohibit testing and reporting of genetic mutations found in these regions. In particular, the US Patent and Trademark Office issued patents on the *BRCA1* and *BRCA2* genes. Although various researchers contributed to the identification of these genes, patent rights were granted to the privately owned biotech firm Myriad Genetics.[98] As the exclusive patent holder, Myriad has opted to strictly enforce its monopoly rights and is the only laboratory in the country where diagnostic testing can be performed. In 2009, the American Civil Liberties Union filed suit against Myriad and the US Patent and Trademark Office, arguing that the patents are illegal because genes are "products of nature." According to the lawsuit, researchers and scientists are prevented from studying, testing, and developing alternative tests because of the strict control of these genes. Several of the patents were overturned in a March 29, 2010 ruling. Judge Robert Sweet stated that purification of DNA does not change the essential characteristic of DNA and is therefore not a patentable product.[99] This ruling has since been overturned and the Supreme Court is scheduled to hear this case in Spring 2013. If the patents are overturned, precedent will be set about how gene patents are issued and genetic counselors, clinicians, and researchers will be able to engage freely in research, testing, and clinical practice involving these genes. Patients would also have access to genetic testing services from multiple, and perhaps more affordable, sources.

New developments are also emerging in the treatment and possibly prevention of *BRCA*-related cancers. Several small studies have evaluated the effect of poly adenosine diphosphate (ADP) ribose polymerases (PARP) inhibitors in combination with chemotherapy for cancer treatment. It appears that PARP inhibitors are particularly effective in patients with *BRCA* mutations.[100,101] Future studies will focus on the use of PARP inhibitors in earlier stage cancers in *BRCA* carriers, cancers in women with triple-negative breast cancers, and *BRCA* carriers in the prevention setting.

Reproductive technology in the form of preimplantation genetic diagnosis is also an option[102] for men and women with a hereditary cancer syndrome, but one that is requested by few patients for adult-onset conditions in which there are viable options for surveillance and risk reduction. The option of sperm selection to increase the likelihood of having a male fetus (or vice versa for a condition that affects mostly males) can be discussed if parents are looking for preconception options. If a *BRCA2* carrier is considering having a child, it is important to assess the spouse's risk of also carrying a *BRCA2* mutation. If the spouse is of Jewish ancestry, or has a personal or family history of breast, ovarian, or pancreatic cancer, *BRCA* testing should be considered and a discussion of the risk of Fanconi anemia in a child with two *BRCA2* mutations should take place.[103]

The combination of technologic advances in genetic testing, new pharmacologic developments for cancer risk reduction, and increased utility for testing in high- and moderate-risk populations will result in a significant expansion in the field of cancer genetic counseling. Maintenance of high standards for thorough genetic counseling, informed consent, and accurate result interpretation will be paramount in reducing potential risks and maximizing the benefits of this technology in the next century.

REFERENCES

1. Peters J. Breast cancer genetics: Relevance to oncology practice. *Cancer Control.* 1995;2(3):195–208.
2. American College of Surgeons, Commission on Cancer. Cancer Program Standards 2012, Version 1.1: Ensuring Patient-Centered Care. http://www.facs.org/cancer/coc/programstandards2012.html. Accessed December 3, 2012.
3. Lubin IM, Caggana M, Constantin C, et al. Ordering molecular genetic tests and reporting results: Practices in laboratory and clinical settings. *J Mol Diagn.* 2008;10(5):459–468.
4. Weeks WB, Wallace AE. Time and money: A retrospective evaluation of the inputs, outputs, efficiency, and incomes of physicians. *Arch Intern Med.* 2003;163(8):944–948.
5. Doksum T, Bernhardt BA, Holtzman NA. Does knowledge about the genetics of breast cancer differ between nongeneticist physicians who do or do not discuss or order BRCA testing? *Genet Med.* 2003;5(2):99–105.

6. Rosenthal ET. Shortage of genetics counselors may be anecdotal, but need is real. *Oncol Times*. 2007;29(19):34,36.]

7. Informed Medical Decisions. Adult Genetics: Genetic counseling for your health concerns. Available at: http://www.informeddna.com/index.php/patients/adult-genetics.html. Accessed August 24, 2009.

8. Informed Medical Decisions. News: Aetna Press Release: Aetna to offer access to confidential telephonic cancer genetic counseling to health plan members. Available at: http://www.informeddna.com/images/stories/news_articles/aetna%20press%20release%20bw.pdf. Accessed August 24, 2009.

9. Claus EB, Schildkraut JM, Thompson WD, et al. The genetic attributable risks of breast and ovarian cancer. *Cancer*. 1996;77:2318–2324.

10. Loman N, Johannsson O, Kristoffersson U. Family history of breast and ovarian cancers and BRCA1 and BRCA2 mutations in a population-based series of early-onset breast cancer. *J Natl Cancer Inst*. 2001;93:1215–1223.

11. Struewing JP, Hartge P, Wacholder S, et al. The risk of cancer associated with specific mutations of BRCA1 and BRCA2 among Ashkenazi Jews. *N Engl J Med*. 1997;336:1401–1408.

12. Eisinger F, Jacquemier J, Charpin C, et al. Mutations at BRCA1: The medullary breast carcinoma revisited. *Cancer Res*. 1998;58:1588–1592.

13. Kandel M, Stadler Z, Masciari S, et al. Prevalence of BRCA1 mutations in triple negative breast cancer. 42nd Annual ASCO Meeting, 2006; Atlanta, Georgia.

14. National Comprehensive Cancer Network Clinical Guidelines in Oncology: Genetics/Familial High-Risk Assessment—Breast and Ovarian Cancer. http://www.nccn.org/professionals/physician_gls/f_guidelines.asp#detection. Accessed November 2, 2012.

15. Risch HA, McLaughlin JR, Cole DE, et al. Population BRCA1 and BRCA2 mutation frequencies and cancer penetrances: A kin-cohort study in Ontario, Canada. *J Natl Cancer Inst*. 2006;98(23):1694–1706.

16. Plon SE, Nathanson K. Inherited susceptibility for pediatric cancer. *Cancer J*. 2005;11(4):255–267.

17. Matloff ET, Brierley KL, Chimera CM. A clinician's guide to hereditary colon cancer. *Cancer J*. 2004;10(5):280–287.

18. Pilarski R. Cowden syndrome: A critical review of the clinical literature. *J Genet Couns*. 2009;18(1):13–27.

19. Varga EA, Pastore M, Prior T, et al. The prevalence of PTEN mutations in a clinical pediatric cohort with autism spectrum disorders, developmental delay, and macrocephaly. *Genet Med*. 2009;11(2):111–117.

20. Gorlin RJ. Nevoid basal-cell carcinoma syndrome. *Medicine*. 1987;66(2):98–113.

21. Schneider K. *Counseling About Cancer: Strategies for Genetic Counseling*. 2nd ed. New York, NY: Wiley-Liss; 2001.

22. Love RR, Evans AM, Josten DM. The accuracy of patient reports of a family history of cancer. *J Chronic Dis*. 1985;38(4):289–293.

23. Alter BP, Rosenberg PS, Brody LC. Clinical and molecular features associated with biallelic mutations in FANCD1/BRCA2. *J Med Genet*. 2007;44(1):1–9.

24. Thompson D, Duedal S, Kirner J, et al. Cancer risks and mortality in heterozygous ATM mutation carriers. *J Natl Cancer Inst*. 2005;97(11):813–822.

25. Korzenik J, Chung DC, Digumarthy S, et al. Case records of the Massachusetts General Hospital. Case 33-2005. A 43-year-old man with lower gastrointestinal bleeding. *N Engl J Med*. 2005;353:1836–1844.

26. American Cancer Society: Cancer Facts and Figures 2009. Atlanta, GA: American Cancer Society, 2009.

27. Olopade O, Weber B. Breast cancer genetics: Toward molecular characterization of individuals at increased risk for breast cancer. Part II. *PPO Updates*. 1998;12(11):1–8.

28. Stratton MR, Rahman N. The emerging landscape of breast cancer susceptibility. *Nat Genet*. 2008;40(1):17–22.

29. Gail MH, Brinton LA, Byar DP, et al. Projecting individualized probabilities of developing breast cancer for white females who are being examined annually. *J Natl Cancer Inst*. 1989;81(24):1879–1886.

30. Claus EB, Risch N, Thompson WD. Autosomal dominant inheritance of early-onset breast cancer. Implications for risk prediction. *Cancer*. 1994;73:643–651.

31. Parmigiani G, Berry D, Agiular O. Determining carrier probabilities for breast cancer susceptibility genes BRCA1 and BRCA2. *Am J Hum Genet*. 1998;62:145–158.

32. Giardiello FM, Brensinger JD, Petersen GM, et al. The use and interpretation of commercial APC gene testing for familial adenomatous polyposis. *N Engl J Med.* 1997;336:823–827.

33. Brierley K, Kim K, Matloff E, et al. Obstetricians' and gynecologists' knowledge, interests, and current practices with regard to providing breast and ovarian cancer genetic counseling. *J Genet Couns.* 2001;10:438–439.

34. Greendale K, Pyeritz RE. Empowering primary care health professionals in medical genetics: How soon? How fast? How far? *Am J Med Genet.* 2001;106:223–232.

35. Wideroff L, Vadaparampil ST, Greene MH, et al. Hereditary breast/ovarian and colorectal cancer genetics knowledge in a national sample of US physicians. *J Med Genet.* 2005;42:749–755.

36. Friedman S. Thoughts from FORCE: Comments Submitted to the Secretary's Advisory Committee on Genetics Health and Society. Available at: http://facingourrisk.wordpress.com/2008/12/03/comments-submitted-to-the-secretarys-advisory-committee-on-genetics-health-and-society/. Accessed April 6, 2010.

37. Walsh T, Casadei S, Coats KH, et al. Spectrum of mutations in BRCA1, BRCA2, CHEK2, and TP53 in families at high risk of breast cancer. *JAMA.* 2006;295(12):1379–1388.

38. U.S. Preventive Services Task Force. Genetic Risk Assessment and *BRCA* Mutation Testing for Breast and Ovarian Cancer Susceptibility. Topic Page. September 2005. Agency for Healthcare Research and Quality, Rockville, MD. Available at: http://www.ahrq.gov/clinic/uspstf/uspsbrgen.htm. Accessed April 6, 2010.

39. King MC, Marks JH, Mandell JB, et al. Breast and ovarian cancer risks due to inherited mutations in BRCA1 and BRCA2. *Science.* 2003;302:643–646.

40. Antoniou A, Pharoah PD, Narod S, et al. Average risks of breast and ovarian cancer associated with BRCA1 or BRCA2 mutations detected in case series unselected for family history: A combined analysis of 22 studies. *Am J Hum Genet.* 2003;72:1117–1130.

41. Ford D, Easton DF, Bishop DT, et al. Risks of cancer in BRCA1 mutation carriers. Breast Cancer Linkage Consortium. *Lancet.* 1994;343:692–695.

42. Piver MS, Jishi MF, Tsukada Y, et al. Primary peritoneal carcinoma after prophylactic oophorectomy in women with a family history of ovarian cancer. *Cancer.* 1993;71:2751–2755.

43. Aziz S, Kuperstein G, Rosen B, et al. A genetic epidemiological study of carcincoma of the fallopian tube. *Gynecol Oncol.* 2001;80:341–345.

44. van Asperen CJ, Brohet RM, Meijers-Heijboer EJ, et al. Cancer risks in BRCA2 families: Estimates for sites other than breast and ovary. *J Med Genet.* 2005;42:711–719.

45. Cancer risks in BRCA2 mutation carriers. The Breast Cancer Linkage Consortium. *J Natl Cancer Inst.* 1999;91(15):1310–1316.

46. Aarnio M, Mecklin JP, Aaltonen LA, et al. Life-time risk of different cancers in hereditary nonpolyposis colorectal cancer (HNPCC) syndrome. *Int J Cancer.* 1995;64:430–433.

47. Schmeler KM, Lynch HT, Chen LM, et al. Prophylactic surgery to reduce the risk of gynecologic cancers in the Lynch syndrome. *N Engl J Med.* 2006;354(3):261–269.

48. Warner E, Plewes DB, Hill KA, et al. Surveillance of BRCA1 and BRCA2 mutation carriers with magnetic resonance imaging, ultrasound, mammography, and clinical breast examination. *JAMA.* 2004;292(11):1317–1325.

49. Kriege M, Brekelmans CT, Boetes C, et al. Efficacy of MRI and mammography for breast-cancer screening in women with a familial or genetic predisposition. *N Engl J Med.* 2004;351(5):427–437.

50. Kuhl C, Weigel S, Schrading S, et al. Prospective multicenter cohort study to refine management recommendations for women at elevated familial risk of breast cancer: The EVA Trial. *J Clin Oncol.* 2010:1450–1457.

51. Powles TJ, Ashley S, Tidy A, et al. Twenty-year follow-up of the Royal Marsden randomized, double-blinded tamoxifen breast cancer prevention trial. *J Natl Cancer Inst.* 2007;99(4):283–290.

52. Cuzick J, Forbes JF, Sestak I, et al. Long-term results of tamoxifen prophylaxis for breast cancer—96-month follow-up of the randomized IBIS-I trial. *J Natl Cancer Inst.* 2007;99(4):272–282.

53. Fisher B, Constantino JP, Wickerman DL, et al. Tamoxifen for the prevention of breast cancer: Report of the National Surgical Adjuvant Breast and Bowel Project P-1 Study. *J Natl Cancer Inst.* 1998;90:1371–1388.

54. King MC, Wieand S, Hale K, et al. Tamoxifen and breast cancer incidence among women with inherited mutations in BRCA1 and BRCA2. National Surgical Adjuvant Breast and Bowel Project (NSABP-P1) Breast Cancer Prevention Trial. *JAMA*. 2001;286:2251–2256.

55. Narod SA, Brunet JS, Ghadirian P, et al. Tamoxifen and risk of contralateral breast cancer in BRCA1 and BRCA2 mutation carriers: A case-control study. Hereditary Breast Cancer Clinical Study Group. *Lancet*. 2000;356:1876–1881.

56. Metcalfe K, Lynch HT, Ghadirian P, et al. Contralateral breast cancer in BRCA1 and BRCA2 mutation carriers. *J Clin Oncol*. 2004;22:2328–2335.

57. Lakhani SR, van de Vijver MJ, Jacquemier J, et al. The pathology of familial breast cancer: Predictive value of immunohistochemical markers estrogen receptor, progesterone receptor, HER-2, and p53 in patients with mutations in BRCA1 and BRCA2. *J Clin Oncol*. 2002;20(9):2310–2318.

58. Hartmann LC, Schaid DJ, Woods JE. Efficacy of bilateral prophylactic mastectomy in women with a family history of breast cancer. *N Engl J Med*. 1999;340:77–84.

59. Matloff ET. The breast surgeon's role in BRCA1 and BRCA2 testing. *Am J Surg*. 2000;180(4):294–298.

60. Turner BC, Harold E, Matloff E, et al. BRCA1/BRCA2 germline mutations in locally recurrent breast cancer patients after lumpectomy and radiation therapy: Implications for breast-conserving management in patients with BRCA1/BRCA2 mutations. *J Clin Oncol*. 1999;17(10):3017–3024.

61. Contant CM, Menke-Pluijmers MB, Seynaeve C, et al. Clinical experience of prophylactic mastectomy followed by immediate breast reconstruction in women at hereditary risk of breast cancer (HB(O)C) or a proven BRCA1 or BRCA2 germ-line mutation. *Eur J Surg Oncol*. 2002;28: 627–632.

62. Forman DL, Chiu J, Restifo RJ, et al. Breast reconstruction in previously irradiated patients using tissue expanders and implants: A potentially unfavorable result. *Ann Plast Surg*. 1998;40(4):360–363.

63. Burke W, Daly MB, Garber J, et al. Recommendations for follow-up care of individuals with an inherited predisposition to cancer. II. BRCA1 and BRCA2. Cancer Genetics Studies Consortium. *JAMA*. 1997;277(12):997–1003.

64. McLaughlin JR, Risch HA, Lubinski J, et al. Reproductive risk factors for ovarian cancer in carriers of BRCA1 or BRCA2 mutations: A case-control study. *Lancet Oncol*. 2007;8(1):26–34.

65. Milne RL, Knight JA, John EM, et al. Oral contraceptive use and risk of early-onset breast cancer in carriers and noncarriers of BRCA1 and BRCA2 mutations. *Cancer Epidemiol Biomarkers Prev*. 2005;14(2):350–356.

66. Domchek S, Friebel T, Neuhausen S, et al. Mortality reduction after risk-reducing bilateral salpingo-oophorectomy in a prospective cohort of BRCA1 and BRCA2 mutation carriers. *Lancet Oncol*. 2006;7(3):223–229.

67. Powell CB, Kenley E, Chen LM, et al. Risk-reducing salpingo-oophorectomy in BRCA mutation carriers: Role of serial sectioning in the detection of occult malignancy. *J Clin Oncol*. 2005;23(1):127–132.

68. Finch A, Beiner M, Lubinski J, et al. Salpingo-oophorectomy and the risk of ovarian, fallopian tube, and peritoneal cancers in women with a BRCA1 or BRCA2 mutation. *JAMA*. 2006;296(2):185–192.

69. Kurian AW, Sigal BM, Plevritis SK. Survival analysis of cancer risk reduction strategies for BRCA1/2 mutation carriers. *J Clin Oncol*. 2010;28(2):222–231.

70. ACOG committee opinion. Breast–ovarian cancer screening. Number 176, October 1996. Committee on Genetics. The American College of Obstetricians and Gynecologists. *Int J Gynaecol Obstet*. 1997;56(1):82–83.

71. Hornreich G, Beller U, Lavie O. Is uterine serous papillary carcinoma a BRCA1 related disease? Case report and review of the literature. *Gynecol Oncol*. 1999;75(2):300–304.

72. Levine DA, Lin O, Barakat RR. Risk of endometrial carcinoma associated with BRCA mutation. *Gynecol Oncol*. 2001;80(3):395–398.

73. Goshen R, Chu W, Elit L, et al. Is uterine papillary serous adenocarcinoma a manifestation of the hereditary breast-ovarian cancer syndrome? *Gynecol Oncol*. 2000;79(3):477–481.

74. Boyd J. BRCA: The breast, ovarian, and other cancer genes. *Gynecol Oncol*. 2001;80(3):337–340.

75. Rebbeck TR, Lynch HT, Neuhausen SL, et al. Prophylactic oophorectomy in carriers of BRCA1 or BRCA2 mutations. *N Engl J Med*. 2002;346(21):1616–1622.

76. Kauff ND, Satagopan JM, Robson ME, et al. Risk-reducing salpingo-oophorectomy in women with a BRCA1 or BRCA2 mutation. *N Engl J Med*. 2002;346(21):1609–1615.

77. Rebbeck TR, Friebel T, Wagner T, et al. Effect of short-term hormone replacement therapy on breast cancer risk reduction after bilateral prophylactic oophorectomy in BRCA1 and BRCA2 mutation carriers: The PROSE study group. *J Clin Oncol*. 2005;23(31):7804–7810.

78. Gronwald J, Tung N, Foulkes WD, et al. Tamoxifen and contralateral breast cancer in BRCA1 and BRCA2 carriers: An update. *Int J Cancer*. 2006;118(9):2281–2284.

79. Kash KM, Holland JC, Halper MS, et al. Psychological distress and surveillance behaviors of women with a family history of breast cancer. *J Natl Cancer Inst*. 1992;84(1):24–30.

80. Lerman C, Hughes C, Lemon SJ. What you don't know can hurt you: Adverse psychologic effects in members of BRCA1-linked and BRCA2-linked families who decline genetic testing. *J Clin Oncol*. 1998;16:1650–1654.

81. Croyle RT, Smith KR, Botkin JR, et al. Psychological responses to BRCA1 mutation testing: Preliminary findings. *Health Psychol*. 1997;16(1):63–72.

82. Hamilton JG, Lobel M, Moyer A. Emotional distress following genetic testing for hereditary breast and ovarian cancer: A meta-analytic review. *Health Psychol*. 2009;28(4):510–518.

83. Clayton EW. Removing the shadow of the law from the debate about genetic testing of children. *Am J Med Genet*. 1995;57(4):630–634.

84. ASHG/ACMG. Points to consider: Ethical, legal, and psychosocial implications of genetic testing in children and adolescents. American Society of Human Genetics Board of Directors, American College of Medical Genetics Board of Directors. *Am J Hum Genet*. 1995;57:1233–1241.

85. Ledger GA, Khosla S, Lindor NM, et al. Genetic testing in the diagnosis and management of multiple endocrine neoplasia type II. *Ann Intern Med*. 1995;122(2):118–124.

86. Rhodes M, Bradburn DM. Overview of screening and management of familial adenomatous polyposis. *Gut*. 1992;33(1):125–131.

87. Bluman LG, Rimer BK, Berry DA. Attitudes, knowledge, and risk perceptions of women with breast and/or ovarian cancer considering testing for BRCA1 and BRCA2. *J Clin Oncol*. 1999;17(3):1040–1046.

88. Tsoucalas C. Legal aspects of cancer genetics—screening, counseling, and registers. In: Lynch H, Kullander S, eds. *Cancer Genetics in Women: Vol I*. Boca Raton, FL: CRC Press, Inc.; 1987:9.

89. ASHG. ASHG Statement: Professional disclosure of familial genetic information. *Am J Hum Genet*. 1998;62:474–483.

90. Matloff ET, Shappell H, Brierley K, et al. What would you do? Specialists' perspectives on cancer genetic testing, prophylactic surgery and insurance discrimination. *J Clin Oncol*. 2000;18(12):2484–2492.

91. Hall M. Genetic discrimination. In: North Carolina Genomics & Bioinformatics Consortium; 2003; North Carolina.

92. Leib JR, Hoodfar E, Larsen Haidle J, et al. The new genetic privacy law. *Commun Oncol*. 2008;5:351–354.

93. Hudson KL, Holohan MK, Collins FS. Keeping pace with the times—the Genetic Information Nondiscrimination Act of 2008. *N Engl J Med*. 2008;358(25):2661–2663.

94. Library of Congress entry for the Genetic Information Nondiscrimination Act of 2008 (H.R. 493). Available at: http://thomas.loc.gov/cgi-bin/bdquery/z?d110:h.r.00493. Accessed December 3, 2012.

95. Library of Congress entry for the Health Care and Education Affordability Reconciliation Act of 2010 (H.R. 4872). Available at: http://thomas.loc.gov/cgi-bin/bdquery/z?d111:HR4872. Accessed December 3, 2012.

96. Manley S, Pennell R, Frank T. Insurance coverage of BRCA1 and BRCA2 sequence analysis. *J Genet Couns*. 1998;7(6):A462.

97. Grann VR, Whang W, Jabcobson JS, et al. Benefits and costs of screening Ashkenazi Jewish women for BRCA1 and BRCA2. *J Clin Oncol*. 1999;17(2):494–500.

98. Sevilla C, Julian-Reynier C, Eisinger F, et al. Impact of gene patents on the cost-effective delivery of care: The case of BRCA1 genetic testing. *Int J Technol Assess Health Care*. 2003;19(2):287–300.

99. Kesselheim AS, Mello MM. Gene patenting—is the pendulum swinging back? *N Engl J Med.* 2010;362(20):1855–1858.

100. Fong PC, Boss DS, Yap TA, et al. Inhibition of poly (ADP-ribose) polymerase in tumors from BRCA mutation carriers. *N Engl J Med.* 2009;361(2):123–134.

101. Iglehart JD, Silver DP. Synthetic lethality—a new direction in cancer-drug development. *N Engl J Med.* 2009;361(2):189–191.

102. Offit K, Kohut K, Clagett B, et al. Cancer genetic testing and assisted reproduction. *J Clin Oncol.* 2006;24(29):4775–4782.

103. Offit K, Levran O, Mullaney B, et al. Shared genetic susceptibility to breast cancer, brain tumors, and Fanconi anemia. *J Natl Cancer Inst.* 2003;95(20):1548–1551.

2 Whole-genome and Whole-exome Sequencing in Hereditary Cancer

Impact on Genetic Testing and Counseling

Julianne M. O'Daniel and Kristy Lee

The past few years have seen a whirlwind of technologic advances in terms of genetic testing. Tumbling laboratory costs have placed whole-genome sequencing (WGS) and whole-exome sequencing (WES) at the forefront of new genetic technologies, gaining attention from clinicians and health care administrators who want to tap into these cutting-edge technologies for their patients. Similar to all new health technologies, WGS and WES present both challenges and opportunities. In this chapter, we hope to present a practical examination of these new technologies in the application to hereditary cancer.

WHOLE-GENOME SEQUENCING/WHOLE-EXOME SEQUENCING TECHNOLOGIES

Although there are several different technology platforms, the basic premise of current sequencing technology, often referred to as "next-generation" sequencing is to determine the base sequences of huge numbers of DNA segments all performed in parallel, which are then typically aligned to a genomic reference in order to detect genetic variation.[1] In both WGS and WES, the DNA sample is first sheared randomly into small fragments, the length of which may vary based on the sequencing platform. Since the original sample contains multiple copies of genomic DNA, the random shearing results in the same segment of DNA being fragmented in different ways. This is important for the alignment step below. These fragments are then amplified through a polymerase chain reaction step similar to traditional sequencing. The result is a library containing hundreds of copies of each of the fragments.

At this stage, WES requires two additional steps to enable focused analysis of the exome, which represents less than 2% of the human genome. The library is enriched for the exonic regions by using oligonucleotide probes that hybridize to, or capture, the specified exon targets.[2] The uncaptured DNA fragments are washed away, and an amplification step follows to maximize the amount of captured exonic fragments.

23

Several kits are commercially available to capture the exome in this fashion. When choosing a kit or testing laboratory, it is important to consider how the exonic regions are defined and covered by the hybridization probes as that will affect the purity and completeness of your exome coverage.[2]

The next step for both WGS and WES is the concurrent sequencing of the whole library or the enriched library, respectively (massively parallel sequencing). Dependent on the technology-specific chemistry, the sequencing instrument uses the library fragments to determine the sequence, which is then captured base-by-base by the instrument.

At this stage, quality scores are also calculated pertaining to both individual and sequences of base calls. These scores are frequently reported as Q scores and represent the logarithmic chance that the call is incorrect. For example, Q20 equates to a 1 in 100 chance the call is wrong, Q30 equates to a 1 in 1,000 chance, and Q40 is approximately a 1 in 10,000 chance. The result from this step is a digital file of short sequences, or reads, with their quality scores called the fastq file.

The reads must then be aligned computationally to a human reference genome to produce an assembly of the individual's genome or exome sequence (Fig. 2.1). Using a reference sequence to guide assembly is referred to as "resequencing," as opposed to de novo sequencing, which does not align to a known reference. In most cases, the publicly available human genome reference sequence is used. Since the fragments were randomly sheared, a number of reads should align to most of the bases of the reference. This overlap helps ensure accurate alignment and variant identifications. The number of times a specific reference base position is matched with a base in the

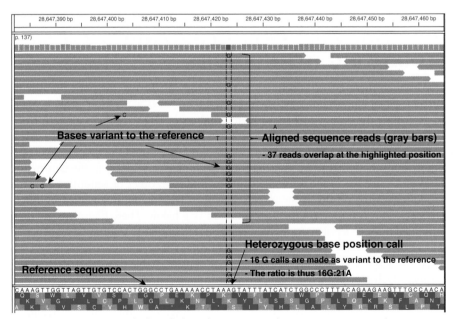

FIGURE 2.1. Computer display of aligned sequence reads at a given position in the genome.

aligned reads is called the depth of coverage. In other words, if five reads overlap the base position, then the coverage is 5× at that position.

A separate algorithm considers the base calls and quality scores of all reads overlapping a specific position in the reference sequence to make a consensus base call at that location in the individual's genome. For example, if the five overlapping reads all have a G at that position, then the call would be a homozygous G/G. However, if two of the reads have a T and three have a G, then it might mean the individual is heterozygous T/G at that position, or it may be that the T's (or G's for that matter) are incorrect. The higher the depth of coverage and the higher the quality of the individual base calls, the higher the confidence that the base called at that position is correct.[3] Higher coverage is imperative for determining heterozygous calls or when low levels of mosaicism may be important, such as in tumor samples. The generally reported coverage for clinical WGS/WES testing ranges from a genome-wide average coverage of approximately 30 to 80 times with WES at the higher end of the spectrum. The enrichment/capture step for WES does not perform at a uniform efficiency across the entire exome, leading to a broader spread of coverage depths as compared with WGS, and thus the need for higher average depth of coverage.[2]

The final and arguably most complicated step is that of clinical interpretation. At this stage, the identified variants are examined against available databases to determine their functional impact and possible clinical significance.[4,5] These analyses generally require automated searches initially to collect frequency data and functional consequence predictions as well as comparisons to reported pathogenic variants in clinical databases such as the Human Gene Mutation Database (http://www.hgmd.cf.ac.uk). Following the automated annotation; however, a manual review is essential to identify which variants may be truly pathogenic based on available clinical evidence often collected in multiple locus-specific databases and which variants may explain either the patient's phenotype or potentially an unrelated condition.[4]

Comparison of Whole-genome Sequencing to Whole-exome Sequencing

Although both WGS and WES are clinically available, there are important differences to consider. The largest difference is the amount and content of the data. WGS includes sequence information for all areas covered in the genome, whereas WES is focused on less than 2% of the genome that is known to code for protein and will not report changes in promoter or regulatory regions. With that in mind, you should expect a lot more data with WGS: Approximately, 120 Gb for a 30× WGS compared with approximately 5 to 10 Gb from WES. Although both methodologies can provide greater than 90% of the entire exome sequence, the method by which WES targets or captures only the exon information leads to slightly less coverage of the entire exome as compared with WGS methods.[6] However, because of the vastly smaller amount of genomic sequence, throughput and depth of coverage are frequently much greater with WES. In regard to clinical testing, there is not much difference in regard to cost with WES ranging from $4,000 to $15,000 and WGS from $7,500 to $10,000.

Current Limitations

WGS/WES has both technical and clinical challenges. Because of several factors, including alignment programs, short read length, and genome complexity, the ability to use WGS/WES to detect variations larger than a few base pairs is limited, although there has been progress in this area. Currently next-generation sequencing technologies have difficulty accurately calling indels (insertions and deletions), trinucleotide repeats, and copy-number variations. To confidently identify these types of variations, a second testing technology is often required. Thus, interpretation and test reports will be focused on single base-pair, substitution variants. Another challenge is the ability to fully and accurately interpret the resulting sequence information. This is complicated by the currently limited accuracy and completeness of the reference human genome as well as the lack of clinical-grade databases for interpretation.[2,4] Ongoing efforts are attempting to address these limitations.

CLINICAL WHOLE-GENOME SEQUENCING/ WHOLE-EXOME SEQUENCING APPLICATIONS

The use of WGS/WES in the clinical setting has already begun, and there is as much excitement surrounding the availability of such testing as there are questions and hesitations. WGS/WES testing has the potential to greatly improve our ability to determine the molecular causation in most Mendelian diseases, and early guidelines for clinical use were recently published by the American College of Medical Genetics and Genomics.[7] Researchers have already shown the value of WGS/WES as a tool for identifying candidate genes for genetic conditions with a defined phenotype including Freeman–Sheldon syndrome as well as autosomal dominant retinitis pigmentosa, one of the most genetically heterogeneous Mendelian conditions.[6,8]

Hereditary cancer syndromes, similar to other Mendelian diseases, have significant genetic heterogeneity, which often necessitates the need to order multiple gene tests. WGS/WES has the potential to enable testing of all possible target genes at once, eliminating the extended time and added cost of sequential gene testing, if needed. This may be particularly helpful in complex disorders such as cancer, where patients may harbor multiple variants that modify their risk. Walsh et al.[9] demonstrated this complexity, identifying 2 germline mutations in 3 of 360 ovarian cancer patients. In addition to one germline mutation in either *BRCA1* or *BRCA2*, one of the three participants had a mutation in *CHEK2* and the other two had mutations in the *MRE11A* gene, which only recently became available for clinical testing. Most clinicians would have felt comfortable with the explanation of the patient having a *BRCA1* or *BRCA2* mutation and would not have pursued additional testing to unearth a second hereditary risk factor for cancer. This information is not only helpful for the individual patient, as they may be at increased risk for additional cancers, but the information is critically important for other family members. Currently, if a patient's relative has negative genetic testing for a known familial mutation in *BRCA1* or *BRCA2*, that relative (depending on details of the family history) would likely be informed that he/she is not at an elevated risk of developing cancer. In cases like this example, that information could be very wrong.

Another hope is that by expanding our knowledge of genes and genetic variants associated with hereditary cancer syndromes, we will have the opportunity to understand more about the natural history of these conditions and possibly guide therapeutics. As WGS/WES becomes more affordable and more widely available, we will continue to identify additional disease-causative genes. We will also likely learn about novel phenotypes associated with variants in previously identified genes.

Cancer Genome Sequencing

Beyond germline variants for hereditary cancer syndromes, WGS/WES is also being applied for therapeutic guidance. This includes the identification of relevant pharmacogenetic variants and investigation of targeted gene–disease–drug interactions, as well as analysis of the patient's cancer genome to identify "driver" variants and possible therapeutic targets.[10,11] Although germline testing can be used for some situations such as for *HER2* gene amplification in breast and upper gastrointestinal cancers, therapeutics based on the molecular characteristics of the tumor require the much more complicated cancer sequence be analyzed.

Cancer genome sequencing typically involves sequencing both the cancer and germline genomes from an individual. A comparison is performed between the two sequences bioinformatically to subtract the variants found in the germline sequence, leaving only the variants that are unique to the tumor sample and thus assumed to have been somatically acquired. These cancer-specific variants are then analyzed using cancer databases such as COSMIC (http://www.sanger.ac.uk/genetics/CGP/cosmic/) to determine which ones may be playing driving roles in the growth of the cancer. Additional gene pathway analysis is necessary to determine potential therapeutic suggestions among available drugs (approved or in trial).

Unlike germline sequencing, cancer sequences are rarely diploid and frequently harbor multiple cell lines. Thus, accurate variant calling against such a complex, mosaic background is a challenge. In addition, the cancer genome is undergoing constant evolution, and thus resequencing and analysis should be considered for continual therapy modification as needed.[11]

COUNSELING IMPACT

Although the therapeutic possibilities are promising and could affect standard care for all cancer patients, the earliest impact of WGS/WES testing will be felt in the hereditary cancer clinic.[11] These clinics are typically staffed by genetic counselors who assist patients and families through complex risk assessment and testing choices. One of the primary aims of genetic counseling is to facilitate informed patient decision making and psychosocial adjustment in regard to genetic information.[12] This process generally includes the following elements: Contracting, risk assessment, pretest counseling, results and risk communication, and follow-up. To better comprehend the impact of using WGS/WES in the clinical setting, it may be helpful to consider the different aspects of the genetic counseling session when incorporating WGS/WES testing.

Contracting

When first meeting a patient, the genetic counselor will ascertain the patient's understanding about why they were referred and determine the expectations, questions, and concerns that need to be addressed during the session. It is during this initial conversation that the counselor can often get a sense of the level of concern that the patient has regarding his/her chance of having an inherited risk of developing cancer. Given the popularity of genomic technology in the media, this initial discussion can also help identify and correct patient expectations regarding testing and the limited availability of genome-guided treatments for his/her cancer.

Risk Assessment

A personal and targeted family history about cancer is the primary tool used in the initial risk assessment, testing recommendations, and results interpretation. The family history should include at least a three- to four-generation pedigree with notation of individuals with cancer, age at onset, and any possible environmental risk factors.[13] Testing recommendations are based on recognizable patterns or clustering of cancers in the family. Missing or incorrect information, such as "female" cancer or stomach as opposed to pancreatic cancer, can result in insufficient, excessive, or simply incorrect testing being ordered.

Even as WES/WGS is incorporated into the clinical setting, obtaining the personal history and a detailed pedigree will continue to be a necessity for interpreting the results for the patient and providing appropriate risk assessment for other relatives. The option of WGS/WES; however, may increase testing access and represent a significant benefit to patients such as those with limited or no family history as in adoption, or for patients who do not clearly meet testing criteria, or fit a precise cancer pattern. Imagine the example of a patient with a personal history of ovarian cancer and a family history of both colon and breast cancer in first-degree relatives. The testing differential must, at a minimum, include genes for both Lynch syndrome (hereditary nonpolyposis colorectal cancer) and hereditary breast and ovarian cancer (HBOC), at least seven genes. WGS/WES enables targeted informatics analysis of genes associated with Lynch syndrome and HBOC as well as analysis of any other genes that are less commonly associated with these hereditary cancers to provide a comprehensive and cost-effective approach.[9]

Pretest Counseling

If testing is considered appropriate, the counselor then seeks to help the patient make an informed choice about proceeding with a testing strategy or not. There are numerous elements to consider, including:

- Clinical features, inheritance pattern, and likelihood of a hereditary cancer syndrome;
- Medical management guidelines based on such a syndrome;
- Genetic testing strategies including suspected genes, turnaround time, and cost;
- Types of results that may be returned, that is, positive (a deleterious mutation), negative, or a variant of unknown significance (VUS); and
- Potential impact testing information may have in terms of medical care, daily life (job, insurance), self-concept, and family relationships.

If the patient decides to proceed with testing, the counselor and patient also discuss how results will be communicated, that is, via a clinic appointment or telephone call.

WGS/WES will change several aspects of this counseling. Rather than discussing different test options with different gene coverage, turnaround times, and costs, counseling can focus on one test and a strategy for analyzing various genes that may explain the suspicion for a hereditary cancer syndrome. The added gene analysis; however, is likely to increase the turnaround time as compared with single-gene or small gene panel tests. For breast cancer patients who require surgery as part of their treatment, waiting 2 to 3 months for a WGS/WES test result to determine whether they wish to have bilateral mastectomies versus a lumpectomy is impractical. Thus, timelines are important considerations in test choice.

Further explanation of test limitations would include a focus on the technology, outlining difficulties with detection of certain types of rearrangements. Many groups also feel it is necessary to confirm any significant variant via traditional Sanger sequencing before using it clinically. This confirmatory testing may or may not be included with the original WGS/WES test ordered. A comparison and contrast of WES/WGS versus traditional small gene panel or single-gene sequencing is outlined in Table 2.1.

Another limitation is our scientific knowledge. Similar to single-gene tests, it is possible to learn a patient has variants for which a conclusive clinical interpretation cannot be made—the elusive VUS. The chance for discovering one or more VUS; however, is higher with WGS/WES, because of the increased number of genes that may be analyzed including those that have only recently been found to contribute to hereditary cancers. Although access to information about these genes is clearly a benefit, the increased number of VUS may be a challenge.

Arguably one of the most significant impacts of WGS/WES on the genetic counseling session will be discussing the full range of possible results that could be learned. It is important to first learn what options the laboratory provides regarding results return. Several WGS/WES testing laboratories are enabling providers to tailor reports for how comprehensive the test should be. The laboratory sequences the entire genome/exome, but can focus the analysis bioinformatically to scrutinize data from a subset of clinically targeted genes. This allows the laboratory to drastically decrease the number of variants to analyze, as well as only report findings related to the referral indication. Testing may be offered in tiers where, for example, tier 1 may include the analysis of only 20 genes and, if uninformative, tier 2 would

TABLE 2.1	Comparison of Traditional Single-gene, Small Panel Gene Sequencing Versus WGS/WES in Hereditary Cancer	
	Traditional Cancer Sequencing	**WGS/WES**
Scope	One gene/gene panel providing information about the referral indication	All genes providing information about the referral indication and possible secondary findings
Turnaround time	Range, 1–12 wks	Range, 6–16 wks
Sample required	5–10 mL of blood in EDTA tube	5–10 mL of blood in EDTA tube
Cost	$1,000–$16,000 or higher depending on size of test panel	$5,000–$15,000
Report	Report includes only information pertinent to gene(s) requested	Report includes results pertinent to clinical indication and may include significant secondary findings
Amended/ updated report	Laboratory issued update for change in VUS interpretation	Report interpretation will evolve over time; no standard policies regarding responsibility for reanalysis and updates
Appointment(s) required	Usually one appointment	Likely Q2 appointments
Patient follow-up	May require referrals to specialists if a diagnosis is made; may have to consider additional tests	May require referrals to multiple specialists if multiple diagnoses are made; may have to consider confirmational tests; data may need to be reanalyzed

expand analysis to data from all genes. This distinction is important to discuss with the patient before testing, because of the combined clinical and research potential of WES/WGS. It remains controversial, for example, whether suspicious variants in highly promising candidate genes that are not currently known to cause cancer susceptibility in humans should be reported as part of a clinical test. It could certainly be argued that such research analyses should not be billed as part of a clinical diagnostic test.

It is also important to learn about options for inclusion/exclusion of findings unrelated to the clinical question. Although occasionally referred to as "unexpected," these "incidental" or "secondary" findings are intrinsic to WGS/WES and should be expected. There are currently no standard guidelines for the return of secondary findings from WGS/WES studies, although, of note, the American College of Medical Genetics and Genomics has appointed a workgroup to provide guidance for laboratories in this area. Regardless, laboratories will have different policies concerning the analysis and return of such information. If available, these options are typically outlined in the testing laboratory's consent. The clinician ordering a WGS/WES test must therefore be aware of the laboratory's policy and discuss the potential findings with the patient in advance. Patient choice regarding whether to learn about certain results will be an important aspect of pretest counseling.

Berg et al.[14] suggest secondary finding results be categorized at the laboratory level into medically actionable results (called Bin 1 results), clinically valid but not directly actionable results (Bin 2), and results of no known clinical significance (Bin 3). They suggest that Bin 1 results be returned to all patients, as these results would directly and favorably impact medical management. Patients could choose whether they wish to receive Bin 2 results, which would include results such as carrier status for autosomal recessive or X-linked traits, pharmacogenomic variants, and other single-nucleotide polymorphisms shown to confer an increased disease risk but not yet shown to be of clear medical benefit. They recommend that Bin 3 results not be returned until they can be confidently interpreted and have been shown to possess clinical validity. With this or a similar system, a counselor can help a patient decide what types of results are of value to them and plan for how and when the different types of results will be communicated.

Thus, additional questions for the pretest counseling include the following:

- Will the patient be given the option to receive results unrelated to the clinical question?
- Will the patient be given options about which types of findings to receive?
- What information does the patient need to decide whether to learn secondary results?
- Will parents be given results options if the patient is a minor?
- How and when will results be discussed?
- Which results will be stored in the medical record and/or plans for future access to additional results or the complete data?

Lastly, another important difference concerns reimbursement for this broad genomic test. Although the cost of testing is comparable or more economical than single-gene and stepwise testing, a patient's out-of-pocket cost may be much higher. Clinicians routinely ordering traditional genetic testing find that private third-party payers often pay the entire or at least a significant portion of the cost of genetic tests, whereas payment from public payers, such as Medicaid, varies.[15] Although success stories are growing, most third-party payers have not yet developed policies regarding coverage of WGS/WES, and reimbursement is not a guarantee.

All of these considerations must be taken into account not only for the patient, but also for the clinician deciding whether to offer WGS/WES versus more traditional genetic tests.

Results and Risk Communication

Typically, the patient with suspected HBOC is offered full sequencing and rearrangement analysis for *BRCA1/2* genes. If this genetic testing is negative, the ordering provider interprets the results in the context of the patient's personal and family history, and performs a posttest risk assessment. The patient is typically informed that there is a small remaining chance that (1) the test was unable to identify a mutation in the *BRCA1/2* genes, or (2) there could be a mutation in another gene conferring an increased risk of cancer that was not analyzed by this test. Alternatively, if the a priori risk of a mutation was small, it may be determined that his/her cancer most likely developed by chance and is not related to a hereditary cancer syndrome. In the last case, the genetic counselor may suggest that another informative relative has genetic testing for the *BRCA1/2* genes.

The promise of WGS/WES is that we will be able to detect more hereditary cancer families by looking beyond the most common and most easily tested genes. As mentioned; however, this broader scope will also increase the chance of VUS results. Although uncertainty is nothing new to genetics, it can be a very difficult issue for patients to understand and emotionally digest. A time frame for reanalysis of VUS results should be discussed. The counselor should contact the laboratory for their policy on reanalysis and updates to facilitate this discussion and create a plan with the patient.

WGS/WES may also significantly impact the logistics of results communication. The amount and complexity of results will increase, and preparation time for the counselor to familiarize themselves with the results and newly identified risks or conditions will also increase. Depending on laboratory reporting policies and patient preference, the results may contain information about conditions not typically addressed in the hereditary cancer clinic. Counselors will need to decide how to manage these secondary results, either through increased professional education and expanded practice expertise, or through referral to a general medical genetics colleague or other appropriate specialists.

Many cancer genetic counselors currently provide results to their patients over the telephone. Depending on the amount and complexity of the results from WGS/WES, it is likely that genetic counselors, especially in the early phases of implementing WGS/WES in the clinic, would need to counsel patients during a clinic appointment. In addition, patients may not be emotionally prepared to learn about variants beyond the initial clinical indication (hereditary cancer) at the first session. Further sessions or interactions may be necessary to address these. Thus, a counselor's workload could be greatly impacted, potentially increasing wait times for new patient referrals. On the other hand, the need for two or more results communication appointments could also potentially increase clinic revenues.

Long-term Patient Follow-up

Traditionally, a patient with a negative test result is asked to recontact the genetics clinic should there be any changes in their personal and/or family history of cancer or to learn about new genetic testing options. Similarly, patients receiving a VUS are also asked to recontact the counselor periodically to learn about any new information that may be available concerning their variant. However, in clinical practice, we find that it is uncommon to be recontacted by patients to update family or personal information, or to learn of updates in genetic testing or their VUS.

The need for revisiting results is also true of WES/WGS. The speed at which the field continues to gain new knowledge regarding the clinical impact of VUS or the identification of novel disease genes is not known. It is certain, however, that the interpretation of WGS/WES data will change over time. Therefore, it will be essential to revisit this information periodically. Questions remain such as how often should the data be reanalyzed? Whose responsibility is it to reinterpret data? Should this be a service provided by the laboratory that performed the test and at what cost to the patient? Should this reinterpretation be ordered by the provider and billed to the patient's insurance company? Or should the burden again be on the patient to contact his/her provider to have his/her data reinterpreted (even though this latter model does not generally work well)? Although several WGS/WES laboratories currently offer reanalysis and updates free of charge, this practice is not expected to continue as testing volumes increase and resources become limited. These are issues that will need to be addressed as the use of WGS/WES becomes more commonplace in the clinic.

SUMMARY

Offering WGS/WES in the clinical setting offers many advantages to traditional single-gene and small panel sequencing tests. Through enabling the analysis of essentially all human genes in one comprehensive test, WGS/WES not only can cut down on the cost of genetic testing for many genetic conditions, but also could arguably cut down on the time it takes to make a diagnosis in the patient. The broad scope of testing can also afford new options to the clinician and patient when the clinical differential is complex or when the family history is limited.

The clinical application of WGS/WES will also pose challenges. In addition to potentially longer testing turnaround time, especially in the early initiation period of WGS/WES, pretest counseling must expand to incorporate the types of results that could be learned from this type of testing and the information patients may need to make informed decisions about their disclosure options. The increased amount and complexity of results may necessitate longer genetic counseling sessions and possibly require genetic counselors to adopt multiple in-person sessions versus telephone consultation models for results disclosure. Finally, as knowledge increases regarding previously identified gene variants and newly discovered genotype/phenotype correlations, our understanding of a patient's genomic data should improve. Therefore, we will need to develop practice policies to guide how often genomic data should be reviewed and who should be responsible for ordering and paying for periodic reanalysis of the data.

As a new clinical technology, WGS/WES will undoubtedly change the way genetic counselors and other clinicians approach genetic testing. It is important to openly assess the limitations and challenges to afford our patients the greatest benefit from this testing in practice.

ACKNOWLEDGMENTS

The authors thank and acknowledge Mark Ross, PhD, of Illumina, Inc.; Allyn McKonkie-Rosell, PhD, and Robin King, MS, of Duke University; James P. Evans, MD, PhD, and Jonathan S. Berg, MD, PhD, of UNC Chapel Hill; and Michael J. Friez, PhD, of Greenwood Genetic Center for their invaluable contributions and insight.

REFERENCES

1. Metzker ML. Sequencing technologies—the next generation. *Nat Rev Genet.* 2010;11:31–46.
2. Bamshad MJ, Ng SB, Bigham AW, et al. Exome sequencing as a tool for Mendelian disease gene discovery. *Nat Rev Genet.* 2011;12:745–755.
3. Ajay SS, Parker SC, Abaan HO, et al. Accurate and comprehensive sequencing of personal genomes. *Genome Res.* 2011;21:1498–1505.
4. Ashley EA, Butte AJ, Wheeler MT, et al. Clinical assessment incorporating a personal genome. *Lancet.* 2010;375:1525–1535.
5. Fernald GH, Capriotti E, Daneshjou R, et al. Bioinformatics challenges for personalized medicine. *Bioinformatics.* 2011;27:1741–1748.
6. Ng SB, Turner EH, Robertson PD, et al. Targeted capture and massively parallel sequencing of 12 human exomes. *Nature.* 2009;461:272–276.
7. The American College of Medical Genetics and Genomics. Policy statement: Points to consider in the clinical application of genomic sequencing. Available at: http://www.acmg.net/StaticContent/PPG/Clinical_Application_of_Genomic_Sequencing.pdf. Accessed on June 23, 2012.
8. Zuchner S, Dallman J, Wen R, et al. Whole-exome sequencing links a variant in DHDDS to retinitis pigmentosa. *Am J Hum Genet.* 2011;88:201–206.
9. Walsh T, Casadei S, Lee MK, et al. Mutations in 12 genes for inherited ovarian, fallopian tube, and peritoneal carcinoma identified by massively parallel sequencing. *Proc Natl Acad Sci U S A.* 2011;108:18032–18037.
10. Ross JS, Cronin M. Whole cancer genome sequencing by next-generation methods. *Am J Clin Pathol.* 2011;136:527–539.
11. Meldrum C, Doyle MA, Tothill RW. Next-generation sequencing for cancer diagnostics: A practical perspective. *Clin Biochem Rev.* 2011;32:177–195.
12. National Society of Genetic Counselors' Definition Task Force, Resta R, Biesecker BB, et al. A new definition of genetic counseling: National Society of Genetic Counselors' Task Force report. *J Genet Couns.* 2006;15:77–83.
13. Riley BD, Culver JO, Skrzynia C, et al. Essential elements of genetic cancer risk assessment, counseling, and testing: Updated recommendations of the national society of genetic counselors. *J Genet Couns.* 2012;21:151–161.
14. Berg JS, Khoury MJ, Evans JP. Deploying whole genome sequencing in clinical practice and public health: Meeting the challenge one bin at a time. *Genet Med.* 2011;13:499–504.
15. Wang G, Beattie MS, Ponce NA, et al. Eligibility criteria in private and public coverage policies for BRCA genetic testing and genetic counseling. *Genet Med.* 2011;13:1045–1050.

3 Direct-to-consumer Personal Genome Testing and Cancer Risk Prediction

Cecelia A. Bellcross, Patricia Z. Page, and Dana Meaney-Delman

A 32-year-old woman presents for her annual physical examination. The patient indicates her sister was diagnosed with breast cancer at age 39 years. The clinician refers the patient for genetic counseling and schedules her for a baseline mammogram. The patient goes online and discovers she can learn her "genetic risk" for breast cancer for a few hundred dollars. She is very reassured when her results come back indicating she has a "7.2% lifetime risk of developing breast cancer, which is 40% less than for females of European ancestry." On the basis of these results, she cancels her mammogram. At her next annual visit, her breast examination reveals a concerning lump in her left breast. The patient is ultimately diagnosed with a stage IIB triple-negative invasive ductal carcinoma. The delayed cancer genetics evaluation reveals a strong paternal family history of breast and ovarian cancer, and she is found to carry a *BRCA1* mutation.

A 35-year-old man sees an ad for a $99 special on personal genome testing and sends in his sample. The report he receives back indicates he is at increased risk for prostate cancer. He talks with his parents to ask about prostate cancer in the family and learns instead that several individuals in his mother's family had early colon cancer. Intrigued by this, he asks his doctor about a connection between colon and prostate cancer, and the doctor refers him to a cancer genetic specialist who works with the family and ultimately determines they carry a Lynch syndrome gene mutation.

A 25-year-old with a low risk of breast cancer—based on family history and other traditional risk factors—is given the "one size fits all perfect gift" of a personal genome scan that will tell her about her genetic risk for more than "200 diseases and conditions." When she learns her breast cancer risk is "50% greater than the average women" and is in the "red zone," she schedules a consultation with a breast surgeon and requests a mammogram. She is recommended to have a repeat mammogram in 6 months to follow microcalcifications. However, because of her anxiety, a biopsy is performed, and result of which is negative. While waiting for her biopsy results, she tells her sister that she had a positive genetic test for breast cancer, whose physician then orders *BRCA1/2* testing.

35

Although the above scenarios are hypothetical, they are quite plausible and are used to illustrate some of the concerns—and possible benefits—associated with direct-to-consumer (DTC) availability of genomic-based tests, which provide risk information for health conditions such as cancer.

In this chapter, we describe the history and methodologic considerations behind DTC genomic profiling, using examples that focus on cancer risk prediction. We explore the literature regarding consumer and provider knowledge and utilization of DTC genetic testing, and the controversy that has surrounded this industry. In addition, we address policy recommendations and regulatory actions, and the changing landscape of the DTC genetic testing market in response. Finally, we take a brief look at public health implications of DTC genetic testing and the future of genomic-based medicine.

DEFINITION, HISTORY, AND METHODOLOGIC CONSIDERATIONS
What is DTC Genetic Testing?

DTC genetic testing refers to genetic tests that are marketed to the public, where the consumer is able to order the test online or by phone, usually without the assistance of a health care provider. Although the term DTC genetic testing has been used in many contexts, our focus will be tests that scan for multiple, common DNA variants associated with disease, as opposed to tests for rare single-gene conditions or DTC marketing.

According to the Genetics and Public Policy Center, as of August 2011, there were 27 companies offering DTC genetic testing for more than 250 health conditions and traits.[1] Along with information about ear wax type, dancing ability, or risk-taking tendencies, one can learn about genetic risks for multiple, common, and serious health conditions such as Alzheimer disease, diabetes, heart disease, and cancer. These companies vary in the types of tests they offer, and how their risks are calculated, but share the commonality that although the tests are performed in a Clinical Laboratory Improvement Amendment certified laboratory, those involving genomic risk profiling have not undergone research-based evaluation of clinical validity or utility and are not Food and Drug Administration regulated.

The data from the Genetics and Public Policy Center included information on 11 companies offering DTC genetic testing for a total of 44 different types of cancer.[1] Nine of these companies did not require involvement of a health care provider to order testing. Table 3.1 provides information on the five companies that still offer testing in this manner, along with information on the types of cancers included and approximate cost.

The Development of the DTC Genetic Testing Industry

DTC genetic testing was a natural entrepreneurial offshoot of the Human Genome Project. In particular, the advent of genome-wide association studies (GWASs)—

TABLE 3.1	Cancer Risk Prediction Tests Offered by DTC Genetic Testing Companies Without Involvement of a Health Care Provider (As of April 15, 2012)	
Company Name	**Cancers Screened by Genomic Risk Profiling**	**Cost**
23andMe[2]	Basal cell, bladder, breast, breast cancer modifiers, breast/ovarian, colorectal, chronic lymphocytic leukemia, esophageal, esophageal squamous cell, esophageal linked with alcohol and smoking, follicular lymphoma, Hodgkin lymphoma, kidney, larynx, lung, melanoma, meningioma, myeloproliferative neoplasms, nasopharyngeal, neuroblastoma, oral and throat, ovarian, pancreatic, prostate, sarcoma, squamous cell stomach, testicular, thyroid	$207
deCODE[3]	Basal cell, bladder, brain glioma, breast, chronic lymphocytic leukemia, colorectal, lung, ovarian, pancreatic, prostate, testicular, thyroid	$500
GenePlanet[4]	Breast, endometrial, gastric, lung, prostate	$525
Accu-Metrics[5]	Basal cell, bladder, breast, colorectal, lung, prostate, thyroid	$989
Map My Gene[6]	Acute lymphoblastic leukemia, acute myelogenous leukemia, adenocarcinoma, bladder, breast, cervical, cholangiocarcinoma, chronic lymphocytic leukemia, chronic myelogenous leukemia, colon, endometrial, gall bladder, gastric, laryngeal, bronchial, liver, melanoma, myeloma, nasopharyngeal, oral, osteosarcoma, ovarian, prostate, retinoblastoma, renal, rectal, small cell lung, thyroid, tongue, urothelial	$2,200 (100 diseases)

which first appeared in the literature in 2005 and have risen almost exponentially since—sought to find genetic markers associated with common diseases, in part to fulfill the promise of the Human Genome Project to provide personalized genomic medicine.[7] These studies use millions of "single-nucleotide polymorphisms" (SNPs) that have been found throughout the human genome. Essentially, a case-control approach is used, where the genomes of 100s to 1,000s of individuals with a particular condition (e.g., breast cancer) and a population of controls without the condition are scanned for SNPs that show differential distribution between the two groups, resulting in odds ratios for the associated genotypes.

Early GWASs were plagued by multiple erroneous assumptions that discredited most of the initial results. However, over time, more rigorous methodology, involving much larger sample sizes, higher levels of statistical significance, replication, and control for population stratification, was used. These studies have resulted in identification of more than 1,400 SNPs with "true" associations for more than 237 human traits and diseases, including breast, prostate, colon, lung, thyroid, and many other cancers.[8]

The rise of DTC genetic testing very closely followed the early influx of GWAS publications, with many companies entering the market in 2008.[9] These companies not only capitalized on this research, but also recognized the limited access to genetic testing in the existing health care infrastructure and the desire of consumers for convenience, privacy, and the right to own their own genetic information.[9]

Although the success of GWASs in identifying SNP-based disease associations cannot be argued, the initial promise of this approach in allowing for "personalized genomic medicine" has yet to be realized, despite the claims of the DTC testing companies. This is in part because the vast majority of SNPs are associated with very low odds ratios for common diseases—typically in the range of 1.1 to 1.4—and thus have minimal impact on absolute risk.[10–13] Furthermore, identified SNPs account for only a small proportion (5% to 10%) of the known heritability of most common diseases.[13–15] Finally, much remains unknown regarding the impact of both gene–gene interactions and gene–environment interactions on an individual's predisposition to disease.[16]

DTC Genomic Profiling for Cancer Risk

Most cancer genetic testing available DTC is performed using genomic profiles, which involve testing for multiple SNPs that have been associated with a specific cancer. The most common method used to calculate the person's disease risk involves conversion of the odds ratios of the genotype at each SNP to relative risks, then combining them in a simple multiplicative model. This overall relative risk is then compared with the general population risk for this cancer, to provide a percent increase and/or a revised absolute risk (Fig. 3.1). This method is highly dependent on the background population risks used, and assumes all SNP effects are independent.

Although most of the companies use well-validated SNPs, they do not use all the same ones in the same way. This means that the disease risk estimates provided may differ from company to company, with one predicting an increased and the other an average or decreased risk. Evidence of this phenomenon has been reported in several publications and attributed to differences in the number/type of SNPs, variation in risk modeling approaches, and average general population risks used.[17–19] Table 3.2 illustrates the differences in the number of SNPs used and their reported effects for the two largest DTC genomic profiling companies (23andMe[2] and deCODE[3]) for some common cancers.

Perhaps, even more concerning are data that suggest that as new disease-associated SNPs are added to a specific disease profile, a person's risk may be reclassified.[16,20] Both 23andMe and deCODE provide consumers with ongoing updates,

---

Calculating a Consumer's risk for cancer based on Four SNPs

◉ Calculate genotype OR for each SNP based on known allele OR
  - T allele OR = 1.15
  - TT genotype OR - $1.15 \times 1.15 = 1.3$

◉ Convert OR to RR using Hardy–Weinberg
  - Allows risk to be compared to general population risk

◉ Multiply genotype RR for each SNP to obtain overall RR
  - SNP1 (TT) RR = 1.3
  - SNP2 (AG) RR = 0.8
  - SNP3 (AA) RR = 1.1
  - SNP4 (CT) RR = 1.05

  Overall RR compared to general population risk: $1.3 \times 0.8 \times 1.1 \times 1.05 = 1.2$

◉ Calculate absolute risk/percent increase
  - If general population risk is 10%
  - Absolute risk = $10\% \times 1.2 = 12\%$
  - Percent increase = $(12–10/10) \times 100 = 20\%$ increase

---

OR, odds ratio; RR, relative risk; SNP, single-nucleotide polymorphism; T/G/S/C, single-nucleotide bases.

FIGURE 3.1. Calculating a consumer's risk for cancer based on four SNPs.

such that a person who originally received a "lower than average" result for a specific cancer may find themselves at "average" or "above average" risk in the future. Although the possibility of risk reclassification is disconcerting, so too is the finding by Singleton et al.[21] that only half of the websites of companies offering genomic risk profiling discussed how consumers would receive updated risk information, or even that their risks could change.

It is also important to clarify that the cancer risk estimates provided do not adjust for family history of the cancer or take into account other known risk factors. For example, a man who is morbidly obese, smokes two packs of cigarettes a day, and has a father with colon cancer at age 50 years will be given the same predicted risk for colon cancer as a man without these risk factors who has the same SNP profile.

Value of Genomic Risk Profiling for Cancer

All of the above issues underline the importance of considering both clinical validity and utility when interpreting the results of SNP-based genomic profiles as a measure of disease risk. Specifically, how accurate is the risk prediction provided by the SNP profile, and will this information result in changes in medical management or health

TABLE 3.2	**Comparison of Two Companies' SNP profiles for Breast, Colon, Ovarian, and Prostate Cancer**

Cancer	Company	Number of SNPs Used	Sample Report SNP Effects
Breast cancer	23andMe	7	"Established report" with SNP genotype ORs ranging from 0.82–1.04
	deCODE	Up to 17[a] (Note: includes SNP for *CHEK2* 1100delC mutation associated with twofold RR)	SNP genotype RRs ranging from 0.83–1.42
Breast and ovarian cancer (*BRCA1/2* Ashkenazi Jewish mutations)	23andMe	3	Lifetime risks associated with *BRCA1/2* mutations are discussed
Ovarian cancer	23andMe	2	"Preliminary report" with both SNP genotype ORs of 1.2
	deCODE	1	SNP genotype RR of 1.13
Colorectal cancer	23andMe	4	"Established report" with SNP genotype ORs ranging from 0.8–1.19
	deCODE	Up to 8[a]	SNP genotype RRs ranging from 0.91–1.16
Prostate cancer	23andMe	12	"Established report" with SNP genotype ORs ranging from 0.64–1.3
	deCODE	Up to 29[a]	SNP genotype RRs ranging from 0.81–1.17

[a]Depending on ancestry.
OR, odds ratio; RR, relative risk.

behaviors that improve outcome? The accuracy of the risk prediction can be measured by the area under the receiver operating characteristic curve (AUC), which plots sensitivity against the false-positive rate. A test that predicts no better than chance will have an AUC of 0.5—essentially a flip of the coin—whereas a test with an AUC of 1 can perfectly predict who will and will not develop the disease. Unfortunately, few studies have been conducted that provide the data needed to assess the clinical validity of most cancer risk prediction tests based on genomic profiling. Those that have been published; however, suggest these profiles have limited predictive ability.

For example, Wacholder et al.[22] reported an AUC of only 0.597 for a breast cancer profile involving 10 SNPs. Even adding these 10 SNPs to the Gail risk model for breast cancer only slightly improved its predictive ability from an AUC of 0.58 to 0.62.[22,23] Similarly, in the case of prostate cancer, Zheng et al.[24] reported an AUC of 0.61 using age, geographic region, and family history, which rose only to 0.63 when the five strongest SNPs were added to the model. Although AUC data are not available for many of the cancers listed in Table 3.1, the use of a small number of SNPs with odds ratios typically less than 1.4 would suggest similarly poor predictive accuracy. Furthermore, the question of whether the use of genomic profiling leads to appropriate alterations in medical management or behavior that actually results in improved health outcomes (i.e., clinical utility) remains, at this point, essentially unanswered.[25]

It should be noted that although the majority of testing performed by DTC genetic testing companies focuses on these SNPs with low cancer-associated odds ratios, there are exceptions.

For example, 23andMe evaluates three SNPs that are essentially markers for the three *BRCA1/2* Ashkenazi Jewish founder mutations. In sharp contrast to the other breast cancer risk SNPs, identification of one of these *BRCA1/2*-related mutations is highly predictive of disease, with odds ratios for breast and ovarian cancer of 10- to 20-fold and mean lifetime risks of 65% and 40%, respectively.[26] The significance of being negative for the three *BRCA1/2*-associated SNPs is primarily relevant for individuals of Jewish ancestry. Those of other ethnic groups would require full sequence analysis of these genes, which is not available DTC. Thus, DTC genomic profiling for cancer risk may result in the unexpected revelation of a significant hereditary cancer risk or false reassurance that such a risk has been ruled out. Some companies also test for SNPs in genes that have been suggested as modifiers of *BRCA1/2* penetrance, which could be misinterpreted as actual *BRCA* mutations.

CONSUMER ISSUES ASSOCIATED WITH DTC GENETIC TESTING
Awareness, Attitudes, and Utilization

Despite the widespread availability of DTC genetic testing for the past several years, it is unclear the extent to which consumers are either aware of or accessing DTC genetic testing for health reasons. In a 2008 cross-sectional survey of US consumers, whereas 22% of individuals were aware of DTC genetic testing for health risks, only 0.3% had actually accessed such tests.[27] A 2008 study in the United Kingdom found only 13% were aware of internet-based personal genome testing.[28] Data obtained from the 2009 Behavior Risk Factor Surveillance System of four co-operating states (combined $n = 16,439$) demonstrated awareness of DTC genomic profiling for health risks ranged from 15.8% to 29.1%, although fewer than 1% of participants in each state reported having used the testing.[29] Even in one study of social networkers, almost half of the participants (47%) were aware of DTC genetic testing, yet only 6% had ever undergone the testing.[30,31] Although 23andMe reports that more than 100,000 individuals have accessed their test,[32] a 2010 publication, which used the website traffic of three largest companies as a proxy for test uptake, concluded that the demand for genomic profiling was relatively low.[33]

Data from the Multiplex Initiative[34] provide an important look at issues of utilization within the context of a research setting. This project was designed to mirror the approach used by commercial DTC genetic testing companies, but uses web content that focuses on health literacy and risk communication.[35,36] Testing was provided at no cost, and those who chose to pursue received education from a research coordinator regarding the risks and benefits of testing. Among 1,959 people who were eligible and completed the baseline survey, 612 (31%) visited the website to consider testing. Of those who registered a decision ($n = 528$), almost half decided against undergoing testing.

Much of the existing literature regarding consumer attitudes and utilization of DTC genetic testing is based on data obtained on so-called early adopters, who generally have confidence in their ability to understand genetics and navigate the Internet and health care system and perceive that results will influence their health behaviors.[36,37] Another group that appears particularly interested in DTC genetic testing is of those who are simply interested in "setting the trend," many of whom proudly blog about their results.[38] While relaying optimism about the promises of genomic research, they may express skepticism about the current technology. Yet, other early adopters express belief in the importance of the information to their health, as well as curiosity and fascination with the science.[39] Some would-be consumers are more cynical and report that DTC companies are "just trying to sell something" and that this approach is merely a "marketing ploy," intended to generate revenue for the company without a direct benefit to the consumer.[40]

Several studies have examined characteristics associated with awareness of and/or interest in online personalized genomic risk assessment. As expected, Internet-savvy individuals are more likely to be aware of testing.[36,41] Other predictors of consumer awareness of DTC genetic testing include white race, higher levels of education, greater income, older age, female sex, and numeracy variables.[27,42] In a UK study of the public, only 5% indicated a hypothetical interest in testing that costs £259, but 50% expressed interest in a free test.[28] Individuals with higher levels of education and those of white race have also been shown to be more willing to pursue testing, with effects influenced by socioeconomic status, affiliation with a health care system, and cost.[36,43,44] In the Multiplex Initiative, further predictors of test utilization included motivation to change health behaviors, confidence in genetics knowledge, and perceived severity of the health conditions involved.[31,36]

Understandings, Perceptions, and Expectations

Previous studies have shown that general genetic concepts are often misunderstood by the general public, and DTC genomic profiling with its use of multiple low-risk variants adds an additional layer of complexity.[45] Genetic literacy—the ability to understand or interpret genetic and genomic information—varies greatly in the population and presents a challenge to the "one size fits all" approach of DTC genetic testing companies.

A recent study involving the Coriell Personalized Medicine Collaborative—a project that provides SNP-based disease risk information at no cost to early adopters with high literacy levels—demonstrated a reasonable understanding of genomic risk information.[46] However, DTC genetic testing is marketed to the general population, who likely has lower levels of health literacy, not to mention genetic literacy. In their study of social networkers, McGuire et al.[30] reported that less than half were confident in their ability to comprehend their results or the risks/ benefits of DTC genetic testing.

In another study, more than 30% of participants reported at least one misconception about DTC genetic testing.[47] Of particular concern is that some individuals may believe the DTC test results are definitive and ignore the information provided by their family history.[37] Even if individuals do not fully trust the DTC results, when a discrepancy exists between the results of the DTC genetic testing and the interpretation of familial risk, it can create significant confusion. As illustrated in a recent case report, extensive education and counseling may be required to assist patients in these circumstances, and it remains uncertain to what extent a true understanding of the meaning of their results can be achieved.[37]

In addition, consumers appear to have somewhat unrealistic expectations of DTC genetic testing, presuming that on presentation of their results to their clinicians an evidence-based individualized health plan can be devised. In one study, more than 90% of DTC testers were planning to share their results with their physicians, and 67% expected clinical recommendations to follow.[47] McGuire et al.[30] found that 78% of consumers planned to share their results with their medical providers, with 34% believing the results represented a medical diagnosis. In a qualitative study from the Coriell Personalized Medicine Collaborative, 25 of 60 participants reported sharing their DTC results with their health care providers, and of these, 15 expected their physicians to change their health care plan or advise them of mechanisms to reduce their risk.[46] Recently, Leighton et al.[48] conducted a study of the general public's response to DTC tests and found that 86.9% of respondents would seek information about their tests from their personal physicians, believing that future medical management would be affected by these tests.

Behavioral Change

If DTC genetic testing is to demonstrate clinical value, it must motivate individuals to change their behavior. Although this remains in debate, most studies published to date suggest DTC genetic testing as ineffective in promoting significant behavioral or lifestyle changes.[49–51] In a meta-analysis of five studies conducted by the Cochrane Collaboration, communicating DNA-based risk of disease was not found to affect smoking rates.[51] The Cochrane review also reported that two studies assessing physical activity and one study assessing medication or vitamin use found no impact of reporting genomic-based disease risks. In contrast, two studies examining dietary intake did find genomic test results to influence behavior. Among participants in the qualitative Coriell study, only one of three of DTC test recipients reported making a lifestyle change, although an additional third indicated they planned to do so.[46] In a recent survey of 1,048 DTC customers, 16% had changed their use of a medication or supplement, one-third said they were being more careful about their diet, and 14% said they were exercising more.[50] However, these behaviors appeared to be strongly influenced by the participant's subjective interpretation of risk, as well as their family history and self-perceived health status.

There is some evidence that consumer access to DTC genomic profiling leads to increased screening or laboratory tests, which may or may not be medically appropriate.[37,50] The likelihood of consumers obtaining additional medical interventions appears to be strongly influenced by whether they share their results with their health care provider.[50] Among 1,048 consumers of DTC genomic profiling tests, 28% reported sharing the results with their health care provider. Of these, 26% indicated they had received additional laboratory tests, as opposed to 2% of the consumers who had not shared their results.[50] Although on the surface this appears a beneficial outcome of DTC genetic testing, if the only indication for additional medical evaluation is the genomic profiling result, the cost of additional clinician visits and resulting medical interventions may far outweigh any positive impacts on the individual's health. Support for this concern is suggested by Giovanni et al.,[52] who estimated that the potential downstream costs of referrals and additional testing following DTC results ranged from as low as $40 to as high as $26,000.

Psychological Consequences

The psychological consequences of DTC genetic testing have just begun to be explored. Some authors cite heightened and undue anxiety as a potential negative consequence of DTC genetic testing.[53] Based on experience from a recent clinical scenario involving a DTC test, the author concluded that DTC genetic testing may be detrimental to mental health in the absence of genetic counseling, causing anxiety, confusion, and misinformation.[54] In addition, Gollust et al.[47] found that 30% of study subjects were concerned about the "worry" that resulted from the DTC genetic testing information, particularly learning about a disease for which they did not want to know their risk. In 2010, Bloss et al.[43] reported that 47% of the DTC participants expressed psychological concerns about testing, with greater concern among young participants, women, those employed by a health care organization, and those with higher baseline anxiety. However, in a later study by the same author, there was no significant difference in pretest and posttest anxiety, suggesting that any psychological changes may be short term.[49] Furthermore, in the qualitative study of participants from the Coriell Personalized Medicine Collaborative, the most common emotional responses to testing results were actually reassurance and acceptance.[46] Further research is needed to determine the extent to which these findings are applicable to the average consumer of DTC genetic testing services.

PROVIDER KNOWLEDGE AND ATTITUDES ABOUT DTC GENETIC TESTING

Primary Care

Although many DTC genetic testing participants expect their providers to be fully versed in genetics and genomics, staying abreast of this rapidly changing field presents a challenge for the average health care provider. Studies from both Canada and the United States have documented the inability of primary care physicians to interpret genetic results and their lack of confidence in this regard.[55–57] A systematic review by Scheuner et al.[58] in 2008 concluded that primary care providers, despite some genetics training, are ill prepared to discuss genetic/genomic results and are unable to translate advances in genomics into clinically relevant practice. DTC genomic profiling, which provides risk information potentially more complicated to interpret than single-gene tests for hereditary disease susceptibility, may find physicians ill prepared to counsel their patients about the results. In a survey of North Carolina primary care physicians, only 39% were even aware of DTC genetic testing, and 85% felt unprepared to answer patient questions with regard to these tests.[59] Although 43% of respondents believed that DTC genetic testing had some clinical utility, more than 75% recognized a need for additional expertise in test interpretation.[59] Even among physicians who belong to a group that routinely offers genomic risk profiling as part of their practice, of 154 providers who had ordered genomic risk profiling for either themselves or a patient, 60% expressed concerns about the clinical utility of testing.[44]

The above data are particularly relevant in light of a 2008 survey of 1,880 US health care providers, only 42% of whom reported being aware of DTC genomic testing for health risks. Of this group, 42% reported having had a patient inquire about DTC genomic testing, whereas 15% reported they had a patient present with the test results for discussion the past year.[27] Among the providers aware of DTC genomic testing, 52% indicated that personal genome results were somewhat or very likely to influence their care of patients. Among those whose patients had provided DTC genetic test results, 75% reported having used this information to alter their patient's medical management.[27] It is unclear if these changes in care are due to a belief of the provider in achieving a clinical benefit or the result of patient pressure to increase surveillance.

Genetics Professionals

A few studies have examined the knowledge and attitudes of genetic professionals toward DTC genetic testing, or how often they are involved with patients who have accessed such testing. In 2010, Giovanni et al.[52] surveyed three genetic professional organizations in the United States, asking about consultations that related to DTC genetic test results. Although the response rate was low, participants reported having seen patients both who were self-referred and who were referred by another clinician. Although 52.3% of these genetics professionals found the information gained from the DTC results "clinically useful," this appeared primarily related to *BRCA1/2* results, which are in general no longer available DTC. In contrast, a small study of genetic professionals who themselves underwent genomic profiling found their perception of the current or future importance of such results to medical practice decreased after testing.[60] A larger study by Hock et al.[61] involving 312 members of the National Society of Genetic Counselors found 83% had received two or fewer inquiries regarding DTC genetic testing, whereas only 14% had received requests for discussion or interpretation of test results. Recently, Brett et al.[62] published a similar study of members of the Human Genetics Society of Australasia, in which 11% reported seeing at least one patient subsequent to his/her receipt of DTC genetic testing results. Surprisingly, only 7% of respondents to this survey reported that they felt confident about interpreting and explaining the results. In a study that contrasted the public's perception of a DTC genomic risk profile for colon cancer with that of genetic counselors, the latter were significantly less likely to believe the results would be medically helpful.[48] Although more data are needed, these combined results suggest that few consumers of DTC genetic testing are seeking the input of genetic providers, who, although not confident about their ability to interpret results, may perceive them as less than clinically useful.

CONTROVERSY, POLICY AND REGULATION, MARKET CHANGES, AND PUBLIC HEALTH ISSUES

Controversy

Many publications have addressed the pros and cons as well as ethical issues associated with DTC genetic testing.[12,63–73] Although a thorough review of the multiple arguments for and against DTC genetic testing is beyond the scope of this chapter, the key issues are outlined in Table 3.3. It should be noted that several of these arguments, both pro and con, are currently theoretical in nature, and more research is required to validate the claims on both sides of the aisle.

Perhaps, one of the most significant criticisms of the DTC genetic testing companies revolves around their marketing practices. The websites of many DTC companies include seemingly contradictory statements about the intended purposes and value of their tests. A company may claim that the tests are for educational or entertainment purposes, while overtly stating that the information can be used to improve your health. These websites also emphasize the value of risk assessment for an individual's physician in determining what preventive actions should be taken to protect his/her health,[21,55–57,59] and inconsistently acknowledge the importance of family history in assessing cancer risk.

TABLE 3.3	Pros and Cons of DTC Genetic Testing

Pros	Cons
Increase in consumer awareness and knowledge of genetics	Limited evidence of clinical validity/unknown clinical utility
Increased access to genetic testing/information	False or misleading claims that may lead to anxiety or false reassurance
Greater patient autonomy	Inadequate counseling/consent
Enhanced patient privacy	Misinterpretation of test results (by providers as well as consumers)
Opportunity for participation in genetic research	Consumer pursuit of unnecessary or inappropriate medical care or purchase of expensive health products
DTC availability and associated convenience may increase clinical uptake of genetic testing	Increased health care costs associated with unnecessary provider visits or medical tests/procedures
Potential for motivating healthy behaviors	Failure to seek appropriate preventive care if falsely reassured
Diminishes issues of genetic exceptionalism	Lack of adequate government oversight/regulation
Encourages genetic innovation and entrepreneurialism	Bypasses ethical and privacy protections inherent within the health care system (e.g., genetic testing of minors for adult onset conditions)

From: Eng C, Sharp RR. Bioethical and clinical dilemmas of direct-to-consumer personal genomic testing: The problem of misattributed equivalence. *Sci Transl Med.* 2010;2:17cm5; McGuire AL, Diaz CM, Wang T, et al. Social networkers' attitudes toward direct-to-consumer personal genome testing. *Am J Bioeth.* 2009;9:3–10; Hogarth S, Javitt G, Melzer D. The current landscape for direct-to-consumer genetic testing: Legal, ethical, and policy issues. *Annu Rev Genomics Hum Genet.* 2008;9:161–182; Gollust SE, Wilfond BS, Hull SC. Direct-to-consumer sales of genetic services on the internet. *Genet Med.* 2003;5:332–337; Mykitiuk R. Caveat emptor: Direct-to-consumer supply and advertising of genetic testing. *Clin Invest Med.* 2004;27:23–32; Annes JP, Giovanni MA, Murray MF. Risks of presymptomatic direct-to-consumer genetic testing. *N Engl J Med.* 2010;363:1100–1101; Caulfield T, Ries NM, Ray PN, et al. Direct-to-consumer genetic testing: Good, bad or benign? *Clin Genet.* 2010;77:101–105; McGuire AL, Evans BJ, Caulfield T, et al. Science and regulation. Regulating direct-to-consumer personal genome testing. *Science.* 2010;330:181–182; Samuel GN, Jordens CF, Kerridge I. Direct-to-consumer personal genome testing: Ethical and regulatory issues that arise from wanting to "know" your DNA. *Intern Med J.* 2010;40:220–224; Howard HC, Avard D, Borry P. Are the kids really all right? Direct-to-consumer genetic testing in children: Are company policies clashing with professional norms? *Eur J Hum Genet.* 2011;19:1122–1126; and Caulfield T, McGuire AL. Direct-to-consumer genetic testing: Perceptions, problems, and policy responses. *Annu Rev Med.* 2012;63:23–33.

Although many of the company websites have done an exceptional job with presentation, including the use of colorful diagrams to illustrate risk comparisons and easily navigated web pages, these sites are tailored to those with a high educational level and are thus likely to confuse consumers with lower health literacy.[74] Of great concern, both 23 and Me and deCODE's websites use the relative rarity of single-gene cancer susceptibility syndromes as a marketing ploy, which is easily misinterpreted. The following two quotes from deCODE's website education on ovarian cancer exemplify this point: "Scientists already know that variants in the *BRCA1* and *BRCA2* genes significantly increase a woman's chances of developing ovarian cancer. However, these variants are rare and account for less than 5% of all ovarian cancers," and "The deCODEme Complete Scan identifies validated ovarian risk variants of the more common type and uses them to provide a personalized interpretation of the associated genetic risk for the disease."[3] The clear implication is that the deCODEme test will be more useful to the majority of people, a claim without established clinical validity.

A further illustration of the potentially misleading information provided on DTC genetic testing websites is provided in an analysis by Singleton et al.[21] They reviewed websites of 23 companies offering health-related DTC genetic testing and found that statements of testing benefits outweighed those addressing risks and limitations by a ratio of 6:1. Although 96% of the websites emphasized the potential for the genetic test to prevent disease or reduce morbidity/mortality, only 30% indicated there are current limitations to the predictive ability of the tests, and 65% did not mention any risks associated with genetic testing.[21]

Policy Recommendations and Regulations Regarding DTC Genetic Testing

In recognition of the issues noted above, several professional societies as well as advisory bodies have issued recommendations and opinion statements regarding DTC genetic testing over the last several years.[75] A consistent message of these documents is a concern for misinterpretation of genetic test results, the lack of involvement of an appropriately trained professional, and the need for federal regulation to protect consumers.[70,76–81] In part, the issues raised by these groups led to a 1-year investigation of DTC genetic testing by the US General Accounting Office. The investigation revealed evidence of deceptive marketing practices, consumer privacy concerns, and inaccurate or misleading medical advice from company consultants.[82] In July 2010, testimony at the General Accounting Office hearing led to a report that concluded that tests provided by the DTC genetic testing companies were "misleading and of little or no practical use."[83] Last year, the American Medical Association issued a letter to the FDA urging it to recommend genetic testing be conducted only under the supervision of a qualified genetics provider.[84] Although the FDA has indicated it will be tightening regulations on the industry, and warning letters have been issued to several DTC companies, there has yet to be any substantial regulatory changes enacted.[73,85,86] However, some states do have legal requirements mandating physician involvement in the ordering of genetic tests,[9] and many European countries have specific DTC genetic testing legislation, whereas others have banned the practice outright.[73,87]

One step toward greater transparency regarding genetic tests being offered to the public is the Genetic Test Registry, a project initiated in 2010 by the National Center for Biotechnology Information.[88] The Genetic Test Registry is intended to be a central place for clinicians and the public to access detailed information on genetic tests, including methodology, purpose, validity, price, and ordering information. Although the concept is promising, as the project has unfolded several challenges to its successful implementation have been identified.[89,90] Currently, the information is voluntarily added by test providers, and unfortunately, at the time of writing, none of the DTC companies listed in Table 3.1 have chosen to participate. It remains unclear whether regulatory agencies, such as the FDA, will require participation in the future or instill other mechanisms of oversight.

Changes in the DTC Genetic Testing Market

Likely in response to these recommendations and calls for greater regulation, there has been a recent trend by some DTC genetic testing companies to change their service models. Although some companies appear to have stopped offering health-related testing altogether, others that formerly did not require clinician involvement to order testing or receive results of genomic risk profiling tests are now doing so.[9,91] There is, however, a great deal of variation in this process, with some only requiring physician involvement in the ordering—with convenient referral to a physician already participating in their program—whereas others release results only to the consumer's provider.[91] Some companies are also working to promote their services within corporate wellness programs and partnering with the limited number of Genomic Medicine Institutes in the country to serve as resources for consumers and providers.[91]

Although requiring involvement of a health care provider may decrease the number of inappropriate tests performed and ideally allow for more integration of family history, it does not adequately address the issue of the clinician's ability to accurately interpret and act on test results, or improve the clinical validity of the testing. Nor does it address the possibility that physicians are merely ordering the tests at the request of their patients, without adequately researching the implications. Thus, although a positive step, these changes may ultimately prove to be an inadequate attempt to respond to previous criticism by the FDA and the medical community.

Whether to placate critics or provide for greater legitimacy in the eyes of the consumer, several DTC genetic testing companies are now emphasizing the role of genetic counseling in the testing process. In some cases, they have hired genetic counselors directly, making them available to answer questions or concerns expressed by clients using a customer service model. Having a genetic counselor available to answer questions, although likely helpful to clients in some circumstances, is not the equivalent of a comprehensive pretest genetic counseling session, which involves an exploration of family history and a detailed explanation of the risks, benefits, and implications of testing, as well as possible psychological and emotional ramifications. Furthermore, whether the services are being offered by qualified individuals is uncertain as illustrated by a company whose "official" genetic counselor is a nutritionist.[92] Even when legitimate board-certified genetic counselors are involved, if they are an employee of the company, one may question their ability to provide an unbiased opinion as to the risks, benefits, and limitations of a given test. Furthermore, although companies may be providing or contracting genetic counseling services, these services often come at a price, and consumer uptake has been reported to be low.[49] All of the above notwithstanding, a company that actively employs genetic counselors has been successful in their efforts to increase consumer utilization of their genetic counseling service after return of DTC genomic profiling results.[85]

Potential Public Health Implications of DTC Genetic Testing

Given the relatively low awareness and uptake of DTC genetic testing, the public health implications of DTC genetic testing are largely theoretical at this time, although significant concerns have been raised.[64,93] Key concerns focus on disparities related to access and ability to understand or benefit from the results. In addition, if consumers begin widely using DTC genetic testing, this could lead to a diversion of health care and research dollars toward follow-up and evaluation of DTC genetic tests and away from potentially more productive cancer prevention efforts.[94] Alternatively, if genomic risk profiling is ultimately shown to improve health, either through inducing positive lifestyle changes or increasing patient compliance with recommended screening or prevention strategies, a positive public health impact might be realized. Even this should come to pass, however, disadvantaged populations, who have historically been low users of genetic testing in general[95] and who appear less aware of DTC genetic tests,[29,42] would be less likely to reap the benefits.

CONCLUSIONS

Whether DTC genetic testing that involves SNP-based genomic profiling will ever become the answer to personalized medicine for the masses is at this point very uncertain. It seems thus far that, despite the controversy, its impact has been relatively limited. Both increased regulation and scientific scrutiny of the clinical validity and utility of such tests appear likely to limit widespread use in the future—at least for access without involvement of a health care provider. At this point in time, DTC genomic profiling for cancer risk prediction is clearly of limited use with respect to guiding medical management recommendations, particularly as family history and other established risk factors are not assessed. And while being able to provide tailored cancer screening and prevention strategies for everyone based on their genetic makeup is an attractive approach, personal genomic profiling is unlikely to prove beneficial in this regard even if additional SNPs are identified.[16]

More likely, the future of predictive genetic testing for cancer and other diseases, both common and rare, will focus on whole-genome sequencing. According to the National Human Genome Research Institute, the cost to sequence a human-size genome in 2001 was $100,000,000.[96] In January 2012, Life Technologies announced that they were able to sequence an entire human genome for $1,000 in only 2 hours.[97]

Although such technology allows for identification of rare variants, copy number, and structural variations with potentially large effects on disease risks, it is also accompanied by the finding of multiple genetic variants of unknown clinical significance.

Although this is an important step toward integration of genomics into health care and holds much promise, the sheer volume of information obtained per genome and the complexities of interpretation imply challenges to the researcher, health care provider, and patient that go far beyond those associated with DTC genomic risk profiling.[98] It can only be hoped that the lessons learned over the past decade will provide the necessary awareness to ensure that whole-genome sequencing does not become available to online consumers without either the scientific foundation to demonstrate its utility or the involvement of a knowledgeable health care provider. Inarguably, meeting the educational needs of clinicians, health care systems, and the public will be essential if genomic medicine is to fulfill its promise of improving the health of the population. It remains unclear, however, whether there is the capacity, infrastructure, and will to ensure such educational efforts are successfully accomplished.

REFERENCES

1. Genetics and Public Policy Center. Direct-to-Consumer by Disease, August 2011. Available at: http://www.dnapolicy.org/resources/DTCAug2011by Diseasecategory.pdf. Accessed on April 15, 2012.
2. 23andMe. Available at: https://www.23andme.com/. Accessed on April 15, 2012.
3. deCODE. Cancer Scan. Available at: http://www.decodeme.com/cancer- scan. Accessed on April 15, 2012.
4. GenePlanet. Personal DNA Analysis. Available at: http://www.geneplanet.com/your_personal_dna_analysis. Accessed on April 15, 2012.
5. Accu-Metrics. Complete Genetic Scan. Available at: http://www.accu-metrics.com/complete-genetic-scan.php. Accessed on April 15, 2012.
6. Map My Gene. Disease Susceptibility Gene Test. Available at: http://www.mapmygene.com/product.htm. Accessed on April 15, 2012.
7. Manolio T. Published GWA Reports, 2005-6/2011. Available at: http://www.genome.gov/multimedia/illustrations/Published_GWA_Reports_ 2005-June2011.pdf. Accessed on April 15, 2012.
8. A Catalog of Published Genome-Wide Association Studies. Available at: http://www.genome.gov/GWAStudies/. Accessed on April 15, 2012.
9. Borry P, Cornel MC, Howard HC. Where are you going, where have you been: A recent history of the direct-to-consumer genetic testing market. *J Community Genet*. 2010;1:101–106.
10. Janssens AC, Gwinn M, Bradley LA, et al. A critical appraisal of the scientific basis of commercial genomic profiles used to assess health risks and personalize health interventions. *Am J Hum Genet*. 2008;82:593–599.
11. Magnus D, Cho MK, Cook-Deegan R. Direct-to-consumer genetic tests: Beyond medical regulation? *Genome Med*. 2009;1:17.
12. Eng C, Sharp RR. Bioethical and clinical dilemmas of direct-to-consumer personal genomic testing: The problem of misattributed equivalence. *Sci Transl Med*. 2010;2:17cm5.
13. Khoury MJ, McBride CM, Schully SD, et al. The Scientific Foundation for personal genomics: Recommendations from a National Institutes of Health-Centers for Disease Control and Prevention multidisciplinary workshop. *Genet Med*. 2009;11:559–567.
14. Kraft P, Hunter DJ. Genetic risk prediction—are we there yet? *N Engl J Med*. 2009;360:1701–1703.
15. Manolio TA, Collins FS, Cox NJ, et al. Finding the missing heritability of complex diseases. Nature. 2009;461:747–753.
16. Janssens AC, van Duijn CM. An epidemiological perspective on the future of direct-to-consumer personal genome testing. *Investig Genet*. 2010;1:10.

17. Ng PC, Murray SS, Levy S, et al. An agenda for personalized medicine. *Nature.* 2009;461:724–726.
18. Imai K, Kricka LJ, Fortina P. Concordance study of 3 direct-to-consumer genetic-testing services. *Clin Chem.* 2011;57:518–521.
19. Swan M. Multigenic condition risk assessment in direct-to-consumer genomic services. *Genet Med.* 2010;12:279–288.
20. Mihaescu R, van Hoek M, Sijbrands EJ, et al. Evaluation of risk prediction updates from commercial genome-wide scans. *Genet Med.* 2009;11:588–594.
21. Singleton A, Erby LH, Foisie KV, et al. Informed choice in direct-to-consumer genetic testing (DTCGT) websites: A content analysis of benefits, risks, and limitations. *J Genet Couns.* 2012;21:433–439.
22. Wacholder S, Hartge P, Prentice R, et al. Performance of common genetic variants in breast-cancer risk models. *N Engl J Med.* 2010;362:986–993.
23. Mealiffe ME, Stokowski RP, Rhees BK, et al. Assessment of clinical validity of a breast cancer risk model combining genetic and clinical information. *J Natl Cancer Inst.* 2010;102:1618–1627.
24. Zheng SL, Sun J, Wiklund F, et al. Cumulative association of five genetic variants with prostate cancer. *N Engl J Med.* 2008;358:910–919.
25. Field A, Krokosky A, Terry SF. Direct-to-consumer marketing of genetic tests: Access does not reflect clinical utility. *Genet Test Mol Biomarkers.* 2010;14:731–732.
26. Chen S, Parmigiani G. Meta-analysis of BRCA1 and BRCA2 penetrance. *J Clin Oncol.* 2007;25:1329–1333.
27. Kolor K, Liu T, St Pierre J, et al. Health care provider and consumer awareness, perceptions, and use of direct-to-consumer personal genomic tests, United States, 2008. *Genet Med.* 2009;11:595.
28. Cherkas LF, Harris JM, Levinson E, et al. A survey of UK public interest in internet-based personal genome testing. *PLoS One.* 2010;5:e13473.
29. Kolor K, Foland J, Anderson B, et al. Public awareness and use of direct-to-consumer personal genomic tests from four state population-based surveys, and implications for clinical and public health practice. *Genet Med.* 2012;14:860–867.
30. McGuire AL, Diaz CM, Wang T, et al. Social networkers' attitudes toward direct-to-consumer personal genome testing. *Am J Bioeth.* 2009;9:3–10.
31. McBride CM, Wade CH, Kaphingst KA. Consumers' views of direct-to-consumer genetic information. *Annu Rev Genomics Hum Genet.* 2010;11:427–446.
32. 23andMe. Database Surpasses 100000 Users. Available at: https://www.23andme.com/about/press/23andme_database_100000k_users/. Accessed on April 15, 2012.
33. Wright CF, Gregory-Jones S. Size of the direct-to-consumer genomic testing market. *Genet Med.* 2010;12:594.
34. The Multiplex Initiative. Available at: http://www.multiplex.nih.gov/. Accessed on April 15, 2012.
35. McBride CM, Koehly LM, Sanderson SC, et al. The behavioral response to personalized genetic information: Will genetic risk profiles motivate individuals and families to choose more healthful behaviors? *Annu Rev Public Health.* 2010;31:89–103.
36. McBride CM, Alford SH, Reid RJ, et al. Characteristics of users of online personalized genomic risk assessments: Implications for physician-patient interactions. *Genet Med.* 2009;11:582–587.
37. Sturm AC, Manickam K. Direct-to-consumer personal genomic testing: A case study and practical recommendations for "genomic counseling." *J Genet Couns.* 2012;21:402–412.
38. McGowan ML, Fishman JR, Lambrix MA. Personal genomics and individual identities: Motivations and moral imperatives of early users. *New Genet Soc.* 2010;29:261–290.
39. Su Y, Howard HC, Borry P. Users' motivations to purchase direct-to-consumer genome-wide testing: An exploratory study of personal stories. *J Community Genet.* 2011;2:135–146.
40. Rahm AK, Feigelson HS, Wagner N, et al. Perception of direct-to-consumer genetic testing and direct-to-consumer advertising of genetic tests among members of a large managed care organization. *J Genet Couns.* 2012;21:448–461.
41. Sanderson SC, O'Neill SC, Bastian LA, et al. What can interest tell us about uptake of genetic testing? Intention and behavior amongst smokers related to patients with lung cancer. *Public Health Genomics.* 2010;13:116–124.
42. Langford AT, Resnicow K, Roberts JS, et al. Racial and ethnic differences in direct-to-consumer genetic tests awareness in HINTS 2007: Sociodemographic and numeracy correlates. *J Genet Couns.* 2012;21:440–447.

43. Bloss CS, Ornowski L, Silver E, et al. Consumer perceptions of direct-to-consumer personalized genomic risk assessments. *Genet Med.* 2010;12:556–566.
44. Haga SB, Carrig MM, O'Daniel JM, et al. Genomic risk profiling: Attitudes and use in personal and clinical care of primary care physicians who offer risk profiling. *J Gen Intern Med.* 2011;26:834–840.
45. Myers MF, Chang MH, Jorgensen C, et al. Genetic testing for susceptibility to breast and ovarian cancer: Evaluating the impact of a direct-to-consumer marketing campaign on physicians' knowledge and practices. *Genet Med.* 2006;8:361–370.
46. Gordon ES, Griffin G, Wawak L, et al. "It's not like judgment day": Public understanding of and reactions to personalized genomic risk information. *J Genet Couns.* 2012;21:423–432.
47. Gollust SE, Gordon ES, Zayac C, et al. Motivations and perceptions of early adopters of personalized genomics: Perspectives from research participants. *Public Health Genomics.* 2012;15:22–30.
48. Leighton JW, Valverde K, Bernhardt BA. The general public's understanding and perception of direct-to-consumer genetic test results. *Public Health Genomics.* 2012;15:11–21.
49. Bloss CS, Schork NJ, Topol EJ. Effect of direct-to-consumer genomewide profiling to assess disease risk. *N Engl J Med.* 2011;364:524–534.
50. Kaufman DJ, Bollinger JM, Dvoskin RL, et al. Risky business: Risk perception and the use of medical services among customers of DTC personal genetic testing. *J Genet Couns.* 2012;21:413–422.
51. Marteau TM, French DP, Griffin SJ, et al. Effects of communicating DNA-based disease risk estimates on risk-reducing behaviours. *Cochrane Database Syst Rev.* 2010:CD007275.
52. Giovanni MA, Fickie MR, Lehmann LS, et al. Health-care referrals from direct-to-consumer genetic testing. *Genet Test Mol Biomarkers.* 2010;14:817–819.
53. Offit K. Genomic profiles for disease risk: Predictive or premature? *JAMA.* 2008;299:1353–1355.
54. Dohany L, Gustafson S, Ducaine W, et al. Psychological distress with direct-to-consumer genetic testing: A case report of an unexpected BRCA positive test result. *J Genet Couns.* 2012;21:399–401.
55. Levy DE, Youatt EJ, Shields AE. Primary care physicians' concerns about offering a genetic test to tailor smoking cessation treatment. *Genet Med.* 2007;9:842–849.
56. Freedman AN, Wideroff L, Olson L, et al. US physicians' attitudes toward genetic testing for cancer susceptibility. *Am J Med Genet A.* 2003; 120A:63–71.
57. Powell KP, Christianson CA, Cogswell WA, et al. Educational needs of primary care physicians regarding direct-to-consumer genetic testing. *J Genet Couns.* 2012;21:469–478.
58. Scheuner MT, Sieverding P, Shekelle PG. Delivery of genomic medicine for common chronic adult diseases: A systematic review. *JAMA.* 2008;299:1320–1334.
59. Powell KP, Cogswell WA, Christianson CA, et al. Primary care physicians' awareness, experience and opinions of direct-to-consumer genetic testing. *J Genet Couns.* 2012;21:113–126.
60. O'Daniel JM, Haga SB, Willard HF. Considerations for the impact of personal genome information: A study of genomic profiling among genetics and genomics professionals. *J Genet Couns.* 2010;19:387–401.
61. Hock KT, Christensen KD, Yashar BM, et al. Direct-to-consumer genetic testing: An assessment of genetic counselors' knowledge and beliefs. *Genet Med.* 2011;13:325–332.
62. Brett GR, Metcalfe SA, Amor DJ, et al. An exploration of genetic health professionals' experience with direct-to-consumer genetic testing in their clinical practice. *Eur J Hum Genet.* 2012;20:825–830. doi: 10.1038/ejhg.2012.13.
63. Udesky L. The ethics of direct-to-consumer genetic testing. *Lancet.* 2010;376:1377–1378.
64. Hogarth S, Javitt G, Melzer D. The current landscape for direct-to-consumer genetic testing: Legal, ethical, and policy issues. *Annu Rev Genomics Hum Genet.* 2008;9:161–182.
65. Hawkins AK, Ho A. Genetic counseling and the ethical issues around direct to consumer genetic testing. *J Genet Couns.* 2012;21:367–373.
66. Gollust SE, Wilfond BS, Hull SC. Direct-to-consumer sales of genetic services on the internet. *Genet Med.* 2003;5:332–337.
67. Mykitiuk R. Caveat emptor: Direct-to-consumer supply and advertising of genetic testing. *Clin Invest Med.* 2004;27:23–32.
68. Annes JP, Giovanni MA, Murray MF. Risks of presymptomatic direct-to-consumer genetic testing. *N Engl J Med.* 2010;363:1100–1101.
69. Caulfield T, Ries NM, Ray PN, et al. Direct-to-consumer genetic testing: Good, bad or benign? *Clin Genet.* 2010;77:101–105.

70. McGuire AL, Evans BJ, Caulfield T, et al. Science and regulation. Regulating direct-to-consumer personal genome testing. *Science*. 2010;330:181–182.

71. Samuel GN, Jordens CF, Kerridge I. Direct-to-consumer personal genome testing: Ethical and regulatory issues that arise from wanting to "know" your DNA. *Intern Med J*. 2010;40:220–224.

72. Howard HC, Avard D, Borry P. Are the kids really all right? Direct-to-consumer genetic testing in children: Are company policies clashing with professional norms? *Eur J Hum Genet*. 2011;19:1122–1126.

73. Caulfield T, McGuire AL. Direct-to-consumer genetic testing: Perceptions, problems, and policy responses. *Annu Rev Med*. 2012;63:23–33.

74. Lachance CR, Erby LAH, Ford BM, et al. Informational content, literacy demands, and usability of websites offering health-related genetic tests directly to consumers. *Genet Med*. 2010;12:304–312.

75. Skirton H, Goldsmith L, Jackson L, et al. Direct to consumer genetic testing: A systematic review of position statements, policies and recommendations. *Clin Genet*. 2012;82:210–218. doi: 10.1111/j.1399-0004.2012.01863.x.

76. Hudson K, Burke W, Byers, P. ASHG statement on direct-to-consumer genetic testing in the United States. *Am J Hum Genet*. 2007;81:635–637.

77. American College of Medical Genetics (ACMG) statement on direct-to-consumer genetic testing. April 7, 2008. Available at: http://www.acmg.net/StaticContent/StaticPages/DTC_Statement.pdf. Accessed on April 15, 2012.

78. Human Genetics Commission. A common framework of principles for direct-to-consumer genetic testing services. Available at: http://www.hgc. gov.uk/UploadDocs/DocPub/Document/HGC%20 Principles%20for%20DTC%20genetic%20tests%20-%20final.pdf. Accessed on April 15, 2012.

79. European Society of Human Genetics. Statement of the ESHG on direct-to-consumer genetic testing for health-related purposes. *Eur J Hum Genet*. 2010;18:1271–1273.

80. National Society of Genetic Counselors. Statement on direct-to-consumer genetic testing. Adopted 2007, Revised 2011. Available at: http://www.nsgc.org/Advocacy/PositionStatements/tabid/107/Default.aspx#DTC. Accessed on April 15, 2012.

81. Secretary's Advisory Committee on Genetics Health and Society. Direct-to-consumer genetic testing. Available at: http://oba.od.nih.gov/SACGHS/sacghs_documents.html. Accessed on April 15, 2012.

82. U.S. House of Representatives Committee on Energy and Commerce. Hearing on "Direct-to-Consumer Genetic Testing and the Consequences to the Public Health." Available at: http://democrats.energycommerce.house.gov/index.php?q=hearing/hearing-on-direct-to-consumer-genetic-testing-and-the-consequences-to-the-public-health. Accessed on April 15, 2012.

83. U.S. Government Accountability Office. Direct-to-Consumer Genetic Tests: Misleading Test Results are Further Complicated by Deceptive Marketing and Other Questionable Practices. Available at: http://www.gao.gov/new.items/d10847t.pdf. Accessed on April 15, 2012.

84. AMA Press Release February 23, 2011. AMA to FDA: Genetic Testing Should be Conducted by Qualified Health Professionals. Available at: http://www.ama-assn.org/ama/pub/news/news/genetic-testing-qualified-professionals.page. Accessed on April 15, 2012.

85. Myers MF, Bernhardt BA. Direct-to-consumer genetic testing: Introduction to the special issue. *J Genet Couns*. 2012;21:357–360.

86. Wagner JK. Understanding FDA regulation of DTC genetic tests within the context of administrative law. *Am J Hum Genet*. 2010;87:451–456.

87. Borry P, van Hellemondt RE, Sprumont D, et al. Legislation on direct-to-consumer genetic testing in seven European countries. *Eur J Hum Genet*. 2012;20:715–721.

88. Green RC, Roberts JS, Cupples LA, et al. Disclosure of APOE genotype for risk of Alzheimer's disease. *N Engl J Med*. 2009;361:245–254.

89. Field A, Krokosky A, Terry SF. Answering the hard questions: The Genetic Testing Registry and its request for information. *Genet Test Mol Biomarkers*. 2011;15:1–2.

90. Albuquerque W, Horn EJ, Terry SF. Beast of burden? Comments on the NIH Genetic Testing Registry. *Genet Test Mol Biomarkers*. 2012;16:155–156.

91. Howard HC, Borry P. Is there a doctor in the house? The presence of physicians in the direct-to-consumer genetic testing context. *J Community Genet*. 2012;3:105–112.

92. The Genetic Testing Laboratories, Inc. DNA Predisposition Testing. Available at: http://www.gtldna.com/predisposition.html. Accessed on April 15, 2012.

93. Hesse BW, Arora NK, Khoury MJ. Implications of Internet availability of genomic information for public health practice. *Public Health Genomics.* 2012;15:201–208.

94. McGuire AL, Burke W. An unwelcome side effect of direct-to-consumer personal genome testing: Raiding the medical commons. *JAMA.* 2008;300:2669–2671.

95. Hall MJ, Olopade OI. Disparities in genetic testing: Thinking outside the BRCA box. *J Clin Oncol.* 2006;24:2197–2203.

96. National Human Genome Research Institute. DNA Sequencing Costs: Data from the NHGRI Large-Scale Genome Sequencing Program. Available at: http://www.genome.gov/sequencingcosts/. Accessed on March 29, 2012.

97. DeFrancesco L. Life technologies promises the $1000 genome. *Nat Biotech.* 2012;30:126.

98. Ormond KE, Wheeler MT, Hudgins L, et al. Challenges in the clinical application of whole-genome sequencing. *Lancet.* 2010;375:1749–1751.

4 Adverse Events in Cancer Genetic Testing

Medical, Ethical, Legal, and Financial Implications

Karina L. Brierley, Erica Blouch, Whitney Cogswell, Jeanne P. Homer, Debbie Pencarinha, Christine L. Stanislaw, and Ellen T. Matloff

Over the past decade, cancer genetic counseling and testing have become essential services in progressive cancer care. With this evolution, there has been much debate over who is best suited to provide genetic services. Traditionally, genetic counseling and testing have been provided by individuals with graduate education, specialized training, and board certification in genetics. However, the push in recent years by some professional organizations and genetic testing companies has been to suggest that all health care providers should provide genetic counseling and testing services themselves. The impetus for this push on the part of the genetic testing companies is controversial, in that the aggressive sales representatives from these companies receive financial incentives for every test ordered and every new ordering provider.

Some potential benefits for provision of genetic counseling and testing by all health care providers, and not just specialists, have been proposed.[1,2] These benefits include that established providers have long-term relationships with their patients and thus deeper knowledge of the patient's overall health and that this may allow greater access to genetic services particularly in underserved populations where there are geographical, cultural, or language barriers.[1,2] Conversely, much of the literature over the past decade cites potential barriers, areas of concern, and negative outcomes from genetic counseling and testing being performed by providers without specialized training in this area.[2,3] Besides a handful of well-known lawsuits, little has been published demonstrating actual clinical examples of adverse outcomes resulting from cancer genetic counseling and testing performed by clinicians without specialization in this area.

In 2010, we published the first known national series of cases of this kind.[3] In this chapter, we will discuss additional cases and controversies. Both the cases in this chapter and those published in our previous series were obtained from genetic counselors who participate in the National Society of Genetic Counselors Cancer Special Interest Group listserv. For the current chapter, genetic counselors from the National Society of Genetic Counselors Cancer Special Interest Group were invited in January 2012 to submit cases of adverse outcomes of cancer genetic counseling and testing performed by providers without specialization in this area for inclusion in a case series publication. Cases were chosen for inclusion that illustrated unique themes/major patterns of errors in cancer genetic counseling and testing. Cases included originated from five of the United States (California, Connecticut, Georgia, Massachusetts, and Tennessee). Multiple colleagues informally reported additional cases but were unwilling to formally report them for inclusion, citing fear of pushback from the clinicians involved and/or potential conflicts with the commercial company that performs much of the cancer genetic testing in the United States and is also the largest employer of genetic counselors in the United States.

We will also review the literature on the factors that may contribute to these errors and the potential barriers and areas of concern related to clinicians without extensive knowledge, training, or certification in genetics providing cancer genetic counseling and testing.

THEMES IN CLINICAL CASE REPORTS
Wrong Testing Ordered

In many of the reported cases, the wrong genetic test was ordered. In some cases, this led to inaccurate medical management recommendations, and in others, unnecessary testing and expenditure of health care dollars.

Wrong Testing Ordered, Resulting in Inaccurate Medical Management Recommendations

In one case, a 19-year-old unaffected female patient of Italian ancestry presented to a gastroenterologist for reflux and gastrointestinal symptoms. The doctor elicited a family history of polyposis in the patient's father and documented that he had "screened the patient for an APC gene mutation" (associated with familial adenomatous polyposis [FAP]). The patient's blood work from that visit indicated a normal complete blood count and F5L screen (i.e., a normal assay for activated protein C, also abbreviated "APC"). A colonoscopy was neither ordered, nor was the patient referred to genetics. Notes from the patient's follow-up care with this physician make no further mention of genetics or FAP. A year later, the patient was seen by a new physician and referred for a colonoscopy and cancer genetic counseling. Testing ordered by the genetic counselor revealed that the patient carried a detectable *APC* gene mutation, and the patient was found to have polyposis upon colonoscopy. The original gastroenterologist in this case ordered the wrong test and apparently closed the case based on a false-negative result. Ninety-three percent of patients with classic FAP go on to develop colorectal cancer by the age of 50 years without colectomy.[4] The average age at diagnosis of colon cancer in untreated individuals with FAP is 39 years.[4]

In another case, a 63-year-old unaffected woman of English, not Jewish, ancestry was seen by her primary care physician because of her concerns about her family history, which included a sister diagnosed with ovarian cancer and a mother who died of early-onset breast cancer. The primary care physician ordered testing for the three *BRCA* mutations that are common among individuals of Jewish ancestry, which was negative. The patient received a copy of the test results with a note from her physician, "BRCA (smiley face)." The sister with ovarian cancer later had full sequencing of the *BRCA1* and *BRCA2* genes and was found to carry a *BRCA2* mutation (not the one common among Ashkenazi Jews, as expected on the basis of their ancestry). Five years later, the original patient was referred to a cancer genetic counselor by her radiologist to make sure she had had the correct testing. The genetic counselor ordered testing for the familial *BRCA2* mutation identified in the sister, and the patient, fortunately, tested true negative. However, if she had carried the mutation, many serious adverse consequences (including cancer diagnoses) could have resulted for her and her at-risk adult children from her not knowing her correct *BRCA* status for many years.

In a third case, an oncologist referred a 23-year-old woman of Mexican, not Jewish, ancestry who was recently diagnosed with bilateral breast cancer for genetic counseling. The referral read "genetic counseling and *BRCA* testing for surgical decision making." Upon taking the patient's family history, the counselor learned that the patient had a sibling who was diagnosed with a glioblastoma at age 14 years and died at age 16 years. Based on the patient's personal history of very early-onset bilateral breast cancer and family history of a childhood brain tumor, the genetic counselor instead ordered testing for mutations in the p53 gene associated with Li–Fraumeni syndrome. The patient was found to carry a p53 mutation, and therefore, learned she was not a good candidate for chest wall irradiation. The patient had previously been counseled by her physician that she would need a prophylactic bilateral salpingo-oophorectomy at age 23 years because of the association of *BRCA* mutations and ovarian cancer, and this suggestion (which would have been controversial, even in a *BRCA* carrier) was difficult to counter with the patient even after a p53 mutation had been identified.

Unnecessary Testing/Misuse of Health Care Dollars

Ordering the wrong genetic testing can also lead to the unnecessary expenditure of thousands of dollars, which is then charged to the insurance company and/or the patient. In one such example, a patient was seen by his surgeon based on the fact that his sister carried a known *MSH2* mutation associated with Lynch syndrome. The surgeon ordered full sequencing of the *MSH2* gene through his office's laboratory, and the charge for this testing with the laboratory send-out fees was $4,700. The patient's insurance, justly, denied payment for this test. The patient was then seen by a cancer genetic counselor when his daughter decided to pursue testing. He was very upset when he learned that the appropriate testing (for the single familial mutation) would have cost $475. The patient was also angry that, despite all of this extra expense, his doctor had given him little pertinent Lynch syndrome information except that he carried the same mutation that his sister carried; he had not been given detailed information about his cancer risks, screening recommendations, and risks and recommendations for other family members.

Results Misinterpreted

Misinterpretation of genetic test results was another common error observed in our series of cases. Many of the cases of result misinterpretation involved variants of uncertain significance, which are among the more difficult results to interpret. However, other cases demonstrated that result misinterpretation occurred in simple, straightforward cases.

Result Misinterpretation, Resulting in an Advanced Cancer Diagnosis

A 46-year-old woman of Polish, not Jewish, ancestry was referred to cancer genetic counseling because of her recent diagnosis of stage III ovarian cancer and strong family history of breast cancer (Fig. 4.1). She initially reported that one of her relatives who had breast cancer had *BRCA* testing in a different country and tested negative. At the end of her appointment, she recalled that she had *BRCA* testing through her gynecologist's office 16 months earlier at age 45 years and was told it was "normal." However, after discussing that she would now meet the testing company's criteria for large rearrangement testing (BART) in *BRCA1/2* at no additional cost, the patient chose to proceed with testing. Upon receiving the request for this additional testing, the laboratory sent the genetic counselor a fax indicating that the patient would not qualify for free BART rearrangement testing because her initial testing was positive for a deleterious mutation in *BRCA1*. The counselor contacted the ordering gynecologist to determine what had occurred and what the patient had been told about her results. The gynecologist was shocked, and very upset, to learn that the patient carried a mutation and to realize that she had misinterpreted the result, which was clearly printed in capital letters in a box at the top of the page. The gynecologist had noticed only the wording listed next to the *BRCA2* gene and a targeted rearrangement panel that indicated that no mutation was detected in that gene. The gynecologist contacted the patient about this error, and the patient was then seen for follow-up genetic coun-

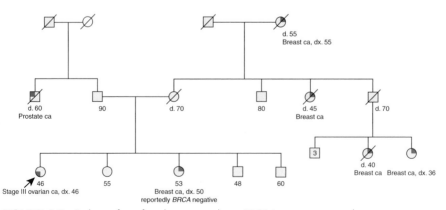

FIGURE 4.1. Pedigree for a female patient whose *BRCA1* positive test result was misinterpreted as negative, resulting in an advanced ovarian cancer diagnosis.

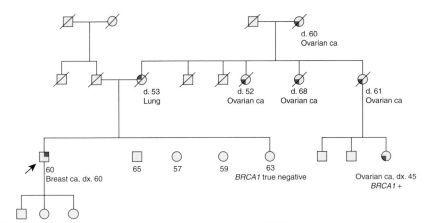

FIGURE 4.2. Pedigree for a male patient whose sister's *BRCA* negative test result was misinterpreted leading to a delay in testing and an advanced male breast cancer diagnosis.

seling. The patient and her husband were painfully aware that if her results had been read correctly 16 months earlier, she could have had a prophylactic BSO and probably avoided a likely fatal advanced ovarian cancer diagnosis. The patient and her husband indicated that they planned to sue her gynecologist.

Another case in which the significance of test results was misinterpreted demonstrates how inaccurate information given to one patient can impact multiple other family members. A 60-year-old man of Irish ancestry diagnosed with breast cancer was seen for cancer genetic counseling based on his personal history and his family history that included five cases of ovarian cancer (Fig. 4.2). One of his maternal cousins with ovarian cancer carried a known *BRCA1* mutation. The patient reported that his sister was tested for this familial *BRCA1* by her gynecologist and learned that she did not carry this mutation. She was told that since she did not have this mutation, none of her siblings (including this gentleman) would carry this mutation, and none of them needed testing. After his cancer diagnosis, this gentleman had testing and learned that he carried the familial *BRCA1* mutation. He was angry that his sister and their family had been given misinformation about their risks. He indicated that he would have sought care for the lump he had found behind his nipple much sooner if he had known he was at increased risk, and this may have allowed him to be diagnosed at an earlier stage, avoid chemotherapy, and to have a better prognosis.

Result Misinterpretation, Leading to Unnecessary Prophylactic Surgery

A 42-year-old patient with a confirmed diagnosis of FAP and an *APC* gene mutation was referred for genetic counseling by her gastroenterologist because she had had genetic testing several years earlier through her colorectal surgeon, but had never had formal genetic counseling. When the genetic counselor took the

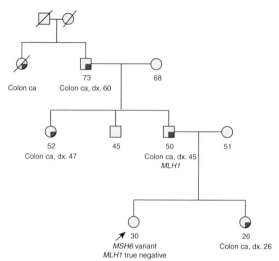

FIGURE 4.3. Pedigree for a female patient whose *MSH6* variant of uncertain significance test result was misinterpreted as a deleterious mutation leading to recommendations for unnecessary prophylactic surgery.

patient's personal history, she learned that the patient had had a total hysterectomy and bilateral salpingo-oophorectomy at age 41 years based on her surgeon's assessment that she "was at an increased risk for cancer there" because of her genetic test results. The surgeon had apparently confused the cancer risks associated with FAP with the ovarian and uterine cancer risks seen with Lynch syndrome. This patient had undergone unnecessary surgery and premature menopause because of this misinformation.

One of the more common result misinterpretations in this, and previous, case series was a variant of uncertain significance being falsely interpreted as a known disease-causing mutation. In one case, a 30-year-old woman was referred to a cancer genetic counselor after being tested by her gastroenterologist and told that she carried an *MSH6* mutation (Fig. 4.3). The patient sobbed through her appointment with the genetic counselor indicating that her doctor had told her that she would need to have a hysterectomy, and therefore, would not be able to have children. She had never had a diagnosis of cancer but had a strong family history of colon cancer including her father, sister, paternal aunt, and paternal grandfather diagnosed at ages 45, 26, 47, and 60 years, respectively (Fig. 4.3). Upon reviewing her test results, the genetic counselor discovered that the patient actually carried a variant of uncertain significance. Many of the affected relatives were living, so genetic testing was recommended in an affected relative. Her father had genetic counseling and testing, and learned that he carried a deleterious *MLH1* mutation. The patient subsequently had testing and learned that she did not carry the *MLH1* mutation identified in her father that was responsible for the cancers in her family. She was thus not at increased risk for colon, uterine, and ovarian cancer, and did not need to have a prophylactic hysterectomy.

Inadequate Genetic Counseling

In some cases, inadequate genetic counseling was the main error that occurred and included incomplete information about implications and options for the patient and/or their family members and practices that go against widely accepted ethical principles in cancer genetic counseling and testing.

Ethical Issues

The parents of a 7-year-old healthy girl of Ashkenazi Jewish ancestry, at the urging of a relative who is a physician, obtained a test kit from a genetic testing company and requested that their daughter's pediatrician order *BRCA* testing based on their Jewish ancestry and the father's family history of ovarian cancer. The pediatrician complied with their request, and the child was found to carry a *BRCA1* mutation. When the parents were seen for genetic counseling, they were upset to learn that this information would also directly impact whichever parent carried the mutation in terms of increased cancer risk and that either of them could carry this mutation and should have testing since they were both of Jewish ancestry. Upon learning the future impact of this mutation for their daughter and the fact that her medical management in childhood would not change based on this information, they left indicating that they wished they had not had her tested at this time. When there is no immediate medical benefit (i.e., interventions that can be offered in childhood), it is almost universally recommended that testing for adult-onset conditions be deferred until adulthood when the individual can make an informed decision about testing because there are potential risks or concerns about testing in childhood including adverse psychosocial reactions, discrimination, and stigmatization.[5–9] This recommendation is also based on the ethical principles of respecting the autonomy of the child and their right not to know.[5–9]

POTENTIAL FACTORS CONTRIBUTING TO ERRORS IN CANCER GENETIC COUNSELING AND TESTING

The literature regarding medical errors across all specialties suggests that certain factors increase the likelihood that errors will occur, including case complexity, time pressures, inadequate experience, insufficient knowledge or training, and poor communication.[10–12] Several of these factors may make these errors more likely among providers without extensive knowledge, training, or certification in genetics than among cancer genetics professionals, including lack of familiarity and inadequate knowledge and training.[10–12] Numerous national and international studies have shown that many providers have inadequate knowledge of genetics to prepare them for providing genetic counseling and testing.[2,13–18] These studies have consistently shown significant deficiencies among nonspecialists in knowledge essential for providing cancer genetic counseling and testing, including inheritance patterns, risk factors for hereditary cancer syndromes, and gene penetrance.[13–18] Even in a recent study of medical residents (who presumably would have the most current education and training in genetics), significant deficits in knowledge of key concepts, including associated cancer risks and inheritance patterns, were identified.[17]

These deficiencies in knowledge are likely related to the fact that the majority of medical professionals have little formal training in genetics.[2,18] A survey of gynecologists found that 65% had no formal classroom or clinical training in genetic testing in gynecologic practice.[18] Even among the youngest physicians (aged ≤40 years), who were likely to have the most modern training, the majority (62.4%) reported not having received formal training in genetics.[18] In 2004, a survey of US and Canadian medical schools found that 62% provided 20 to 40 hours of medical genetics course work, and 18% provided less than 20 hours.[19] Most of this instruction took place during the first year of medical school and focused on general concepts, not practical application.[19]

Time pressures probably also contribute to errors in cancer genetic counseling and testing performed by clinicians without extensive training and knowledge in this area. Genetic counseling and testing are complex and time-consuming processes that minimally involve obtaining a detailed personal and three-generation family medical history and providing thorough pretest informed consent and posttest result disclosure and interpretation.[20,21] Professional guidelines suggest that the informed consent process should include a discussion of what testing to consider, whom to test in the family, possible test results and their implications for the individual and family members, options for cancer screening and risk reduction, economic considerations, and psychosocial considerations.[20,21] Thus, in busy clinic settings where primary care physicians and gynecologists have an average of 20 minutes or less per patient encounter,[22] it is unrealistic and unfair to ask these providers to add a service as complex as cancer genetic counseling and testing to an already busy appointment. In fact, many physicians self-report lack of time as a barrier to providing genetic counseling and testing services.[2,16,23]

In addition to having inadequate knowledge and time to provide genetic counseling and testing services, experts cite concerns that many physicians have insufficient familiarity with the unique, complex ethical, and psychosocial issues that are often part of the genetic counseling process (e.g., the impact of results on the entire family, policies regarding testing minors for adult-onset conditions, and concerns about genetic discrimination).[2,24–27] Numerous professional guidelines uniformly discourage testing minors for adult-onset disorders (including hereditary cancer syndromes) unless there are immediate medical interventions available in childhood that will reduce morbidity or mortality.[5–9] Yet, a 2010 survey of primary care physicians showed that 31% would "unconditionally" recommend testing a healthy 13-year-old girl for her mother's *BRCA* mutation.[26] One of the case examples presented above where a pediatrician ordered *BRCA* testing on a 7-year-old girl provides a parallel clinical illustration of this study.

Clinicians without extensive training and knowledge in genetics may also not be sufficiently aware of current policy guidelines and laws in order to accurately inform patients about insurance coverage for testing, existing protections against genetic discrimination, and whether they are an appropriate candidate for testing.[24,25,27] A 2009 survey of family physicians showed that more than half (54.5%) had no awareness of the Genetic Information Nondiscrimination Act (GINA) of 2008, a national law that provides protection against genetic discrimination by health insurers and employers.[27] Even among those physicians who reported having some basic knowledge of GINA, many were not aware of the particular areas protected (i.e., group health insurance, private individual health insurance, employment) by GINA and the limitations of GINA (i.e., no protections regarding life or long-term care insurance).[27]

A secondary concern raised by these cases is the waste of health care dollars on unnecessary testing and procedures. Particularly in the current economy, rising health care costs are a significant subject of attention from the government, physician groups, employers, and the general public.[28] US health care costs have been consistently increasing at a rapid pace, twice that of inflation. In 2010, US health care expenditures reached $2.6 trillion dollars or 17.6% of the gross domestic product.[29] Many experts agree that health care costs are significantly higher than necessary and that waste, overuse, and inappropriate or unnecessary care are some of the major contributors to this excess.[28,29] In addition to the cases in this series, two recent studies demonstrate how unnecessary genetic testing may be contributing to excess health care spending. One survey of 1,500 physicians asked them to distinguish between clinical scenarios representing cases where the risk was sufficiently increased to warrant *BRCA* testing and cases where the risk was low and testing was not warranted on the basis of published guidelines.[30] Although 25% of the physicians had ordered *BRCA* testing in the past year, 45% chose at least one low-risk scenario as warranting testing, and only 19% were able to correctly identify which scenarios warranted tested and which did not.[30] In another recent study, physicians were asked whether to recommend testing and which testing they would order for at-risk relatives of a patient based on the patient carrying a deleterious mutation or a variant of uncertain significance.[31] The majority (82%) would inappropriately order testing when the result was a variant of uncertain significance, and in both situations, most would inappropriately choose to order comprehensive sequencing, which would result in at least a ninefold increase in unnecessary testing costs.[31] These findings were independent of physicians' experience or specialty.[31] In response to this expensive problem, several insurance companies are now tracking the number of inappropriate requests for genetic testing, requiring prior notification or authorization for genetic testing, encouraging or requiring genetic counseling by providers with expertise and/or board certification in genetics before testing, and covering care by telemedicine genetic counseling services for their members.[32–35]

Numerous lawsuits have found health care providers negligent with regard to genetic testing, including several involving hereditary cancer syndromes.[36,37] Physicians appear to be the most common target of these lawsuits in which they were found negligent for failing to collect a sufficient family history, refer to a genetic counselor or geneticist, recognize the possibility of a hereditary cancer syndrome, recommend appropriate testing, recommend suitable risk reduction options, and/or warn at-risk relatives.[36] In two similar lawsuits from the past decade, women who were diagnosed with ovarian cancer and ultimately died of their disease, and their families successfully sued their physicians for failing to refer them for genetic counseling and testing and/or advise them about their options for risk reduction based on their strong family histories of breast and ovarian cancer.[37] A number of other cases have found physicians negligent in recognizing and appropriately advising patients regarding hereditary colon cancer in their families.[38]

Over the past decade, direct-to-consumer marketing for genetic tests has become more widespread targeting both physicians and consumers. Although there is no direct evidence to suggest that these campaigns have contributed to an increase in adverse events in cancer genetic counseling and testing, experts have voiced potential concerns. One concern is that genetic testing practice patterns of primary care providers may be more strongly influenced by direct marketing, lay press, and threats of malpractice than by expert protocols and journal articles.[2] Direct-to-consumer marketing campaigns by the testing company that holds the exclusive patents on testing for the *BRCA1* and *BRCA2* genes have been a particular focus of controversy. This company has openly stated that in order to grow their revenue they expanded their sales force and focused on urging gynecologists and oncologists to provide cancer genetic counseling and testing in their offices rather than referring patients to a genetic counselor.[35] The testing company insists that community physicians are prepared to perform genetic counseling, and their sales force provides "genetic counseling education" for office physicians and their staff.[35] However, this is contrary to the bulk of the available data that suggest that most providers lack the time, knowledge, and awareness to provide adequate genetic counseling. It also conflicts with the Commission on Cancer Program Standards, which directly state that "educational seminars offered by commercial laboratories about how to perform genetic testing are not considered adequate training for cancer risk assessment and genetic counseling."[21] There is clearly a conflict of interest here because the individuals providing the "education" work for a commercial company that profits from the testing.

Another disturbing possibility is that physicians may be delegating the genetic counseling and testing process to office staff. A survey of New York obstetrician–gynecologists showed that, in many cases, office staff, including secretaries, were accountable for completing genetic test requisitions, reviewing test results, and giving test results to patients.[39] Forty-four percent of physicians in the study reported that secretaries filled out genetic test requisitions, 59% reported that secretaries review the results, and 86% report that secretaries communicated results to patients over the phone.[39] These findings raise questions about what steps are taken to ensure that office personnel are properly equipped and capable of performing these tasks, particularly, if sales representatives from testing companies are providing the "genetic counseling education" to physicians' office staff.

Recent advances in technology have led to the development of more complicated genetic and genomic testing options, including multiple gene panels, as well as whole-exome and whole-genome sequencing. Although these new testing options offer the promise of many benefits in terms of "personalized medicine" and advances in the diagnosis and treatment of both rare and common diseases, they have generated new concerns and heightened existing concerns about the potential medical, legal, social, and ethical challenges of genetic testing.[40–43] Whole-exome and whole-genome tests generate massive amounts of data, including potentially hundreds or thousands of variants per individual.[40,41] The significance of these variants and the function and clinical impact of many of the genes containing these variants are unknown.[40,43] The interpretation of how these genetic changes impact health is likely to be far more complex, involving weaker associations, lower-penetrance mutations, and interactions between multiple genes and the environment.[42,43] Unfortunately, our ability to generate massive amounts of genetic data has far outpaced our ability to analyze and interpret the clinical significance of these data.[40] Thus, using this information clinically to care for patients poses significant challenges even for providers with extensive knowledge and experience in medical genetics. The amount and complexity of these data also poses significant ethical and legal challenges, including what constitutes informed consent, the potential for incidental findings, what information to disclose to patients, how the data should be stored and shared, who owns the data, and implications for the patient and family members.[40–42]

The cases illustrated here demonstrate that errors with major medical, legal, financial, and ethical implications are occurring today in relatively straightforward genetic testing scenarios. As the field becomes more, and not less, complex, it is unrealistic and unfair to expect the average clinician to provide genetic counseling and testing services alone.

ACKNOWLEDGMENTS

The authors thank Mary E. Freivogel, MS, CGC, for her contribution to this chapter.

REFERENCES

1. Guttmacher AE, Jenkins J, Uhlmann WR. Genomic medicine: Who will practice it? A call to open arms. *Am J Med Genet.* 2001;106:216–222.
2. Greendale K, Pyeritz RE. Empowering primary care health professionals in medical genetics: How soon? How fast? How far? *Am J Med Genet.* 2001;106:223–232.
3. Brierley KL, Campfield D, Ducaine W, et al. Errors in delivery of cancer genetics services: Implications for practice. *Conn Med.* 2010;74:413–423.
4. Jasperson KW, Burt RW. APC-associated polyposis conditions. Available at: http://www.ncbi.nlm.nih. gov/books/NBK1345/. Accessed on April 3, 2012.
5. Borry P, Stultiens L, Nys H, et al. Presymptomatic and predictive genetic testing in minors: A systematic review of guidelines and position papers. *Clin Genet.* 2006;70:374–381.
6. American Academy of Pediatrics: Committee on Bioethics. Ethical issues with genetic testing in pediatrics. *Pediatrics.* 2001;107:1451–1455.
7. Berliner JL, Fay AM. Risk assessment and genetic counseling for hereditary breast and ovarian cancer: Recommendations of the National Society of Genetic Counselors. *J Genet Couns.* 2007;16:241–260.
8. ASHG Board of Directors and ACMG Board of Directors. ASHG/ACMG report: Points to consider: Ethical, legal, and psychosocial implications of genetic testing in children and adolescents. *Am J Hum Genet.* 1995;57:1233–1241.
9. American Society of Clinical Oncology. American Society of Clinical Oncology policy statement update: Genetic testing for cancer susceptibility. *J Clin Oncol.* 2003;21:2397–2406.
10. Reason J. Understanding adverse events: Human factors. *Qual Health Care.* 1995;4:80–89.
11. Mahlmeister LR. Human factors and error in perinatal care. *J Perinat Neonatal Nurs.* 2010;24:12–21.
12. Wilson RM, Harrison BT, Gibberd RW, et al. An analysis of the causes of adverse events from the Quality in Australian Health Care Study. *Med J Aust.* 1999;170:411–415.

13. Wideroff L, Vadaparampil ST, Greene MH, et al. Hereditary breast/ovarian and colorectal cancer genetics knowledge in a national sample of US physicians. *J Med Genet.* 2005;42:749–755.

14. Doksum T, Bernhardt BA, Holtzman NA. Does knowledge about the genetics of breast cancer differ between nongeneticist physicians who do or do not discuss or order BRCA testing? *Genet Med.* 2003;5:99–105.

15. Domanska K, Carlsson C, Bendahl PO, et al. Knowledge about hereditary nonpolyposis colorectal cancer; mutation carriers and physicians at equal levels. *BMC Med Genet.* 2009;10:30.

16. Suther S, Goodson P. Barriers to the provision of genetic services by primary care physicians: A systematic review of the literature. *Genet Med.* 2003;5:70–76.

17. Ready KJ, Daniels MS, Sun CC, et al. Obstetrics/gynecology residents' knowledge of hereditary breast and ovarian cancer and Lynch syndrome. *J Cancer Educ.* 2010;25:401–404.

18. Wilkins-Haug L, Hill L, et al. Gynecologists' training, knowledge, and experiences in genetics: A survey. *Obstet Gynecol.* 2000;95:421–424.

19. Thurston VC, Wales PS, Bell MA, et al. The current status of medical genetics instruction in U.S. and Canadian medical schools. *Acad Med.* 2007;82:441–445.

20. Riley BD, Culver JO, Skrzynia C, et al. Essential elements of genetic cancer risk assessment, counseling, and testing: updated recommendations of the National Society of Genetic Counselors. *J Genet Couns.* 2012;21:151–161.

21. Commission on Cancer. Cancer Program Standards 2012: Ensuring Patient-Centered Care v.1.0. Available at: www.facs.org/cancer/coc/cocprogramstandards2012.pdf. Accessed on April 3, 2012.

22. Weeks WB, Wallace AE. Time and money: A retrospective evaluation of the inputs, outputs, efficiency, and incomes of physicians. *Arch Intern Med.* 2003;163:944–948.

23. Wood ME, Stockdale A, Flynn BS. Interviews with primary care physicians regarding taking and interpreting the cancer family history. *Fam Pract.* 2008;25:334–340.

24. Brandt R, Zonera A, Sabel A, et al. Cancer genetics evaluation: Barriers to and improvements for referral. *Genet Test.* 2008;12:9–12.

25. Lowstuter KJ, Sand S, Blazer KR, et al. Influence of genetic discrimination perceptions and knowledge on cancer genetics referral practice among clinicians. *Genet Med.* 2008;10:691–698.

26. O'Neill SC, Peshkin BN, Luta G, et al. Primary care providers' willingness to recommend BRCA1/2 testing to adolescents. *Fam Cancer.* 2010;9:43–50.

27. Laedtke AL, O'Neill SM, Rubinstein WS, et al. Family physicians' awareness and knowledge of the Genetic Information Non-discrimination Act (GINA). *J Genet Couns.* 2012;21:345–352.

28. Swensen SJ, Kaplan GS, Meyer GS, et al. Controlling healthcare costs by removing waste: What American doctors can do now. *BMJ Qual Saf.* 2011;20:534–537.

29. Sherman D. Stemming overtreatment in U.S. healthcare may cut costs of care. Available at: http://www.reuters.com/article/2012/02/16/us-health-overtreatment-idUSTRE81F15Y20120216. Accessed on April 3, 2012.

30. Bellcross CA, Kolor K, Goddard KAB, et al. Awareness and utilization of BRCA1/2 testing among U.S. primary care physicians. *Am J Prev Med.* 2011;40:61–66.

31. Plon SE, Cooper HP, Parks B, et al. Genetic testing and cancer risk management recommendations by physicians for at-risk relatives. *Genet Med.* 2011;13:148–154.

32. Informed Medical Decisions. News: Aetna Press Release: Aetna to offer access to confidential telephonic cancer genetic counseling to health plan members. Available at: http://www.informeddna.com/images/stories/news_articles/aetna%20press%20release%20bw.pdf. Accessed on August 24, 2009.

33. Ray T. Lack of Physician Education, Genetic Counseling Could Ruin Value Proposition of PGx Testing, Insurer Says. *Pharmacogenomics Reporter.* Available at: http://www.genomeweb.com/dxpgx/lack-physician-education-genetic-counseling-could-ruin-value-proposition-pgx-tes. Accessed on August 24, 2009.

34. Ray T. United Healthcare issues prior notification requirement for Myriad's BRACAnalysis Test. *Pharmacogenomics Reporter.* Available at: http://www.genomeweb.com/united-healthcare-issues-prior-notification-requirement-myriads-bracanalysis-tes. Accessed on April 3, 2012.

35. Ray T. Myriad defends policy of urging docs to genetically counsel BRACAnalysis customers. *Pharmacogenomics Reporter.* Available at: http://www.genomeweb.com/dxpgx/myriad-defends-policy-urging-docs-genetically-counsel-bracanalysis-customers. Accessed on April 3, 2012.

36. Lindor RA, Marchant GE, O'Connor SD. A review of medical malpractice claims related to clinical genetic testing. *J Clin Oncol.* 2011;29(suppl); abstract 6073.
37. Miletich S, Armstrong K, Mayo J. Life-or-death question, but debate was hidden for years. *The Seattle Times.* October 19, 2006. Available at: http://community.seattletimes.nwsource.com/archive/?date=200 61019&slug=virginiamason19m. Accessed on April 3, 2012.
38. Lynch HT, Paulson J, Severin M, et al. Failure to diagnose hereditary colorectal cancer and its medico-legal implications: A hereditary nonpolyposis colorectal cancer case. *Dis Colon Rectum.* 1999;42:31–35.
39. Lubin IM, Caggana M, Constantin C, et al. Ordering molecular genetic tests and reporting results: Practices in laboratory and clinical settings. *J Mol Diagn.* 2008;10:459–468.
40. Raffan E, Semple RK. Next generation sequencing—implications for clinical practice. *Br Med Bull.* 2011;99:53–71.
41. Ku C-S, Cooper DN, Polychronakos C, et al. Exome sequencing: Dual role as a discovery and diagnostic tool. *Ann Neurol.* 2012;71:5–14.
42. Li C. Personalized medicine—the promised land: Are we there yet? Clin Genet. 2011;79:403–412.
43. Gonzaga-Jauregui C, Lupski JR, Gibbs RA. Human genome sequencing in health and disease. *Annu Rev Med.* 2012;63:35–61.

5 Genetic Testing by Cancer Site

Breast

Kristen M. Shannon and Anu Chittenden

Women in the United States have a 12% lifetime risk of developing breast cancer.[1] Although only about 5% to 10% of all cases of breast cancer are attributable to a highly penetrant cancer predisposition gene, individuals who carry a mutation in one of these genes have a significantly higher risk of developing breast cancer, as well as other cancers, over their lifetime compared with the general population. The ability to distinguish those individuals at high risk allows health care providers to intervene with appropriate counseling and education, surveillance, and prevention with the overall goal of improved survival for these individuals. This chapter focuses on the identification of patients at high risk for breast cancer and provides an overview of the clinical features, cancer risks, causative genes, and medical management for the most clearly described hereditary breast cancer syndromes.

IDENTIFICATION OF HIGH-RISK INDIVIDUALS

An accurate and comprehensive family history of cancer is essential for identifying individuals who may be at risk for inherited breast cancer. As with any family history, it is important to gather a three-generation family history with information on both maternal and paternal lineages.[2,3] Particular focus should be on individuals with malignancies (affected), but those family members without a personal history of cancer (unaffected) should also be included. It is also important to include the presence of nonmalignant findings in the proband and family members, as some inherited cancer syndromes have other physical characteristics associated with them (e.g., trichilemmomas with Cowden syndrome [CS]).

When taking the family history, the accuracy of the information obtained from an individual patient should be considered. Many factors can influence an individual's knowledge of his/her family history, and errors in the reporting of family history have been documented.[4,5] A recent study indicates that individuals are often confident that a family member has had cancer but are typically unsure of the details surrounding that diagnosis.[6,7] Reports of breast cancer tend to be accurate, whereas reports of ovarian cancer are less trustworthy.[8,9] It is important to note that family histories can change over time, with clinically relevant diagnoses arising in family members especially between the ages of 30 and 50 years.[10] Finally, the physical examination of the proband and family members can be incredibly helpful in the identification of some inherited breast cancer syndromes, such as CS.

GENETIC TESTING

Although some published guidelines for genetic testing exist, much of the time the decision to offer genetic testing is based on clinical judgment. The National Comprehensive Cancer Network (NCCN) provides guidelines for individuals whom should be offered genetic testing for some of the genes mentioned in this text (NCCN 2011). In the end, however, it is up to the individual provider's judgment as to whether genetic testing is indicated.

Genetic testing for breast cancer susceptibility is rapidly changing. The classic method includes pursuing genetic testing for individual cancer predisposition gene(s) that the clinical suspects may be the cause of breast cancer in the family. In this scenario, finding the appropriate laboratory to perform the testing is very important because laboratory techniques (as well as sensitivity of the technique) vary. Most genetic testing includes sequencing of the gene in question. However, there are emerging data that suggest deletion/duplication studies are imperative for genetic testing as the mutational spectra include various rare, yet important genomic rearrangements.[11]

Recent changes in genetic testing and specifically the advent of next-generation sequencing tests, have led various genetic testing companies to establish "panel" testing for multiple breast cancer susceptibility genes. In this scenario, up to 14 different breast cancer susceptibility genes are analyzed from 1 blood specimen. These genes vary in clinical significance from the very highly penetrant breast cancer susceptibility gene *TP53* to the low penetrant breast cancer gene *CHEK2*. How this testing will evolve and the role it will play in clinical care remains to be seen.

BRCA1 AND *BRCA2*
Description

Mutations in the *BRCA1* and *BRCA2* genes give rise to the "classic" inherited breast cancer syndrome "hereditary breast and ovarian cancer (HBOC) syndrome." The vast majority of cases of HBOC are due to mutations in the *BRCA1* and *BRCA2* genes,[12,13] which were cloned in 1994 and 1995, respectively.[14,15] *BRCA1* and *BRCA2* mutations are rare in most populations, occurring in approximately 1 of 400 individuals, but much more common in the Ashkenazi Jewish population in which 1 of 40 individuals carries 1 of 3 main disease-causing mutations: 2 in *BRCA1* (185delAG and 5382insC) and the 6174delT mutation in BRCA2.[16,17] Other founder mutations have been identified, but the utility of these in the United States population is minimal.[18,19]

There has been a great deal of research into the tumor biology associated with *BRCA1/2* mutation carriers. *BRCA2*-associated breast cancers are similar in phenotype and clinical behavior in comparison to sporadic cancers.[20,21] *BRCA1*-related breast cancers are often of higher histologic grade, show an excess of medullary histopathology, and are more likely than sporadic tumors to be "triple negative" (i.e., estrogen receptor–negative, progesterone receptor–negative, and are less likely to demonstrate HER2/neu overexpression).[22] Serous papillary ovarian carcinoma is a key feature of hereditary cancers in *BRCA1* mutation carriers; it is less common in *BRCA2* carriers. Endometrioid and clear-cell subtypes of ovarian cancer have been observed,[23] but borderline ovarian tumors do not seem to be a part of the phenotype.[24] Both primary tumors of the fallopian tubes and peritoneum occur with increased frequency in mutation carriers.[25] The prognosis of ovarian cancer in *BRCA1* and *BRCA2* carriers is better than age-matched controls.[23,26,27]

Identifying *BRCA1/2* Carriers

Identifying those individuals at highest risk for harboring a mutation in *BRCA1* or *BRCA2* is of utmost importance so that they can benefit from surveillance and prevention options. There exist various models designed to estimate the likelihood of identifying a mutation in the *BRCA1* or *BRCA2* gene[13,28–31]; these models have strengths and limitations that health care providers need to be familiar with to use and interpret them appropriately.[32–34] The BRCAPRO model, likely the most often used in clinical cancer genetics, estimates the probability that an individual is a carrier of a *BRCA* mutation using family history and Bayes' theorem.[28] It is important when using these risk models to understand the limitations of these risk calculations and to place risk estimates into the appropriate context. It is important to note that risk estimates calculated by different models may vary, a factor that complicates the use of quantitative thresholds for making screening recommendations.[35] The health care provider should use clinical judgment in conjunction with estimates from models to provide the most precise risk assessment for an individual patient.

Cancer Risks

The penetrance associated with mutations in *BRCA1* and *BRCA2* remains an active area of research. The risks of developing specific cancers can be found in Table 5.1. The range of breast cancer risk is influenced by the population under study: Higher risk estimates have come from studies with affected families and somewhat lower risk estimates from studies in populations. Also, the risk of ovarian cancer is not the same for all *BRCA2* mutations, with mutations in the central ovarian cancer cluster region conferring a higher lifetime risk.[42] Other factors, such as birth cohort, oral contraceptive use, age at first pregnancy, and exercise, have all been shown to influence penetrance risk in populations.[36] There has been a report of increased risk of gallbladder and bile duct cancer, stomach cancer, and melanoma with *BRCA2* mutation, none of which seem to be clinically actionable.[37,43]

TABLE 5.1	BRCA 1/2 Cancer Risks	
Cancer Site	BRCA1 Mutation (%)	BRCA2 Mutation (%)
Female breast	50–80	40–70
Ovarian	<40	<20
Prostate	<30	<39
Pancreatic	1.3–3.2	2.3–7

From: Ford D, Easton DF, Stratton M, et al. Genetic heterogeneity and penetrance analysis of the BRCA1 and BRCA2 genes in breast cancer families. The Breast Cancer Linkage Consortium. *Am J Hum Genet.* 1998;62:676–689; King MC, Marks JH, Mandell JB. Breast and ovarian cancer risks due to inherited mutations in BRCA1 and BRCA2. *Science.* 2003;302:643–646; Ozcelik H, et al. Germline BRCA2 6174delT mutations in Ashkenazi Jewish pancreatic cancer patients. *Nat Genet.* 1997;16:17–18; Antoniou A, et al. Average risks of breast and ovarian cancer associated with BRCA1 or BRCA2 mutations detected in case series unselected for family history: A combined analysis of 22 studies. *Am J Hum Genet.* 2003;72:1117–1130; Risch HA, et al. Prevalence and penetrance of germline BRCA1 and BRCA2 mutations in a population series of 649 women with ovarian cancer. *Am J Hum Genet.* 2001;68:700–710; The Breast Cancer Linkage Consortium. Cancer risks in BRCA2 mutation carriers. *J Natl Cancer Inst.* 1999;91:1310–1316; Thompson D, Easton DF. Cancer incidence in BRCA1 mutation carriers. *J Natl Cancer Inst.* 2002;94:1358–1365.

Management

The current recommendations for the screening of women at risk for HBOC is based on the best available evidence and is expected to change as more specific features of *BRCA1*- and *BRCA2*-related disease become available. The current screening recommendations for women are listed in Table 5.2.

Risk-reduction mastectomies are an appropriate consideration for women at the highest hereditary risk for breast cancer. Studies have shown a 90% to 95% reduction in breast cancer risk following prophylactic mastectomy.[44–47] The evidence for the use of tamoxifen or raloxifene as a chemopreventive agent in *BRCA* carriers is limited; however, tamoxifen has been shown to reduce the risk of contralateral breast cancers in *BRCA* carriers.[48,49] Two recent studies support the role of risk-reducing salpingo-oophorectomy: The hazard ratio for ovarian cancer for women who underwent prophylactic surgery and that for those who chose close surveillance were 0.15 and 0.04, respectively.[50,51] Women should be informed about the potential for the subsequent development of peritoneal carcinomatosis, which has been reported up to 15 years after risk-reducing bilateral salpingo-oophorectomy.[25,52] Combination oral contraceptives containing estrogen and progestin result in a protective effect against ovarian cancer in some studies, but not in others.[53–55]

Male *BRCA* mutation carriers are advised to undergo training in breast self-examination with regular monthly practice and semiannual clinical breast examinations, and workup of any suspected breast lesions is recommended. The NCCN Guidelines also recommend that a baseline mammogram be considered, with an annual

TABLE 5.2	NCCN Guidelines for Management of *BRCA1/2* Carriers

Women

- Breast self-examination training and education starting at age 18 y
- Clinical breast examination, every 6–12 mo, starting at age 25 y
- Annual mammogram and breast magnetic resonance imaging screening starting at age 25 y, or individualized based on earliest age at onset in the family
- Discuss option of risk-reducing mastectomy on case-by-case basis and counsel regarding degree of protection, reconstruction options, and risks
- Recommend risk-reducing salpingo-oophorectomy, ideally between 35 and 40 y and upon completion of childbearing, or individualized based on earliest age at onset of ovarian cancer in the family; counseling includes a discussion of reproductive desires, extent of cancer risk, degree of protection for breast and ovarian cancer, management of menopausal symptoms, possible short-term hormone replacement therapy to a recommended maximum age at natural menopause, and related medical issues
- For those patients who have not elected risk-reducing salpingo-oophorectomy, consider concurrent transvaginal ultrasound (preferably days 1–10 of menstrual cycle in premenopausal women) and CA-125 (preferably after day 5 of menstrual cycle in premenopausal women), every 6 mo starting at age 35 y or 5–10 y before the earliest age at first diagnosis of ovarian cancer in the family
- Consider chemoprevention options for breast and ovarian cancer, including discussing risks and benefits
- Consider investigational imaging and screening studies, when available (e.g., novel imaging technologies and more frequent screening interval(s) in the context of a clinical trial

Men

- Breast self-examination training and education starting at the age of 35 y
- Clinical breast examination, every 6–12 mo, starting at the age of 35 y
- Consider baseline mammogram at the age of 40 y; annual mammogram if gynecomastia or parenchymal/glandular breast density on baseline study
- Adhere to screening guidelines for prostate cancer

mammogram if gynecomastia or parenchymal/glandular breast density is identified on baseline study.[56] The NCCN Guidelines recommend that male *BRCA* mutation carriers should adhere to the current prostate cancer screening guidelines.[56,57]

Psychosocial Considerations

The psychosocial needs of *BRCA*-positive women have been studied fairly widely. Studies have shown that although there is slight worsening of distress symptoms following cancer genetic counseling in *BRCA1/BRCA2* mutation carriers, these symptoms were minimal, did not affect everyday life activities, and had almost disappeared at 1-year follow-up.[58–62] Approximately, 20% of *BRCA1/2* mutation carrier women experience high distress after learning their test result.[63,64] Factors that are related to high posttest distress include a high level of pretest anxiety, higher pretest perceived risk, and whether they are opting for prophylactic surgery to reduce their risk.[59,63,65] It is important to note, however, that even in women who experienced distress after receipt of genetic test information, women do not "regret" their decision to be tested.[66] It has been suggested that health care providers consider including a brief pretest psychological assessment before initiating genetic testing for *BRCA1* and *BRCA2*[67] so that these women can be targeted for more comprehensive support once test results are available.[68]

The anxiety-associated symptoms reported by *BRCA1/2* carriers include sleeplessness and "bad mood."[60,69,70] One other psychosocial issue reported by single women with *BRCA1/2* mutations is that they experience increased urgency at finding a life partner capable of handling the emotional strain of the cancer world and open to pursuing multiple paths toward parenthood.[71]

Various studies have suggested that existing social support networks are inadequate for *BRCA1/2* mutation carriers and that formal services are unavailable or underutilized.[66,70,72] To address this lack of formal support services, a retreat for *BRCA1/2* carriers that includes educational updates about medical management, genetic privacy, and discrimination and addresses psychological and family issues may provide a valuable opportunity for *BRCA* carriers and their families to receive updated medical information, share personal experiences, provide and receive support, and change health behaviors.[73]

Distress in male *BRCA* carriers has not be studied quite as widely, but one study noted that high distress after disclosure of the result was reported by 1 of 4 male mutation carriers.[74]

TP53

Description

Germline mutations in the *TP53* gene give rise to a disease called Li–Fraumeni syndrome (LFS), which is a rare cancer predisposition syndrome thought to be responsible for ~1% of breast cancers.[75] LFS is often thought of as a hereditary predisposition to cancer in general, involving many tumor types and occurring at any point in an

TABLE 5.3	Tumors Reported to be Associated with LFS	
Wilms Tumor	**Bladder Cancer**	**Prostate Cancer**
Malignant phyllodes tumor	Hepatoblastoma	Pancreatic cancer
Lung cancer	Lymphomas	Neuroblastoma
Choroid plexus tumor	Nasopharyngeal cancer	Testicular cancer
Colorectal cancer	Ureteral tumors	Ovarian cancer
Stomach cancer	Laryngeal cancer	Melanoma
Gonadal germ cell tumors	Teratomas	

From: Gonzalez KD, et al. Beyond Li Fraumeni syndrome: Clinical characteristics of families with p53 germ-line mutations. *J Clin Oncol.* 2009;27:1250–1256; Nichols KE, et al. Germ-line p53 mutations predispose to a wide spectrum of early-onset cancers. *Cancer Epidemiol Biomarkers Prev.* 2001;10:83–87; Hwang SJ, et al. Germline p53 mutations in a cohort with childhood sarcoma: Sex differences in cancer risk. *Am J Hum Genet.* 2003;72:975–983; Kleihues P, et al. Tumors associated with p53 germline mutations: A synopsis of 91 families. *Am J Pathol.* 1997;150:1–13; Olivier M, et al. Li-Fraumeni and related syndromes: Correlation between tumor type, family structure, and TP53 genotype. *Cancer Res.* 2003;63:6643–6650; Birch JM, et al. Relative frequency and morphology of cancers in carriers of germline TP53 mutations. *Oncogene.* 2001;20:4621–4628; Strong LC, Williams WR, Tainsky MA. The Li-Fraumeni syndrome: From clinical epidemiology to molecular genetics. *Am J Epidemiol.* 1992;135:190–199.

individual's lifetime, including childhood. The majority of cases of LFS are due to mutations in the *p53* gene.[76–79] The component tumors of LFS include bone sarcomas (primarily osteosarcomas and chondrosarcomas), soft-tissue sarcomas, breast cancer, brain tumors, leukemia, and adrenocortical carcinomas.[80] The classic component tumors are thought to account for 63% to 77% of cancer diagnoses in individuals with LFS.[80–83] Breast cancer is the most common tumor in *p53* mutation carriers (24% to 31.2%), followed by soft-tissue sarcomas (11.6% to 17.8%), brain tumors (3.5% to 14%), osteosarcomas (12.6% to 13.4%), and adrenocortical tumors (6.5% to 9.9%).[84,85] Other tumors that have been argued to be component tumors of LFS are listed in Table 5.3.

There are some data regarding common histology of LFS component tumors. Breast cancers are most commonly invasive ductal carcinomas.[80] Rhabdomyosarcomas account for 55% of soft-tissue sarcomas, followed by fibrosarcomas (13%) and then malignant fibrous histiocytomas.[84] For LFS-associated brain tumors, 69% are astrocytic (astrocytoma or glioblastoma), followed by medulloblastoma/primitive neuroectodermal tumors (17%).[84]

Identifying LFS

Li et al.[80] first defined LFS in 1988 at which point clinical criteria were established, now known as classic LFS criteria (Table 5.4). In 1994, Birch et al.[77] went on to define less stringent criteria (Table 5.4) in an attempt to capture families with *p53* mutations

TABLE 5.4	Clinical Criteria for Classic Li–Fraumeni Syndrome

LFL Syndrome and Chompret Criteria

Classic LFS criteria
- Proband diagnosed with a sarcoma before 45 y of age and
- A first-degree relative[a] with cancer diagnosed before 45 y of age and
- A first- or second-degree relative[b] on the same side of the family with cancer diagnosed before 45 y of age or a sarcoma at any age

LFL syndrome criteria
- Proband with any childhood cancer or sarcoma, brain tumor, or adrenocortical carcinoma diagnosed before 45 y of age and
- First- or second-degree relative with a component LFS cancer (sarcoma, breast cancer, brain tumor, leukemia, or adrenocortical carcinoma) diagnosed at any age and
- One first- or second-degree relative on the same side of the family with any cancer diagnosed before age 60 y

Chompret criteria
- Proband diagnosed with a narrow spectrum cancer (sarcoma, brain tumor, breast cancer, or adrenocortical carcinoma) before the age of 36 y, and at least one first- or second-degree relative affected by a narrow-spectrum tumor (other than breast cancer if the proband was affected by breast cancer) before 46 y or a relative with multiple primary tumors at any age
- A proband with multiple primary tumors, two of which belong to the narrow spectrum and the first of which occurred before 36 y, regardless of family history
- A proband with adrenocortical carcinoma, regardless of age at diagnosis or family history

[a]First-degree relative is defined as parent, sibling, or child.
[b]Second-degree relative is defined as grandparent, aunt, uncle, niece, nephew, or grandchild.

who did not necessarily conform to the classic criteria. Families who met the broader criteria of Birch et al.[77] were referred to as "LFS-like (LFL)" families. Both classic and LFL criteria are based on family history and fail to recognize potential *p53* mutation carriers who have de novo germline *p53* mutations. Although the de novo rate is not well defined for *p53*, one study showed as high as a 24% rate.[88]

More recently in 2001, Chompret et al.[89] developed criteria for identifying patients likely to carry *p53* mutations (Table 5.4) and included criteria that address families who display a collection of component tumors but also address individuals whose personal histories are suggestive of *p53* mutation even in the absence of a suggestive family history. The Chompret criteria were designed to include individuals who may potentially carry de novo *p53* mutations.

Fifty to seventy percent of individuals who meet the classic definition of LFS will have a mutation in *p53*.[77,89–92] Individuals who meet the LFL criteria are less likely to be *p53* mutation carriers, estimated at 21% to 40%.[79,90] Twenty percent of individuals meeting the Chompret criteria will be identified as *p53* mutation carriers.[89]

Cancer Risks

Typically, LFS-associated tumors occur at significantly younger ages than when they occur sporadically. However, depending on tumor type, the mean age at diagnosis varies from childhood well into adulthood.[84] Understanding cancer risk for LFS is somewhat complicated as the ranges of risk vary greatly between studies and depend largely on study population. When pooling studies that examine overall cancer risk in *p53* mutation carriers (both female and male), the risk of developing cancer by ages 15 to 20 years is 12% to 42%, by ages 40 to 45 years is 52% to 66%, by age 50 years is 80%, and by age 85 years is 85%.[82,83,88,93] When separating out the sexes, it is apparent that female *p53* mutation carriers have generally a higher lifetime cancer risk in comparison to males.[83,88,94]

Individuals with a diagnosis of LFS are also at markedly increased risk of developing multiple primary tumors. Hisada et al.[95] found that, following a first cancer diagnosis, there is a 57% risk for a second primary tumor within 30 years of the first diagnosis, followed by a 38% risk for a third primary tumor within 10 years of the second cancer diagnosis. In addition, it has been widely observed that second, third, and so on primary cancers commonly occur in the radiation field of previously treated cancers.[76,80,88,95]

Psychosocial Issues

The psychosocial effects of being a member of an LFS family and/or being affected with LFS have not been widely studied.[96,97] The nature of the disease itself leads to unique psychosocial implications with individual members of LFS families often experiencing many cancer diagnoses (and deaths) in their immediate and extended family. These cancer diagnoses will be throughout the life span, with many parents having to deal with a child's diagnosis and many children needing to deal with a parent's diagnosis. It is likely that these repeated experiences of grief and stress pose a significant psychological burden for the members of LFS families.[98] Although no data exist, this psychosocial burden may also impact the individuals' relationships with their family members including, but not limited to, children and spouses.

Because of the rarity of the syndrome, many individuals with LFS may feel isolated. Other inherited syndromes, in general, and inherited cancer syndromes, in particular, have "support groups" that can help with the coping process when an individual is diagnosed with the disease. Unfortunately, no such group exists in the United States today. An online discussion group/support group for individuals with LFS is available (http://listserv.acor.org/SCRIPTS/WA-ACOR.EXE?OK=53111E8B&L=LI-FRAUMENI). Members of the listserv include patients with LFS, health care providers, and spouses and friends of individuals with LFS. The listserv serves as a place not only to share information about the disease but also to discuss fears, anxiety, grief, and other psychological manifestations of the disease.

(PTEN)
Description

CS is a rare hereditary cancer syndrome that is characterized by overgrowth in different organ systems. The incidence of CS is thought to be about 1 in 200,000, but it may be underdiagnosed.[99] CS belongs to the set of syndromes known as the PTEN (phosphatase and tensin homolog) hamartoma tumor syndromes.[100] *PTEN* mutations are found in the vast majority of patients with CS, although mutations in other genes such as *BMPR1A* and the succinate dehydrogenase genes have been reported in a small number of patients who have features of CS but do not meet diagnostic criteria (CS-like).[101,102]

Diagnostic Criteria/Testing Criteria

Traditionally, one of the hallmark features of CS is the development of multiple hamartomas of the skin and mucosa. A thorough physical examination, including head circumference measurement and examination for skin manifestations, is an important component of assessing for CS. However, a lack of hamartomas does not exclude CS; diagnostic criteria are complicated.[103] The NCCN's most recent guidelines (v.1.2011) for testing for CS are in Table 5.5; they will be updated shortly.

Identifying CS

In 2011, the Cleveland Clinic made available an online calculator for risk of a *PTEN* mutation in adults, as well as a set of pediatric criteria (http://www.lerner.ccf.org/gmi/ccscore/). Risk estimates were based on data from the largest prospective cohort of patients collected with a potential diagnosis of CS. Information on physical findings, specific cancer diagnoses, intestinal polyps, and other benign conditions is collected. If a patient has a risk of mutation greater than 3%, testing for *PTEN* is recommended.[104]

Cancer Risks

The highest risk of cancer associated with CS is for female breast cancer. Other cancers that are thought to be a part of the spectrum of cancers seen in CS include thyroid cancer, uterine cancer, and, more recently, renal cell cancer, melanoma, and colorectal cancer have also been reported. The magnitude of risk for the cancers associated with CS varies widely.[104,105] A recent article from Cleveland Clinic estimated the lifetime risks of cancer to be much higher than previously reported; however, it is likely that there is significant ascertainment bias present in this cohort.[104] A comparison of two publications reviewing the cancer risks associated with CS is presented in Table 5.6.

TABLE
5.5
NCCN Guidelines: Testing Criteria for CS

NCCN Guidelines for Testing (v.1.2011)—CS

Individual from a family with a known *PTEN* mutation

or

Individual with a personal history of
- Bannayan–Riley–Ruvalcaba (BRR) syndrome
- Adult Lhermitte-Duclos disease (dysplastic gangliocytoma of the cerebellum)
- Autism spectrum disorder and macrocephaly
- ≥2 biopsy proven trichilemmomas
- ≥2 major criteria (one must be macrocephaly)
- ≥3 major criteria, without macrocephaly
- One major and ≥3 minor criteria
- ≥4 minor criteria
- Fewer criteria are needed when an individual has a relative with a clinical diagnosis of CS or BRR (any one major criterion or two minor criteria)

Major criteria
- Breast cancer
- Mucocutaneous lesions
  - Biopsy-proven trichilemmoma
  - Multiple palmoplantar keratoses
  - Multifocal or extensive oral mucosal papillomatosis
  - Multiple cutaneous facial papules (often verrucous)
  - Macular pigmentation of glans penis
- Macrocephaly (≥97th percentile, 58 cm in adult women, 60 cm in adult male)
- Endometrial cancer
- Nonmedullary thyroid cancer
- Multiple gastrointestinal hamartomas or ganglioneuromas

Minor criteria
- Other thyroid lesions (e.g., adenoma, multinodular goiter)
- Mental retardation (intelligence quotient ≤ 75)
- Autism spectrum disorder
- Single gastrointestinal hamartoma or ganglioneuroma
- Fibrocystic disease of the breast
- Lipomas
- Fibromas
- Renal cell carcinoma
- Uterine fibroids

TABLE 5.6	**Cancer Risks Associated with CS**

Lifetime Cancer Risks Associated with CS

	Pilarski et al.[105] (2009)	Tan et al.[104] (2012) (%)
Breast cancer risk	25–50%	85
Thyroid cancer	3–10%	35
Endometrial cancer	5–10%	28
Renal cell cancer	Unknown	34
Melanoma	Unknown	6
Colorectal cancer	Unknown	9

Management

CS is a complex diagnosis to make and to receive. Because of the degree of variability in CS, it is difficult for clinicians to make a firm diagnosis except in the most obvious of cases. In situations where there is a high suspicion, a negative genetic test result may be uninformative for the patient and her family. Conversely, a positive result or variant of uncertain significance in an individual without classic features of Cowden can lead to uncertainty regarding how aggressive to be about screening and prevention measures. The NCCN Guidelines for management are in Table 5.7.

Psychosocial Issues

There is a dearth of literature addressing the psychological issues for individuals and families with a clinical and/or genetic diagnosis of CS, possibly due to its rarity. However, there are several factors associated with CS that could add to the psychological burden of having a hereditary syndrome. These include variability in clinical presentation, difficulty screening (especially for breast cancer), disfigurement due to mucocutaneous lesions and surgical procedures, the possibility of intellectual disabilities and/or autism in children, lack of knowledge about how often *PTEN* mutations are found de novo versus inherited in a family, a large number of uncertain variants found through genetic testing, and overall lack of knowledge about the syndrome.

Because of the association of CS with autism and macrocephaly, many children are now undergoing genetic testing for alterations in the *PTEN* gene; a small number of them will be found to have CS or a related disorder.[106] When the child is the index case in the family, testing him/her may provide information for adult family members about cancer risks. In addition, parents may find value in knowing that there is an underlying genetic cause to their child's issues and in finding a community with a shared diagnosis. There is also the hope that the development of targeted therapies may help ameliorate the disease in children and, going forward, in adults.

TABLE 5.7	**NCCN Guidelines for CS Management**

NCCN Guidelines for Management—CS (v.1.2011)

Women

- Breast self-examination training and education starting at the age of 18 y
- Clinical breast examination, every 6–12 mo, starting at the age of 25 y or 5–10 y before the earliest known breast cancer in the family
- Annual mammography and breast magnetic resonance imaging screening starting at the age of 30–35 y or 5–10 y before the earliest known breast cancer in the family (whichever comes first)
- For endometrial cancer screening, encourage patient education and prompt response to symptoms and participation in a clinical trial to determine the effectiveness and necessity of screening modalities
- Discuss option of risk-reducing mastectomy and hysterectomy on a case-by-case basis and counsel regarding degree of protection, extent of cancer risk, and reconstruction options

Men and women

- Annual comprehensive physical examination starting at the age of 18 y or 5 y before the youngest age at diagnosis of a component cancer in the family (whichever comes first), with particular attention to breast and thyroid examinations
- Baseline thyroid ultrasound at the age of 18 y, and consider annually thereafter
- Consider colonoscopy starting at the age of 35 y, then every 5–10 y or more frequently if patient is symptomatic or polyps found
- Consider annual dermatologic examination
- Education regarding the signs and symptoms of cancer

Risk to relatives

- Advise about possible inherited cancer risk to relatives and options for risk assessment and management
- Recommend genetic counseling and consideration of genetic testing for at-risk relatives

The benefit of testing an asymptomatic child whose parent has a known mutation in *PTEN* is still unknown. Although childhood cancers have been reported in CS, these cancers appear to be rare. Some experts argue that thyroid and other screening is warranted in children for the early detection and prevention of related cancers[107];

however, others would say that the psychological burden of screening outweighs any small medical benefit that may be derived from discovering benign lesions that are unlikely to become cancerous at a young age. Testing unaffected children for CS remains controversial.

STK11

Peutz–Jeghers syndrome (PJS) is a rare autosomal dominant gastrointestinal hamartomatous polyposis syndrome. It is estimated that the incidence is approximately 1 in 150,000 in North America and Western Europe.[108,109] Peutz–Jeghers is characterized by the development of Peutz–Jeghers polyps in the intestine in conjunction with pigmentation (brown or bluish spots) around and inside the mouth, nose and lips, and perianal area, as well as other parts of the body. These lesions are often most prominent in childhood and fade with age.

Most families with PJS have mutations in the *STK11* gene, although this gene does not explain all inherited cases of PJS as well as many simplex cases.[110] The lifetime risk

---

TABLE 5.8	Clinical Criteria for PJS and Hereditary Diffuse Gastric Cancer Syndrome

PJS Clinical Diagnostic Criteria

Any one of the following is present
- Two or more histologically confirmed Peutz–Jeghers polyps
- Any number of Peutz–Jeghers polyps detected in one individual who has a family history of PJS in close relative(s)
- Characteristic mucocutaneous pigmentation in an individual who has a family history of PJS in close relative(s)
- Any number of Peutz–Jeghers polyps in an individual who also has characteristic mucocutaneous pigmentation

Beggs et al.[110] (2010)

Hereditary Diffuse Gastric Cancer Clinical Criteria

Any of the following:
- Two gastric cancer cases in a family, one individual aged <50 y with confirmed diffuse gastric cancer (DGC)
- Three confirmed DGC cases in first- or second-degree relatives independent of age
- Simplex case (i.e., a single occurrence in a family) of DGC occurring before the age of 40 y
- Personal or family history of DGC and lobular breast cancer, one diagnosed before the age of 50 y

Fitzgerald et al.[113] (2010)

of breast cancer in females is reported in a wide range, with the most consistent risks being in the 30% to 50% range.[111,112] Other cancers that can be seen in PJS include cancers of the colon, pancreas, stomach, ovary, small intestine, lung, cervix, testes, uterus, and esophagus.[110] Consensus diagnostic criteria were published in 2010 and are listed in Table 5.8.[110] PJS is described in depth in "Genetic Testing by Disease Site: Gastrointestinal."

CDH1

Hereditary diffuse gastric cancer is a rare autosomal dominant hereditary syndrome characterized by diffuse (or signet ring cell pathology) stomach cancer. The incidence of this syndrome is not well known but likely to be rare. The lifetime risk of stomach cancer is thought to be approximately 80% compared with less than 1% in the general population.[114,115] The second most common cancer in families with this syndrome is lobular breast cancer, with a lifetime risk of about 40% in women.[116–120] Cleft lip and palate have also been reported in some families.[121] The International Gastric Cancer Linkage Consortium published clinical criteria in 2010, shown in Table 5.8.[113] The incidence of CDH1 mutations in lobular breast cancer cases is thought to be low in the absence of a family history of gastric cancer.[122] Please see "Genetic Testing by Disease Site: Gastrointestinal" for more detailed information.

MODERATE- AND LOW-PENETRANCE BREAST CANCER GENES

There are several genes that have already been described in families with breast cancer including CHEK2 and ATM. The risk of breast cancer associated with alterations in these genes is thought to be lower than with traditional hereditary breast cancer syndromes; other factors are likely to interact with the effects of changes in these genes and result in a more moderate increase in risk for breast cancer.

Recently, a US group published a study on 12 genes linked to hereditary ovarian cancer, which are also being analyzed in families with hereditary breast cancer.[123–125] More laboratories are beginning to offer genetic testing for panels of genes that are important in DNA repair pathways.[126] There are several categories of these genes.

(1) Category 1—genes functionally related to BRCA1 and BRCA2 (ATM, BARD1, CHEK2, MRE11A, NBN, RAD50, RAD51D)
   - ATM (ataxia telangiectasia mutated)
   - BARD1 (BRCA1-associated RING domain 1)
   - CHEK2 (cell cycle checkpoint kinase 2)
   - MRE11A (meiotic recombination 11 homolog A)
   - NBN (nibrin; aka NBS1)
   - RAD50
   - RAD51D

(2) Category 2—(other) genes in the Fanconi anemia pathway that increase breast cancer risk (*BRIP1, PALB2, RAD51C*)
   - *BRIP1* (*BRCA*-interacting protein C-terminal helicase 1; *FANCJ*)
   - *PALB2* (partner and localizer of *BRCA2*; *FANCN*)
   - *RAD51C* (*FANCO*)
(3) Category 3—genes involved in hereditary colorectal cancer (*MLH1, MSH2, MSH6, PMS2, EPCAM, MYH*)

For many of the genes in categories 1 and 2, risks of breast cancer are not well defined, and it is unclear if women who test negative for a mutation that was found in an affected relative ("true negatives") are really at general population risk.

Lynch Syndrome and *MYH*-associated Polyposis

Lynch syndrome (LS) is the most common hereditary form of colorectal cancer, accounting for about 2% to 3% of colorectal cancer cases. It is caused by mutations in genes involved in DNA mismatch repair, including *MLH1, MSH2, MSH6, PMS2*, and, indirectly, *EPCAM*. LS is typically characterized by the development of relatively early-onset colorectal and uterine cancer; risks for other cancers including stomach cancer, cancer of the small intestine, pancreatic cancer, sebaceous carcinomas, ovarian cancer, cancers of the urinary collecting tract, and rarely brain tumors are thought to be increased.[127] Most studies have not shown a significant increase in breast cancer risk for *MMR* mutation carriers versus noncarriers,[128] although a more recent article studying a cohort of LS families prospectively did show a fourfold increase in breast cancer risk.[129] It is clear that defective mismatch repair can be seen in some breast cancers in women from LS families.[130,131] Whether there is a true increase in risk (and the magnitude of this risk) remains to be seen. Please see "Genetic Testing by Disease Site: Gastrointestinal" for more detailed information.

MYH-associated polyposis (MAP) is the lesser known of the adenomatous polyposis syndromes (vs. familial adenomatous polyposis). *MYH* is involved in base excision repair; without *MYH*, oxidative DNA damage leads to the formation of 8-oxo-G, which mispairs with adenine. This leads to an increase in G:C >T:A transversions in *APC* and other genes.[132] MAP is associated with an attenuated phenotype; fewer adenomas (generally in the range of 10 to 100) and a mixture of polyp types (serrated adenomas, hyperplastic polyps) and duodenal polyps are often seen.[133,134] Extraintestinal manifestations, including breast cancer, have been reported in MAP.[135,136] However, *MYH* does not appear to be a common cause of breast cancer.[137] Please see "Genetic Testing by Disease Site: Gastrointestinal" for more detailed information.

SUMMARY

This chapter has provided a synopsis of the genes linked to the most well-defined syndromes associated with breast cancer and an introduction to breast cancer gene panels. It is important for clinicians to be able to identify the classic breast cancer syndromes, know the relevant genes, and understand the medical management and psychosocial issues associated with the syndromes. The advent of whole genome sequencing and the ability to analyze the estimated 22,000 genes in the human genome with cheap and efficient technology bring the hope that all of the genes involved in hereditary and familial breast cancer will be found. However, making this information clinically relevant will require much more research. Elucidating the interaction of mutations in these genes with modifying factors could help clarify risks in families and lead to targeted screening and prevention measures. It is clear that genetic testing will become more complicated over time and that the interpretation of test results will require continuing education and expertise in the field.

REFERENCES

1. Howlander N, Noone AM, Krapcho M, et al, eds. *SEER Cancer Statistics Review*, 1975–2008. Bethesda, MD: National Cancer Institute; 2011.
2. Bennett RL, et al. Standardized human pedigree nomenclature: Update and assessment of the recommendations of the National Society of Genetic Counselors. *J Genet Couns.* 2008;17:424–433.
3. Bennett RL, et al. Recommendations for standardized human pedigree nomenclature. Pedigree Standardization Task Force of the National Society of Genetic Counselors. *Am J Hum Genet.* 1995;56:745–752.
4. Love RR, Evans AM, Josten DM. The accuracy of patient reports of a family history of cancer. *J Chronic Dis.* 1985;38:289–293.
5. Theis B, et al. Accuracy of family cancer history in breast cancer patients. *Eur J Cancer Prev.* 1994;3:321–327.
6. Reid GT, et al. Family history questionnaires designed for clinical use: A systematic review. *Public Health Genomics.* 2009;12:73–83.
7. Jefferies S, Goldgar D, Eeles R. The accuracy of cancer diagnoses as reported in families with head and neck cancer: A case-control study. *Clin Oncol (R Coll Radiol).* 2008;20:309–314.
8. Murff HJ, Spigel DR, Syngal S. Does this patient have a family history of cancer? An evidence-based analysis of the accuracy of family cancer history. *JAMA.* 2004;292:1480–1489.
9. Chang ET, et al. Reliability of self-reported family history of cancer in a large case-control study of lymphoma. *J Natl Cancer Inst.* 2006;98:61–68.
10. Ziogas A, et al. Clinically relevant changes in family history of cancer over time. *JAMA.* 2011;306:172–178.
11. Walsh T, et al. Spectrum of mutations in BRCA1, BRCA2, CHEK2, and TP53 in families at high risk of breast cancer. *JAMA.* 2006;295:1379–1388.
12. Ford D, et al. Genetic heterogeneity and penetrance analysis of the BRCA1 and BRCA2 genes in breast cancer families. The Breast Cancer Linkage Consortium. *Am J Hum Genet.* 1998;62:676–689.
13. Frank TS, et al. Sequence analysis of BRCA1 and BRCA2: Correlation of mutations with family history and ovarian cancer risk. *J Clin Oncol.* 1998;16:2417–2425.
14. Miki Y, et al. A strong candidate for the breast and ovarian cancer susceptibility gene BRCA1. *Science.* 1994;266:66–71.
15. Wooster R, et al. Identification of the breast cancer susceptibility gene BRCA2. *Nature.* 1995;378:789–792.
16. Struewing JP, et al. The risk of cancer associated with specific mutations of BRCA1 and BRCA2 among Ashkenazi Jews. *N Engl J Med.* 1997;336:1401–1408.
17. Kauff ND, et al. Incidence of non-founder BRCA1 and BRCA2 mutations in high risk Ashkenazi breast and ovarian cancer families. *J Med Genet.* 2002;39:611–614.
18. Thorlacius S, et al. A single BRCA2 mutation in male and female breast cancer families from Iceland with varied cancer phenotypes. *Nat Genet.* 1996;13:117–119.
19. Unger MA, et al. Screening for genomic rearrangements in families with breast and ovarian cancer identifies BRCA1 mutations previously missed by conformation-sensitive gel electrophoresis or sequencing. *Am J Hum Genet.* 2000;67:841–850.

20. Chappuis PO, Nethercot V, Foulkes WD. Clinico-pathological characteristics of BRCA1- and BRCA2-related breast cancer. *Semin Surg Oncol.* 2000;18:287–295.
21. Phillips KA, Andrulis IL, Goodwin PJ. Breast carcinomas arising in carriers of mutations in BRCA1 or BRCA2: Are they prognostically different? *J Clin Oncol.* 1999;17:3653–3663.
22. Rakha EA, Reis-Filho JS, Ellis IO. Basal-like breast cancer: A critical review. *J Clin Oncol.* 2008;26:2568–2581.
23. Boyd J, et al. Clinicopathologic features of BRCA-linked and sporadic ovarian cancer. *JAMA.* 2000;283:2260–2265.
24. Lakhani SR, et al. Pathology of ovarian cancers in BRCA1 and BRCA2 carriers. *Clin Cancer Res.* 2004;10:2473–2481.
25. Levine DA, et al. Fallopian tube and primary peritoneal carcinomas associated with BRCA mutations. *J Clin Oncol.* 2003;21:4222–4227.
26. Cass I, et al. Improved survival in women with BRCA-associated ovarian carcinoma. *Cancer.* 2003;97:2187–2195.
27. Arun B, et al. Response to neoadjuvant systemic therapy for breast cancer in BRCA mutation carriers and noncarriers: A single-institution experience. *J Clin Oncol.* 2011;29:3739–3746.
28. Berry DA, et al. BRCAPRO validation, sensitivity of genetic testing of BRCA1/BRCA2, and prevalence of other breast cancer susceptibility genes. *J Clin Oncol.* 2002;20:2701–2712.
29. Tyrer J, Duffy SW, Cuzick J. A breast cancer prediction model incorporating familial and personal risk factors. *Stat Med.* 2004;23:1111–1130.
30. Couch FJ, et al. BRCA1 mutations in women attending clinics that evaluate the risk of breast cancer. *N Engl J Med.* 1997;336:1409–1415.
31. Shattuck-Eidens D, et al. BRCA1 sequence analysis in women at high risk for susceptibility mutations. Risk factor analysis and implications for genetic testing. *JAMA.* 1997;278:1242–1250.
32. Kang HH, et al. Evaluation of models to predict BRCA germline mutations. *Br J Cancer.* 2006;95:914–920.
33. Barcenas CH, et al. Assessing BRCA carrier probabilities in extended families. *J Clin Oncol.* 2006;24:354–360.
34. James PA, et al. Optimal selection of individuals for BRCA mutation testing: A comparison of available methods. *J Clin Oncol.* 2006;24:707–715.
35. Saslow D, et al. American Cancer Society Guideline for human papillomavirus (HPV) vaccine use to prevent cervical cancer and its precursors. *CA Cancer J Clin.* 2007;57:7–28.
36. King MC, Marks JH, Mandell JB. Breast and ovarian cancer risks due to inherited mutations in BRCA1 and BRCA2. *Science.* 2003;302:643–646.
37. Ozcelik H, et al. Germline BRCA2 6174delT mutations in Ashkenazi Jewish pancreatic cancer patients. *Nat Genet.* 1997;16:17–18.
38. Antoniou A, et al. Average risks of breast and ovarian cancer associated with BRCA1 or BRCA2 mutations detected in case series unselected for family history: A combined analysis of 22 studies. *Am J Hum Genet.* 2003;72:1117–1130.
39. Risch HA, et al. Prevalence and penetrance of germline BRCA1 and BRCA2 mutations in a population series of 649 women with ovarian cancer. *Am J Hum Genet.* 2001;68:700–710.
40. The Breast Cancer Linkage Consortium. Cancer risks in BRCA2 mutation carriers. *J Natl Cancer Inst.* 1999;91:1310–1316.
41. Thompson D, Easton DF. Cancer incidence in BRCA1 mutation carriers. *J Natl Cancer Inst.* 2002;94:1358–1365.
42. Thompson D, Easton D. Variation in cancer risks, by mutation position, in BRCA2 mutation carriers. *Am J Hum Genet.* 2001;68:410–419.
43. van Asperen CJ, et al. Cancer risks in BRCA2 families: Estimates for sites other than breast and ovary. *J Med Genet.* 2005;42:711–719.
44. Hartmann LC, et al. Efficacy of bilateral prophylactic mastectomy in BRCA1 and BRCA2 gene mutation carriers. *J Natl Cancer Inst.* 2001;93:1633–1637.
45. Rebbeck TR, et al. Bilateral prophylactic mastectomy reduces breast cancer risk in BRCA1 and BRCA2 mutation carriers: The PROSE Study Group. *J Clin Oncol.* 2004;22:1055–1062.
46. Meijers-Heijboer H, et al. Breast cancer after prophylactic bilateral mastectomy in women with a BRCA1 or BRCA2 mutation. *N Engl J Med.* 2001;345:159–164.

47. Robson M, et al. Appropriateness of breast-conserving treatment of breast carcinoma in women with germline mutations in BRCA1 or BRCA2: A clinic-based series. *Cancer.* 2005;103:44–51.

48. Narod SA, et al. Tamoxifen and risk of contralateral breast cancer in BRCA1 and BRCA2 mutation carriers: A case-control study. Hereditary Breast Cancer Clinical Study Group. *Lancet.* 2000;356:1876–1881.

49. Gronwald J, et al. Tamoxifen and contralateral breast cancer in BRCA1 and BRCA2 carriers: An update. *Int J Cancer.* 2006;118:2281–2284.

50. Kauff ND, et al. Risk-reducing salpingo-oophorectomy in women with a BRCA1 or BRCA2 mutation. *N Engl J Med.* 2002;346:1609–1615.

51. Rebbeck TR, et al. Prophylactic oophorectomy in carriers of BRCA1 or BRCA2 mutations. *N Engl J Med.* 2002;346:1616–1622.

52. Piver MS, et al. Primary peritoneal carcinoma after prophylactic oophorectomy in women with a family history of ovarian cancer. A report of the Gilda Radner Familial Ovarian Cancer Registry. *Cancer.* 1993;71:2751–2755.

53. Modan B, et al. Parity, oral contraceptives, and the risk of ovarian cancer among carriers and noncarriers of a BRCA1 or BRCA2 mutation. *N Engl J Med.* 2001;345:235–240.

54. Narod SA, et al. Oral contraceptives and the risk of hereditary ovarian cancer. Hereditary Ovarian Cancer Clinical Study Group. *N Engl J Med.* 1998;339:424–428.

55. Narod SA, et al. Oral contraceptives and the risk of breast cancer in BRCA1 and BRCA2 mutation carriers. *J Natl Cancer Inst.* 2002;94:1773–1779.

56. NCCN clinical practice guidelines in oncology. Genetic/familial high-risk assessment: Breast and ovarian cancer; V1.2011. 2011. Available at: http://www.nccn.org. Accessed April 23, 2012.

57. Liede A, Karlan BY, Narod SA. Cancer risks for male carriers of germline mutations in BRCA1 or BRCA2: A review of the literature. *J Clin Oncol.* 2004;22:735–742.

58. DiCastro M, et al. Genetic counseling in hereditary breast/ovarian cancer in Israel: Psychosocial impact and retention of genetic information. *Am J Med Genet.* 2002;111:147–151.

59. Lodder LN, et al. One year follow-up of women opting for presymptomatic testing for BRCA1 and BRCA2: Emotional impact of the test outcome and decisions on risk management (surveillance or prophylactic surgery). *Breast Cancer Res Treat.* 2002;73:97–112.

60. Crotser CB, Boehmke M. Survivorship considerations in adults with hereditary breast and ovarian cancer syndrome: State of the science. *J Cancer Surviv.* 2009;3:21–42.

61. Hamilton JG, Lobel M, Moyer A. Emotional distress following genetic testing for hereditary breast and ovarian cancer: A meta-analytic review. *Health Psychol.* 2009;28:510–518.

62. Reichelt JG, et al. Psychological and cancer-specific distress at 18 months post-testing in women with demonstrated BRCA1 mutations for hereditary breast/ovarian cancer. *Fam Cancer.* 2008;7:245–254.

63. Lodder L, et al. Psychological impact of receiving a BRCA1/BRCA2 test result. *Am J Med Genet.* 2001;98:15–24.

64. Power TE, et al. Distress and psychosocial needs of a heterogeneous high risk familial cancer population. *J Genet Couns.* 20:249–269.

65. O'Neill SC, et al. Distress among women receiving uninformative BRCA1/2 results: 12-month outcomes. *Psychooncology.* 2009;18:1088–1096.

66. Di Prospero LS, et al. Psychosocial issues following a positive result of genetic testing for BRCA1 and BRCA2 mutations: Findings from a focus group and a needs-assessment survey. *CMAJ.* 2001;164:1005–1009.

67. Ertmanski S, et al. Identification of patients at high risk of psychological distress after BRCA1 genetic testing. *Genet Test Mol Biomarkers.* 2009;13:325–330.

68. Roussi P, et al. Enhanced counselling for women undergoing BRCA1/2 testing: Impact on knowledge and psychological distress-results from a randomised clinical trial. *Psychol Health.* 2010;25:401–415.

69. Shochat T, Dagan E. Sleep disturbances in asymptomatic BRCA1/2 mutation carriers: Women at high risk for breast-ovarian cancer. *J Sleep Res.* 19:333–340.

70. Werner-Lin A. Formal and informal support needs of young women with BRCA mutations. *J Psychosoc Oncol.* 2008;26:111–133.

71. Werner-Lin A. Beating the biological clock: The compressed family life cycle of young women with BRCA gene alterations. *Soc Work Health Care.* 2008;47:416–437.

72. Metcalfe KA, et al. An evaluation of needs of female BRCA1 and BRCA2 carriers undergoing genetic counselling. *J Med Genet*. 2000;37:866–874.

73. McKinnon W, et al. Results of an intervention for individuals and families with BRCA mutations: A model for providing medical updates and psychosocial support following genetic testing. *J Genet Couns*. 2007;16:433–456.

74. Lodder L, et al. Men at risk of being a mutation carrier for hereditary breast/ovarian cancer: An exploration of attitudes and psychological functioning during genetic testing. *Eur J Hum Genet*. 2001;9:492–500.

75. Sidransky D, et al. Inherited p53 gene mutations in breast cancer. *Cancer Res*. 1992;52:2984–2986.

76. Malkin D, et al. Germ line p53 mutations in a familial syndrome of breast cancer, sarcomas, and other neoplasms. *Science*. 1990;250:1233–1238.

77. Birch JM, et al. Prevalence and diversity of constitutional mutations in the p53 gene among 21 Li-Fraumeni families. *Cancer Res*. 1994;54:1298–1304.

78. Srivastava S, et al. Germ-line transmission of a mutated p53 gene in a cancer-prone family with Li-Fraumeni syndrome. *Nature*. 1990;348:747–749.

79. Varley JM, et al. Germ-line mutations of TP53 in Li-Fraumeni families: An extended study of 39 families. *Cancer Res*. 1997;57:3245–3252.

80. Li FP, et al. A cancer family syndrome in twenty-four kindreds. *Cancer Res*. 1988;48:5358–5362.

81. Gonzalez KD, et al. Beyond Li Fraumeni syndrome: Clinical characteristics of families with p53 germ-line mutations. *J Clin Oncol*. 2009;27:1250–1256.

82. Nichols KE, et al. Germ-line p53 mutations predispose to a wide spectrum of early-onset cancers. *Cancer Epidemiol Biomarkers Prev*. 2001;10:83–87.

83. Hwang SJ, et al. Germline p53 mutations in a cohort with childhood sarcoma: Sex differences in cancer risk. *Am J Hum Genet*. 2003;72:975–983.

84. Kleihues P, et al. Tumors associated with p53 germline mutations: A synopsis of 91 families. *Am J Pathol*. 1997;150:1–13.

85. Olivier M, et al. Li-Fraumeni and related syndromes: Correlation between tumor type, family structure, and TP53 genotype. *Cancer Res*. 2003;63:6643–6650.

86. Birch JM, et al. Relative frequency and morphology of cancers in carriers of germline TP53 mutations. *Oncogene*. 2001;20:4621–4628.

87. Strong LC, Williams WR, Tainsky MA. The Li-Fraumeni syndrome: From clinical epidemiology to molecular genetics. *Am J Epidemiol*. 1992;135:190–199.

88. Chompret A, et al. P53 germline mutations in childhood cancers and cancer risk for carrier individuals. *Br J Cancer*. 2000;82:1932–1937.

89. Chompret A, et al. Sensitivity and predictive value of criteria for p53 germline mutation screening. *J Med Genet*. 2001;38:43–47.

90. Varley JM, Evans DG, Birch JM. Li-Fraumeni syndrome—a molecular and clinical review. *Br J Cancer*. 1997;76:1–14.

91. Frebourg T, et al. Germ-line p53 mutations in 15 families with Li- Fraumeni syndrome. *Am J Hum Genet*. 1995;56:608–615.

92. Brugieres L, et al. Screening for germ line p53 mutations in children with malignant tumors and a family history of cancer. *Cancer Res*. 1993;53:452–455.

93. Le Bihan C, et al. ARCAD: A method for estimating age-dependent disease risk associated with mutation carrier status from family data. *Genet Epidemiol*. 1995;12:13–25.

94. Wu CC, et al. Joint effects of germ-line p53 mutation and sex on cancer risk in Li-Fraumeni syndrome. *Cancer Res*. 2006;66:8287–8292.

95. Hisada M, et al. Multiple primary cancers in families with Li-Fraumeni syndrome. *J Natl Cancer Inst*. 1998;90:606–611.

96. Dorval M, et al. Anticipated versus actual emotional reactions to disclosure of results of genetic tests for cancer susceptibility: Findings from p53 and BRCA1 testing programs. *J Clin Oncol*. 2000;18:2135–2142.

97. Peterson SK, et al. Psychological functioning in persons considering genetic counseling and testing for Li-Fraumeni syndrome. *Psychooncology*. 2008;17:783–789.

98. Oppenheim D, et al. The psychological burden inflicted by multiple cancers in Li-Fraumeni families: Five case studies. *J Genet Couns*. 2001;10:169–183.

99. Nelen MR, et al. Novel PTEN mutations in patients with Cowden disease: Absence of clear genotype-phenotype correlations. *Eur J Hum Genet.* 1999;7:267–273.

100. PTEN hamartoma tumor syndrome (PHTS). 2011. Available at: http://www.ncbi.nlm.nih.gov/books/NBK1488/. Accessed April 23, 2012.

101. Zhou XP, et al. Germline mutations in BMPR1A/ALK3 cause a subset of cases of juvenile polyposis syndrome and of Cowden and Bannayan-Riley-Ruvalcaba syndromes. *Am J Hum Genet.* 2001;69:704–711.

102. Ni Y, et al. Germline mutations and variants in the succinate dehydrogenase genes in Cowden and Cowden-like syndromes. *Am J Hum Genet.* 2008;83:261–268.

103. Eng C. Will the real Cowden syndrome please stand up: Revised diagnostic criteria. *J Med Genet.* 2000;37:828–830.

104. Tan MH, et al. Lifetime cancer risks in individuals with germline PTEN mutations. *Clin Cancer Res.* 2012;18:400–407.

105. Pilarski R. Cowden syndrome: A critical review of the clinical literature. *J Genet Couns.* 2009;18:13–27.

106. Conti S, et al. Phosphatase and tensin homolog (PTEN) gene mutations and autism: Literature review and a case report of a patient with Cowden syndrome, autistic disorder, and epilepsy. *J Child Neurol.* 2012;27:392–397.

107. Smith JR, et al. Thyroid nodules and cancer in children with PTEN hamartoma tumor syndrome. *J Clin Endocrinol Metab.* 2011;96:34–37.

108. Zbuk KM, Eng C. Hamartomatous polyposis syndromes. *Nat Clin Pract Gastroenterol Hepatol.* 2007;4:492–502.

109. Kutscher AH, et al. Incidence of Peutz-Jeghers syndrome. *Am J Dig Dis.* 1960;5:576–577.

110. Beggs AD, et al. Peutz-Jeghers syndrome: A systematic review and recommendations for management. *Gut.* 2010;59:975–986.

111. Lim W, et al. Relative frequency and morphology of cancers in STK11 mutation carriers. *Gastroenterology.* 2004;126:1788–1794.

112. Hearle N, et al. Frequency and spectrum of cancers in the Peutz-Jeghers syndrome. *Clin Cancer Res.* 2006;12:3209–3215.

113. Fitzgerald RC, et al. Hereditary diffuse gastric cancer: Updated consensus guidelines for clinical management and directions for future research. *J Med Genet.* 2010;47:436–444.

114. Kluijt I, et al. Familial gastric cancer: Guidelines for diagnosis, treatment and periodic surveillance. *Fam Cancer.* 2012;11:363–369.

115. SEER cancer statistics review. *SEER Cancer Statistics Review, 1975–2008.* Howlader N, Krapcho M, Neyman N, et al, eds. November 2010. Posted to the SEER Web site. Bethesda, MD: National Cancer Institute; 2011.

116. Kaurah P, et al. Founder and recurrent CDH1 mutations in families with hereditary diffuse gastric cancer. *JAMA.* 2007;297:2360–2372.

117. Brooks-Wilson AR, et al. Germline E-cadherin mutations in hereditary diffuse gastric cancer: Assessment of 42 new families and review of genetic screening criteria. *J Med Genet.* 2004;41:508–517.

118. Pharoah PD, et al. Incidence of gastric cancer and breast cancer in CDH1 (E-cadherin) mutation carriers from hereditary diffuse gastric cancer families. *Gastroenterology.* 2001;121:1348–1353.

119. Keller G, et al. Diffuse type gastric and lobular breast carcinoma in a familial gastric cancer patient with an E-cadherin germline mutation. *Am J Pathol.* 1999;155:337–342.

120. Oliveira C, et al. Screening E-cadherin in gastric cancer families reveals germline mutations only in hereditary diffuse gastric cancer kindred. *Hum Mutat.* 2002;19:510–517.

121. Frebourg T, et al. Cleft lip/palate and CDH1/E-cadherin mutations in families with hereditary diffuse gastric cancer. *J Med Genet.* 2006;43:138–142.

122. Schrader KA, et al. Germline mutations in CDH1 are infrequent in women with early-onset or familial lobular breast cancers. *J Med Genet.* 2011;48:64–68.

123. Walsh T, et al. Mutations in 12 genes for inherited ovarian, fallopian tube, and peritoneal carcinoma identified by massively parallel sequencing. *Proc Natl Acad Sci U S A.* 2011;108:18032–18037.

124. Ripperger T, et al. Breast cancer susceptibility: Current knowledge and implications for genetic counselling. *Eur J Hum Genet.* 2009;17:722–731.

125. Lalloo F, Evans DG. Familial breast cancer. *Clin Genet*. 2012;82:105–114. doi: 10.1111/j.1399-0004.2012.01859.x.

126. Shuen AY, Foulkes WD. Inherited mutations in breast cancer genes—risk and response. *J Mammary Gland Biol Neoplasia*. 2011;16:3–15.

127. Weissman SM, et al. Genetic counseling considerations in the evaluation of families for Lynch syndrome—a review. *J Genet Couns*. 2011;20:5–19.

128. Watson P, et al. The risk of extra-colonic, extra-endometrial cancer in the Lynch syndrome. *Int J Cancer*. 2008;123:444–449.

129. Win AK, et al. Colorectal and other cancer risks for carriers and noncarriers from families with a DNA mismatch repair gene mutation: A prospective cohort study. *J Clin Oncol*. 2012;30:958–964.

130. Walsh MD, et al. Lynch syndrome-associated breast cancers: Clinicopathologic characteristics of a case series from the colon cancer family registry. *Clin Cancer Res*. 2010;16:2214–2224.

131. Buerki N, et al. Evidence for breast cancer as an integral part of Lynch syndrome. *Genes Chromosomes Cancer*. 2012;51:83–91.

132. Lefevre JH, et al. MYH biallelic mutation can inactivate the two genetic pathways of colorectal cancer by APC or MLH1 transversions. *Fam Cancer*. 2010;9:589–594.

133. Sieber OM, et al. Multiple colorectal adenomas, classic adenomatous polyposis, and germ-line mutations in MYH. *N Engl J Med*. 2003;348:791–799.

134. Boparai KS, et al. Hyperplastic polyps and sessile serrated adenomas as a phenotypic expression of MYH-associated polyposis. *Gastroenterology*. 2008;135:2014–2018.

135. Vogt S, et al. Expanded extracolonic tumor spectrum in MUTYH-associated polyposis. *Gastroenterology*. 2009;137:1976–1985. e1–e10.

136. Nielsen M, et al. Multiplicity in polyp count and extracolonic manifestations in 40 Dutch patients with MYH associated polyposis coli (MAP). *J Med Genet*. 2005;42:e54.

137. Beiner ME, et al. Mutations of the MYH gene do not substantially contribute to the risk of breast cancer. *Breast Cancer Res Treat*. 2009;114:575–578.

6 Genetic Testing by Cancer Site

Ovary

Scott M. Weissman, Shelly M. Weiss, and Anna C. Newlin

Ovarian cancer is responsible for ~3% of all cancers among women, and in 2012, there will be ~22,280 new cases and 15,500 deaths from this cancer; this is the highest death rate for any cancer of the female reproductive system.[1] Given this fact, it is of critical importance to identify women who face an elevated risk for ovarian cancer to allow for early detection or prevention. A number of risk factors (e.g., nulliparity, early menarche, late menopause) for ovarian cancer have been identified and reviewed by others.[2–4] By far, the most important risk factor is family history. Having one first-degree relative with ovarian cancer increases the lifetime risk from 1.4% (average risk) to 5% and at least 7% with two or more first-degree relatives.[5] However, in families with two or more cases of ovarian cancer, there may be a hereditary cause for the cancer, which in turn would result into higher lifetime ovarian cancer risks. Historically, it was believed that ~10% of ovarian cancers were due to an underlying hereditary syndrome, but more recent data indicate that just two syndromes (hereditary breast and ovarian cancer syndrome and Lynch syndrome) account for at least 20% of ovarian cancers, and overall, at least 25% of newly diagnosed cases are due to a hereditary mutation in a single gene[6–8]; this suggests that a much larger proportion of ovarian cancer cases is hereditary in nature than originally thought (Fig. 6.1). This chapter reviews ovarian cancer within the context of known hereditary cancer syndromes. In addition, we address some of the newer genes ovarian cancer has been linked to as clinical genetic testing for some of these genes are quickly becoming available to health care professionals.

HEREDITARY BREAST AND OVARIAN CANCER SYNDROME (THE *BRCA1* AND *BRCA2* GENES)

Hereditary breast and ovarian cancer syndrome due to mutations in the *BRCA1* and *BRCA2* (*BRCA1/2*) genes is the most common cause of hereditary ovarian cancer, including fallopian tube and primary peritoneal cancer. Anywhere from 0.125% to 0.20% of the general population carry mutations in *BRCA1/2* compared

93

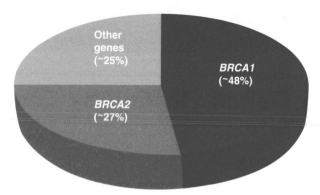

FIGURE 6.1. Genes responsible for hereditary ovarian cancer (including fallopian tube and primary peritoneal cancer). Other genes include *BARD1, BRIP1, CHEK2, MRE11, MSH6, NBN, PALB2, RAD50, RAD51C,* and *TP53*. Data derived from: Walsh T, Casadei S, Lee MK, et al. Mutations in 12 genes for inherited ovarian cancer, fallopian tube, and peritoneal carcinoma identified by massively parallel sequencing. *Proc Natl Acad Sci U S A.* 2011;108:18032–18037.

with 15% of women with a diagnosis of invasive ovarian cancer.[6,8–10] The contribution of the *BRCA1/2* genes to ovarian cancer is even greater in certain ethnicities that have higher *BRCA1/2* mutation prevalence rates (e.g., Polish, Ashkenazi Jewish [AJ], French Canadian). For example, the prevalence of *BRCA1/2* mutations in individuals of AJ ancestry and women of AJ ancestry with ovarian cancer is ~2.3% and ~30% to 40%, respectively.[11–13] Because of the strong connection between ovarian cancer and *BRCA1/2*, multiple professional societies and organizations recommend genetic counseling and testing for any woman with ovarian cancer regardless of age at onset or family history (Table 6.1). The current sensitivity of *BRCA1/2* genetic testing at the commercial laboratory is ~90% for identifying mutations in either gene.

The lifetime risk of developing ovarian cancer differs between the two genes. A number of studies over the years have quantified the lifetime risk[20–26]; however, two large meta-analyses suggest an ~40% and 20% lifetime risk for *BRCA1* and *BRCA2* mutation carriers, respectively.[27,28] In 1997, Gayther et al.,[29] in an effort to determine whether there were any genotype–phenotype correlations associated with *BRCA2* mutations, identified a region in exon 11 of *BRCA2* between nucleotides 3,035 and 6,629 that appeared to confer a further increased risk of ovarian cancer; they coined this region the "ovarian cancer cluster region" (OCCR). A follow-up study of the OCCR in families from the Breast Cancer Linkage Consortium (which included the families from the study by Gayther et al.[29]) further refined the OCCR to nucleotides 3,059 to 4,075 and 6,503 to 6,629, but found that the phenotype of increased ovarian cancer may actually be due to a reduced breast cancer risk.[30] Regardless, the potential difference in ovarian cancer risk was not significant enough to affect management recommendations. In addition to genotype–phenotype associations, researchers have studied other genetic modifiers (e.g., single-nucleotide

TABLE 6.1	Societies or Organizations with Position Statements Recommending *BRCA1/2* Genetic Counseling and/or Testing Related to Ovarian Cancer

Society/Organization	Year	Recommendation
American College of Medical Genetics[14]	2005	≥1 cases of OC and at least one relative on the same side of the family with BC (at any age)
American College of Obstetrics and Gynecology[15]	2009	Genetic risk assessment is recommended for patients with ≥20–25% chance of having a predisposition to OC (FT and PPC included), which include women with a personal history of OC; women with OC and an FDR or SDR with OC, premenopausal BC or both; women with BC ≤50 y and an FDR or SDR with OC Genetic risk assessment is helpful for patients with a 5–10% chance of having a predisposition to OC, which include women at any age with OC, PPC, or FT of high grade, serous histology
American Society of Breast Surgeons[16]	2006	A personal or family history of ovarian cancer (particularly nonmucinous types) should have access to *BRCA* testing
NCCN[17]	2012	Genetic risk assessment should be offered to any woman with BC who has an FDR, SDR, or TDR with epithelial OC, FT, or PPC at any age; any woman with OC, FT, or PPC; any unaffected individual with a family history of >1 OC from the same side of the family *BRCA1/2* genetic testing should be offered to any woman with BC <50 y with >1 FDR, SDR, or TDR with epithelial OC, FT, or PPC at any age; any woman with BC regardless of age when there are >2 FDR, SDR, or TDR with epithelial OC, FT, or PPC at any age; any woman with epithelial OC, FT, or PPC; any individual with PC at any age with >2 FDR, SDR, or TDR with BC and/or OC and/or PC at any age; an unaffected individual who has an FDR or SDR who meet any of the above criteria or a TDR with BC and/or OC/FT/PPC with >2 FDR, SDR, or TDR with BC (one <50 y) and/or OC

(Continued)

Society/Organization	Year	Recommendation
Society of Gynecologic Oncologists[18]	2007	Genetic risk assessment is recommended for patients with ≥20–25% chance of having a predisposition to OC (FT and PPC included), which include women with a personal history of OC and BC; women with OC and an FDR, SDR, or TDR with OC or BC ≤50 y; women with OC at any age who are AJ; women with BC ≤50 y and an FDR, SDR, or TDR with OC
		Genetic risk assessment is helpful for patients with a 5–10% chance of having a predisposition to OC, which include women with OC or BC at any age and ≥2 FDR, SDR, or TDR with BC at any age (particularly if at least one BC is ≤50 y); unaffected women with an FDR or SDR who meet the above criteria
US Preventative Services Task Force[19]	2005	Unaffected women whose family history is suggestive of a *BRCA1/2* mutation should be referred for genetic counseling and evaluation for *BRCA1/2* testing; this includes:
		Non-AJ women—a combination of both BC and OC among FDR and SDR; a combination of ≥2 FDR or SDR with OC regardless of age at onset; an FDR or SDR with both BC and OC at any age
		AJ women—any FDR (or two SDRs on the same side of the family) with OC

OC, ovarian cancer; BC, breast cancer; FT, fallopian tube cancer; PPC, primary peritoneal cancer; PC, pancreatic cancer; FDR, first-degree relative (parent, child, sibling); SDR, second-degree relative (aunt/uncle, grandparent, grandchild, niece/nephew, half-sibling); TDR, third-degree relative (first cousin, great aunt/uncle, great grandparent, great grandchild).

polymorphisms) that can influence ovarian cancer risk in *BRCA1/2* mutation carriers, but these data need maturation before testing for genetic modifiers can be used clinically.[31–34]

The average age at onset of ovarian cancer is between 49 and 53 years for *BRCA1* and 55 and 58 years for *BRCA2* compared with 63 years in the general population.[6,8,35–37] Unlike breast cancer, women with a diagnosis of very early-onset ovarian cancer (<40 years) are significantly less likely to harbor *BRCA1/2* mutations.[8,26,35,38,39] This is in part due to the fact that early-onset ovarian cancers are more likely to be associated with borderline tumors, earlier stages, and more favorable histologic characteristics, none of which are typical of *BRCA1/2*-related ovarian cancer.[40]

BRCA1/2-associated ovarian cancers are almost uniformly epithelial in origin and, for the most part, are invasive and nonmucinous; there are case reports of germ cell and stromal tumors in *BRCA1/2* mutation carriers. Mucinous and borderline tumors individually account for ~2% of ovarian tumors identified in *BRCA1/2* mutation carriers; this percentage is the same for both prospective and retrospective analyses, which are nicely summarized by Evans et al.[41] Compared with sporadic ovarian cancers, *BRCA1/2* ovarian cancers are more often of serous histology, higher grade, and solid type, and have intact p53 staining on immunohistochemistry (IHC).[39,41–44] It is important to note that other histologic findings are seen in mutation carriers (e.g., endometrioid, clear cell, papillary), and one study found more giant cell-type cancers in *BRCA1* mutation carriers compared with controls.[42] Several smaller studies have found that *BRCA1/2*-related ovarian cancers have a better prognosis compared with ovarian cancers in nonmutation carriers.[39,45–48] This finding seems to have been confirmed as a recent large pooled analysis of 26 observational studies comparing 3,879 *BRCA1/2* ovarian cancers and 2,666 noncarriers found the 5-year survival for *BRCA2* carriers was 52%, 44% for *BRCA1* carriers, and 36% for noncarriers.[44] The survival difference remained after adjusting for age at diagnosis, stage, histology, and grade.

One potential reason for the differences in survival may be that *BRCA1/2*-related ovarian cancers respond better to platinum-based agents.[45,48] *BRCA1/2* repair DNA damage through homologous recombination and platinum agents are particularly active in cells deficient in homologous recombination.[48,49] It is through this pathway that another class of drugs called poly(ADP-ribose) polymerase (PARP) inhibitors has been developed to help treat *BRCA1/2*-related cancers. Unlike platinum agents targeting homologous recombination, PARP inhibitors block repair of single-strand DNA breaks through base excision repair, which in turn can lead to double-strand breaks that cannot be repaired by *BRCA1/2*-deficient tumor cells at the same time sparing normal cells.[50–52] A number of phase I and phase II trials have been reported, and clinical trials continue to study PARP inhibitors in both ovarian and breast cancers.[53–56]

Identifying women who have a *BRCA1/2* mutation would ideally lead to women either being diagnosed with ovarian cancer at earlier stages or preventing ovarian cancer altogether. When counseling women who have tested positive for a *BRCA1/2* mutation, it is these central tenets, ovarian cancer screening versus prevention, that guide discussions. Current National Comprehensive Cancer Network (NCCN) guidelines for managing ovarian cancer risk include the recommendation for risk-reducing bilateral salpingo-oophorectomy (RRSO) between the ages of 35 and 40 years when childbearing is complete; for women not choosing RRSO, transvaginal ultrasound, and CA-125 are recommended every 6 months starting at age 30 years or 5 to 10 years before the earliest age at onset of ovarian cancer in the family.[17] Surgical prevention is recommended over screening for two main reasons. First, many women can receive a dual risk reduction with one surgery. RRSO has been shown to reduce ovarian cancer risk by 80% to 95%,[57–60] and breast cancer risk by 50% (for premenopausal women) in *BRCA1/2* mutation carriers.[59–62] Anywhere from 2.5% to 17%[63–65] of women who undergo RRSO are found to have an occult ovarian, fallopian tube, or primary peritoneal cancer upon pathology review, emphasizing the need for a "high-risk" pathologic examination of the tissues.[66] However, after surgery, women may still face an ~4% risk of developing primary peritoneal cancer over the course of 20 years.[57] The second major reason surgery is recommended over screening is that ovarian cancer screening is ineffective at detecting ovarian cancer at early stages[67]; the pros and cons of ovarian cancer screening with transvaginal ultrasound and CA-125 have been reviewed elsewhere.[4] A second option for reducing ovarian cancer risk is through oral contraceptive (OCP) use. OCP use can reduce ovarian cancer risk by ~50% with 5 years of use; the benefit has been shown for both *BRCA1* and *BRCA2* carriers.[68,69] However, it is worth noting that data are conflicting about whether OCP use can increase breast cancer risk, so it is important to take into account a woman's age, family history, and genetic test results before making recommendations to use OCPs.[70–73] Recently, researchers at Stanford created an online decision tool to aid female *BRCA1/2* mutation carriers in conjunction with a health care provider making decisions with respect to cancer screening and surgical prevention[74]; the tool is available at http://brcatool.stanford.edu.

Lynch Syndrome

Approximately 2% to 4% of ovarian cancer is believed to be associated with Lynch syndrome, also referred to as hereditary nonpolyposis colorectal cancer syndrome.[7,75] Lynch syndrome is an autosomal dominant cancer predisposition syndrome characterized by a significantly increased lifetime risk of colorectal cancer (~30% to 70%) and extracolonic malignancies of the endometrium (28% to 60%), stomach (6% to 9%), small bowel (3% to 4%), urinary tract (3% to 8%), central nervous system (4%), hepatobiliary tract (1%), and sebaceous skin lesions (1% to 9%).[76]

Lynch syndrome is caused by germline mismatch repair (MMR) gene mutations in *MLH1*, *MSH2*, *MSH6*, and *PMS2*. Alterations in these four genes account for approximately 36%, 38%, 14%, and 15% of Lynch syndrome, respectively.[77] In addition, germline deletions in *EPCAM* inactivate *MSH2* through epigenetic silencing in a small proportion of individuals with Lynch syndrome.[78] Variations in cancer risk have been noted among the four *MMR* genes. An increased risk for endometrial cancer and slightly decreased risk for colorectal cancer are observed in families with germline *MSH6* mutations compared with families with *MLH1* and *MSH2* mutations.[79] Germline mutations in *PMS2* are associated with the lowest overall risk for Lynch syndrome–associated malignancies.[80]

Lynch syndrome is diagnosed clinically within families meeting either the Amsterdam I or Amsterdam II criteria[81,82] (Table 6.2). Although fulfillment of the Amsterdam criteria is a significant predictor of identifying a germline MMR gene mutation in a family, it is well known that at least 25% of families affected with Lynch syndrome do not meet the Amsterdam criteria.[83]

The lifetime risk of ovarian cancer in Lynch syndrome is estimated to be anywhere between 4% and 11%,[78,84,85] with a mean age of diagnosis at 42.7 years.[75] In this series, approximately one-third of the individuals were younger than 40 years at the time of diagnosis ($n = 80$). Approximately 94% of ovarian tumors in Lynch syndrome are invasive epithelial in origin, with borderline and granulosa cell tumors representing

TABLE 6.2	**Amsterdam Criteria for Clinical Diagnosis of Lynch Syndrome**

Amsterdam I Criteria[81]

- Three affected family members with histologically verified colorectal cancer, one of whom is a first-degree relative of the other two
- Colorectal cancer in at least two successive generations
- At least one of the affected relatives with colorectal cancer is diagnosed at <50 y
- Familial adenomatous polyposis (FAP) has been excluded

Amsterdam II Criteria[82]

- Three affected family members with a Lynch syndrome–associated cancer (colon, endometrial, small bowel, ureter, or renal pelvis), one of whom is a first-degree relative of the other two
- Cancer diagnoses in at least two successive generations
- At least one of the affected relatives with a Lynch syndrome–associated cancer is diagnosed at <50 y
- FAP has been excluded

~4% of cases. Lynch-related ovarian tumors are most frequently, moderately or well differentiated. Of note, synchronous endometrial cancer was identified in 21.5% of cases. In a meta-analysis of 159 cases of MMR-related ovarian cancers, histologic subtypes included serous (32%), endometrioid (29%), mixed (24%), mucinous (19%), and clear cell (18%).[87] In a study of individuals with Lynch-related ovarian cancer compared with individuals with sporadic ovarian cancer, no significant difference was observed in survival rate, although the total number of Lynch-related ovarian cancers was small ($n = 26$).[87]

Lynch syndrome is one of a few hereditary cancer syndromes that have more than one method available to make a genetic diagnosis by identifying MMR deficiency including (1) tumor studies, specifically microsatellite instability (MSI) and IHC, and (2) germline genetic testing (typically includes DNA sequencing and a technology to look for large structural rearrangements). In initiating a genetic evaluation for Lynch syndrome, tumor studies are generally the recommended first-line tests.[78] However, because the majority of available data on performing MSI and IHC pertain to colorectal and endometrial tumors,[76–78] it is not certain whether tumor studies on ovarian cancers as a first-line approach are valid. Approximately 12% of unselected ovarian cancers will have an MSI-high phenotype.[75] In an analysis of 52 ovarian carcinomas in a population who received a diagnosis at younger than 50 years, defects in MMR expression were identified in 10% of cases using MSI and IHC.[88] Domanska et al.[89] evaluated ovarian carcinomas in a population who received a diagnosis at younger than 40 years and found MMR deficiency with IHC in ~6% of cases. If tumor studies are indicative of Lynch syndrome (results show the tumor to be MSI-high and/or loss of ≥1 MMR proteins), germline genetic testing should be offered and will identify a deleterious mutation anywhere from 20% to 70% of the time.[78] Molecular analysis is widely available for the four MMR genes and *EPCAM*. However, if tumor studies are performed on an ovarian cancer, and the results are not indicative of Lynch syndrome, given the paucity of data, Lynch syndrome cannot conclusively be ruled out, and germline genetic testing may still be warranted, depending on the patient's age at onset and family history.

If a tumor specimen is not available, germline genetic testing may be initiated at the outset. A recent abstract showed that up to 4% of unselected ovarian cancers may be found to have a germline mutation in *MLH1*, *MSH2*, or *MSH6*.[7] If a patient with ovarian cancer needs a genetic evaluation for Lynch syndrome, the ideal approach would be for the health care provider to have a detailed discussion about the pros and cons of each testing methodology with the patient, so that the patient and provider can jointly come to a decision about the best approach given the rest of the family history of cancer.

Current ovarian cancer management guidelines for women with Lynch syndrome include prophylactic hysterectomy and bilateral salpingo-oophorectomy after completion of childbearing; there is not enough data to support routine ovarian cancer screening with transvaginal ultrasound and CA-125 blood tests for women, although it may be considered at the "clinician's discretion."[90]

Peutz–Jeghers Syndrome

Peutz–Jeghers syndrome (PJS) is a rare autosomal dominant inherited disorder characterized by gastrointestinal hamartomatous polyposis, mucocutaneous melanin pigmentation, and benign and malignant tumors of the gastrointestinal tract, breast, ovary, cervix, and testis. The incidence of PJS is unknown but has been estimated between 1:8,300 and 1:200,000 births.[91,92]

In contrast to the other hamartomatous syndromes in which polyps occur most commonly in the colon, PJS-related polyps occur most commonly in the small intestine (90%), although they can also occur elsewhere in the gastrointestinal tract including the stomach (25%) and large bowel (33%), and may also develop outside the digestive tract in the uterus, bladder, lungs, and nasal passages.[93] Gastrointestinal polyps can result in chronic bleeding and anemia, and cause recurrent obstruction and intussusception requiring repeated laparotomy and bowel resection. Polyposis usually becomes symptomatic in early adolescence, although intestinal obstruction has been reported in infancy.[94] Polyps may be of mixed histologic types (hyperplastic, adenomatous) but are mostly hamartomatous and may number from one to dozens.

The characteristic mucocutaneous hyperpigmentation presents in childhood as dark blue to dark brown macules around the mouth, eyes, and nostrils; in the perianal area; and on the buccal mucosa. Hyperpigmented macules on the fingers are common and can also occur on the feet and in the axillae. The macules may fade in puberty and adulthood; however, pigmented areas inside the mouth or on the gums tend to persist into adulthood.[95]

In a single individual, a clinical diagnosis of PJS may be made when any one of the following is present[96]:

- Two or more histologically confirmed PJ polyps
- Any number of PJ polyps detected in one individual who has a family history of PJS in close relative(s)
- Characteristic mucocutaneous pigmentation in an individual who has a family history of PJS in close relative(s)
- Any number of PJ polyps in an individual who also has characteristic mucocutaneous pigmentation.

Individuals with PJS are at increased risk for a wide variety of epithelial malignancies (colorectal, gastric, pancreatic, breast, and ovarian cancers). The estimated incidence of cancer among PJS patients was identified as 18-fold higher than that in the general population by Giardello et al.,[97] although a recent meta-analysis by van Lier et al.[98] placed the lower end of the range at close to 10-fold.

Females with PJS are at risk for sex cord tumors with annular tubules (SCTATs), a distinctive benign ovarian neoplasm, the predominant component of which has morphologic features intermediate between those of the granulosa cell tumor and those of the Sertoli cell tumor; focal differentiation into either tumor may occur. Up to 36% of women who have SCTATs are found to have PJS.[99] SCTATs may cause sexual precocity and infertility and are generally considered benign, but may become malignant. Of the 74 cases that formed the basis of the investigation of Young et al.,[99] 27 were associated with PJS; these tumors were all benign and were typically multifocal, bilateral, very small or even microscopic in size, and calcified. Although SCTATs predominate as the ovarian tumors identified in PJS, other histologic findings have been identified including granulosa cell tumors, cystadenomas, nonneoplastic cysts, Brenner tumors, dysgerminomas, and Sertoli cell tumors.[100] Patients have ranged in age from 4.5 to 60 years at the time their ovarian tumors were diagnosed; more than half were 22 years or younger.

In 1998, investigators discovered that mutations in the serine threonine kinase 11 gene (*STK11*, also known as *LKB1* gene) cause PJS.[101,102] Genetic testing for clinical practice is now widely available; mutations in the *STK11* gene are detected in 50% to 90% of individuals with PJS.[103–106] The variability in detection rates is likely due to differences in selection criteria and testing methodologies. The majority of mutations are truncating or missense mutations, which eliminate the kinase function of the protein. However, up to 30% of mutations may be large deletions, which would not be detected by sequencing alone.[107] Therefore, the optimal approach for genetic testing would include both full sequencing and analysis for large deletions and duplications. Although the addition of large deletion analysis to *STK11* testing has greatly increased the mutation detection rate, there is still a very small portion of individuals and families meeting the clinical diagnostic criteria in which a deleterious mutation cannot be identified.[108,109] There are reports of families with a clinical diagnosis of PJS who do not link to 19p13.3, suggesting that there might be another genetic locus causing PJS in rare families.[110]

TABLE 6.3	**Adapted NCCN Guidelines for Peutz–Jeghers Cancer Screening**	

Site	Screening Procedure and Interval	Initiation Age
Breast	Mammogram and breast magnetic resonance imaging (MRI) annually	~25 y old
	Clinical breast examination every 6 mos	
Colon	Colonoscopy every 2–3 y	~Late teens
Stomach	Upper endoscopy every 2–3 y	~Late teens
Pancreas	Magnetic resonance cholangiopancreatography and/or endoscopic ultrasound every 1–2 y	~25–30 y old
	CA-19-9 at similar intervals	
Small intestine	Small-bowel visualization (CT enterography, small-bowel enteroclysis, capsule endoscopy) baseline at 8–10 y with follow-up interval based on findings but at least by age 18 y, then every 2–3 y, although this may be individualized, or with symptoms	~8–10 y old
Ovary	Pelvic examination and Papanicolaou smear annually	~18–20 y old
Cervix	Consider transvaginal ultrasound	
Uterus		
Testes	Annual testicular examination and observation for feminizing changes	~10 y old
Lung	Provide education about symptoms and smoking cessation	
	No other specific recommendations have been made	

From: NCCN clinical practice guidelines in oncology (NCCN Guidelines). Colorectal cancer screening. V2.2012. Available at: http://www.nccn.org/professionals/physician_gls/pdf/colorectal_screening.pdf. Accessed on April 30, 2012.

Current management guidelines for individuals with PJS are reflected in the current NCCN guidelines (Table 6.3)[90] and with respect to ovarian cancer screening include consideration of an annual transvaginal ultrasound starting between the ages of 18 and 20 years. These recommendations reflect expert opinion as no controlled trials have been published on the effectiveness of surveillance in PJS.[96] With respect to uncontrolled data, German investigators recently reported a surveillance strategy that led to the early detection of 50% of all cancers (5/10) diagnosed in 31 PJS patients.[104] Malignancies that occur in PJS, including SCTATs, should be treated in a standard manner, and conservative management of gonadal tumors in females is deemed appropriate.

Newer Genes

RAD51C

RAD51C, a RAD51 paralog, is an integral part of the DNA double-strand break repair through homologous recombination. Biallelic RAD51C mutations have recently been identified in Fanconi anemia patients, and subsequently, monoallelic mutations have been identified in up to 2.9% of highly penetrant breast and ovarian cancer families who previously screened negative for BRCA1/2 mutations.[111–114] RAD51C families show major similarities in ovarian cancer occurrence with families carrying BRCA1/2 mutations. Moreover, as these families show apparently complete segregation of the mutation with the cancer phenotype, the penetrance of RAD51C mutations is predicted to be at least comparable to that of BRCA1/2 mutations.

In comparison to the younger age at onset of BRCA1/2-associated ovarian cancers, the reported mean age at onset for ovarian cancer in women with RAD51C mutations ranges from 57.7 to 60 years (range, 50 to 81 years).[112,115,116] RAD51C-associated ovarian tumors are almost uniformly epithelial in origin and, for the most part, are invasive and nonmucinous.[112,115,116] Other reported histologic findings include invasive endometrioid adenocarcinoma, malignant cystadenoma, and fallopian tube carcinoma.[116]

Two recurrent founder mutations in the RAD51C gene have been identified in Finnish breast and/or ovarian cancer families, suggesting that founder mutations in this gene may exist in other ethnic groups.[116]

RAD51D

Identification of RAD51C mutations in families with breast and ovarian cancer prompted investigations into the role of another RAD51 paralog, RAD51D, in cancer susceptibility. Monoallelic mutations have been identified in up to 0.9% of highly penetrant breast and ovarian cancer families who previously screened negative for BRCA1/2 mutations; it is estimated that ~0.6% of unselected individuals with ovarian cancer will harbor RAD51D mutations.[117] Loveday et al.[117] found that mutations were more prevalent in families with more than one ovarian cancer: Four mutations were identified in 235 families (1.7%) with two or more ovarian cancer cases. Remarkably, three mutations were found in 59 families (5.1%) with three or more ovarian cancer cases.

RAD51D-associated ovarian tumors are almost uniformly epithelial in origin, with one report of a clear-cell ovarian carcinoma.[118] The relative risk of ovarian cancer for RAD51D mutation carriers is estimated to be 6.3, which equates to ~10% cumulative risk by age 80 years.[117]

The current studies, although few in number, clearly show that RAD51D is an ovarian cancer predisposition gene, but further studies in familial and sporadic ovarian cancer series would be of value to further clarify the risks of ovarian cancer. Cells deficient in RAD51D are sensitive to treatment with a PARP inhibitor, suggesting a possible therapeutic approach for cancers arising in RAD51D mutation carriers.[117]

Given the recent identification of their contribution to ovarian cancer susceptibility, *RAD51C*, as well as *RAD51D*, has to be validated in larger mutation positive cohorts to generate reliable estimations of the clinical implications of carrying germline mutations as well as determine appropriate screening and cancer prevention strategies.

CONCLUSIONS

The puzzle of identifying genes causative of hereditary ovarian cancer continues to be deciphered. Historically, *BRCA1* and *BRCA2* have been the only genes considered when evaluating families suggestive of a hereditary ovarian cancer syndrome, but new studies have linked ovarian cancer to other known hereditary syndromes such as Lynch syndrome as well as new genes such as *RAD51C/D*. As genetic testing advances and newer technologies such as next-generation sequencing and whole-exome sequencing are used, additional genes will continue to be discovered. With these discoveries, new insights into ovarian cancer pathogenesis will be understood and hopefully lead to better and more effective treatments such as PARP inhibitors, but more importantly, more women can be identified as being at risk before developing ovarian cancer, leading to increased ovarian cancer prevention.

REFERENCES

1. American Cancer Society. Cancer Facts & Figures 2012. Available at: www.cancer.org/acs/groups/content/@epidemiologysurveilance/documents/document/acspc-031941.pdf. Accessed on April 7, 2012.
2. Nelson HD, Westhoff C, Piepert J, et al. Screening for ovarian cancer: Brief evidence update. Available at: http://www.uspreventiveservicestaskforce.org/uspstf/uspsovar.htm. Accessed on April 7, 2012.
3. Roett MA, Evans P. Ovarian cancer: An overview. *Am Fam Physician.* 2009;80:609–616.
4. Schorge JO, Modesitt SC, Coleman RL, et al. SGO white paper on ovarian cancer: Etiology, screening and surveillance. *Gynecol Oncol.* 2010;119:7–17.
5. Kerlikowske K, Brown JS, Grady DG. Should women with familial ovarian cancer undergo prophylactic oophorectomy? *Obstet Gynecol.* 1992;80:700–707.
6. Pal T, Permuth-Wey J, Betts JA, et al. BRCA1 and BRCA2 mutations account for a large proportion of ovarian carcinoma cases. *Cancer.* 2005;104:2804–2816.
7. Pal T, Mohammad R, Sun P, et al. The frequency of MLH1, MSH2 and MSH6 mutations in a population-based sample of ovarian cancers [abstract]. In: *Proceedings of the 102nd Annual Meeting for the American Association for Cancer Research*; April 2–6, 2011; Orlando, FL. Philadelphia, PA: AACR; 2011. Abstract 5617.
8. Walsh T, Casadei S, Lee MK, et al. Mutations in 12 genes for inherited ovarian cancer, fallopian tube, and peritoneal carcinoma identified by massively parallel sequencing. *Proc Natl Acad Sci U S A.* 2011;108:18032–18037.
9. Wooster R, Bignel G, Lancaster J, et al. Identification of the breast cancer susceptibility gene BRCA2. *Nature.* 1995;378:789–792.
10. Ford D, Easton DF, Peto J. Estimates of the gene frequency of BRCA1 and its contribution to breast and ovarian cancer incidence. *Am J Hum Genet.* 1995;57:1457–1462.
11. Struewing JP, Hartge P, Wacholder S, et al. The risk of cancer associated with specific mutations of BRCA1 and BRCA2 among Ashkenazi Jews. *N Engl J Med.* 1997;336:1401–1408.
12. Moslehi B, Chu W, Karlan B, et al. BRCA1 and BRCA2 mutation analysis of 208 Ashkenazi Jewish women with ovarian cancer. *Am J Hum Genet.* 2000;66:1259–1272.

13. Modan B, Hartge P, Hirsh-Yechezkel G, et al. Parity, oral contraceptives and the risk of ovarian cancer among carriers and non-carriers of a BRCA1 or BRCA2 mutation. *N Engl J Med.* 2001;345:235–240.

14. American College of Medical Genetics Foundation. ACMG genetic susceptibility to breast and ovarian cancer: Assessment, counseling and testing guidelines. Available at: http://www.health.ny.gov/diseases/cancer/obcancer/pp27-35.htm. Accessed on April 21, 2012.

15. American College of Obstetricians and Gynecologists, ACOG Committee on Practice Bulletins—Gynecology, ACOG Committee on Genetics, et al. ACOG Practice Bulletin No. 103: Hereditary breast and ovarian cancer syndrome. *Obstet Gynecol.* 2009;113:957–966.

16. American Society of Breast Surgeons. BRCA genetic testing for patients with and without breast cancer. Available at: http://www.breastsurgeons.org/statements/PDF_Statements/BRCA_Testing.pdf. Accessed on April 21, 2012.

17. NCCN Clinical Practice Guidelines in Oncology (NCCN Guidelines). Genetic/Familial High-Risk Assessment: Breast and Ovarian. Version 1.2012. Available at: http://www.nccn.org/professionals/physician_gls/pdf/genetics_screening.pdf. Accessed on May 9, 2012.

18. Lancaster JM, Powell CB, Kauff ND, et al. Society of Gynecologic Oncologists Education Committee statement on risk assessment for inherited gynecologic cancer predispositions. *Gynecol Oncol.* 2007;107:159–162.

19. U.S. Preventative Services Task Force. Genetic risk assessment and BRCA mutation testing for breast and ovarian cancer susceptibility: Recommendation statement. *Ann Intern Med.* 2005;143:355–361.

20. Easton DF, Bishop DT, Ford D, et al. Genetic linkage analysis in familial breast and ovarian cancer: Results from 214 families. *Am J Hum Genet.* 1993;52:678–701.

21. Ford D, Easton DF, Bishop DT, et al. Risks of cancer in BRCA1-mutation carriers. Breast Cancer Linkage Consortium. *Lancet.* 1994;343:692–695.

22. Easton DF, Ford D, Bishop DT et al. Breast and ovarian cancer incidence in BRCA1-mutation carriers. *Am J Hum Genet.* 1995;56:265–271.

23. Narod SA, Ford D, Devilee P, et al. An evaluation of genetic heterogeneity in 145 breast-ovarian cancer families: Breast Cancer Linkage Consortium. *Am J Hum Genet.* 1995;56:254–264.

24. Ford D, Easton DF, Stratton M, et al. Genetic heterogeneity and penetrance analysis of the BRCA1 and BRCA2 genes in breast cancer families. *Am J Hum Genet.* 1998;62:676–689.

25. The Breast Cancer Linkage Consortium. Cancer risks in BRCA2 mutation carriers. *J Natl Cancer Inst.* 1999;91:1310–1316.

26. Antoniou A, Pharoah PD, Narod S, et al. Average risks of breast and ovarian cancer associated with BRCA1 or BRCA2 mutations detected in a case series unselected for family history: A combined analysis of 22 studies. *Am J Hum Genet.* 2003;72:1117–1130.

27. Chen S, Iversen ES, Friebel T, et al. Characterization of BRCA1 and BRCA2 mutations in a large United States sample. *J Clin Oncol.* 2006;24:863–871.

28. Chen S, Parmigiani G. Meta-analysis of BRCA1 and BRCA2 penetrance. *J Clin Oncol.* 2007;25:1329–1333.

29. Gayther SA, Mangion J, Russell P, et al. Variation of risks of breast and ovarian cancer associated with different germline mutations of the BRCA2 gene. *Nat Genet.* 1997;15:103–105.

30. Thompson D, Easton D. Variation in cancer risks, by mutation position, in BRCA2 mutation carriers. *Am J Hum Genet.* 2001;68:410–419.

31. Chenevix-Trench G, Milne RL, Antoniou AC, et al. An international initiative to identify genetic modifiers of cancer risk in BRCA1 and BRCA2 mutation carriers: The Consortium of Investigators of Modifiers of BRCA1 and BRCA2 (CIMBA). *Breast Cancer Res.* 2007;9:104.

32. Rebbeck TR, Mitra N, Domchek SM, et al. Modification of ovarian cancer risk by BRCA1/2-interacting genes in a multicenter cohort of BRCA1/2 mutation carriers. *Cancer Res.* 2009;69:5801–5810.

33. Jakubowska A, Rozkrut D, Antoniou A, et al. The Leu33Pro polymorphism in the ITGB3 gene does not modify BRCA1/2-associated breast or ovarian cancer risks: Results from a multicenter study among 15542 BRCA1 and BRCA2 mutation carriers. *Breast Cancer Res Treat.* 2009;121:639–649.

34. Ramus SJ, Kartsonaki C, Gayther SA, et al. Genetic variation at 9p22.2 and ovarian cancer risk for BRCA1 and BRCA2 mutation carriers. *J Natl Cancer Inst.* 2011;103:105–116.

35. Risch HA, McLaughlin JR, Cole DE, et al. Prevalence and penetrance of germline BRCA1 and BRCA2 mutations in a population series of 649 women with ovarian cancer. *Am J Hum Genet.* 2001;68:700–710.

36. Frank TS, Deffenbaugh AM, Reid JE, et al. Clinical characteristics of individuals with germline mutations in BRCA1 and BRCA2: Analysis of 10000 individuals. *J Clin Oncol.* 2002;20:1480–1490.

37. National Cancer Institute. SEER stat fact sheets: Ovary. Available at: http://seer.cancer.gov/statfacts/html/ovary.html. Accessed on April 8, 2012.

38. Stratton JF, Thompson D, Bobrow L, et al. The genetic epidemiology of early-onset epithelial ovarian cancer: A population-based study. *Am J Hum Genet.* 1999;65:1725–1732.

39. Boyd J, Sonoda Y, Federici MG, et al. Clinicopathologic features of BRCA-linked and sporadic ovarian cancer. *JAMA.* 2000;283:2260–2265.

40. Friedlander ML, Dembo AJ. Prognostic factors in ovarian cancer. *Semin Oncol.* 1991;18:205–212.

41. Evans DGR, Young K, Bulman M, et al. Probability of BRCA1/2 mutation varies with ovarian histology: Results from screening 442 ovarian cancer families. *Clin Genet.* 2008;73:338–345.

42. Lakhani SR, Manek S, Penault-Llorca F, et al. Pathology of ovarian cancers in BRCA1 and BRCA2 carriers. *Clin Cancer Res.* 2004;10:2473–2481.

43. Mavaddat N, Barrowdale D, Andrulis IL, et al. Pathology of breast and ovarian cancers among BRCA1 and BRCA2 mutation carriers: Results from the Consortium Investigators of Modifiers of BRCA1/2 (CIMBA). *Cancer Epidemiol Biomarkers Prev.* 2012;21:134–147.

44. Bolton KL, Chenevix-Trench G, Goh C, et al. Association between BRCA1 and BRCA2 mutations and survival in women with invasive epithelial ovarian cancer. *JAMA.* 2012;307:382–390.

45. Ben David Y, Chetrit A, Hirsh-Yechezkel G, et al. Effect of BRCA mutations on the length of survival in epithelial ovarian cancers. *J Clin Oncol.* 2002;20:463–466.

46. Cass I, Baldwin RL, Varkey T, et al. Improved survival in women with BRCA-associated ovarian carcinoma. *Cancer.* 2003;97:2187–2195.

47. Chetrit A, Hirsh-Yechezkel G, Ben-David Y, et al. Effect of BRCA1/2 mutations on long term survival of patients with invasive ovarian cancer: The national Israeli study of ovarian cancer. *J Clin Oncol.* 2008;26:20–25.

48. Tan DS, Rothermundt C, Thomas K, et al. "BRCAness" syndrome in ovarian cancer: A case-control study describing clinical features and outcome of patents with epithelial ovarian cancer associated with BRCA1 and BRCA2 mutations. *J Clin Oncol.* 2008;26:5530–5536.

49. Roy R, Chun J, Powell SN. BRCA1 and BRCA2: Different roles in a common pathway of genome protection. *Nat Rev Cancer.* 2012;12:68–78.

50. Bryant HE, Schultz N, Thomas HD, et al. Specific killing of BRCA2-deficient tumors with inhibitors of poly(ADP-ribose) polymerase. *Nature.* 2005;434:913–917.

51. Fong PC, Boss DS, Yap TA, et al. Inhibition of poly(ADP-ribose) polymerase in tumors from BRCA mutation carriers. *N Engl J Med.* 2009;361:123–134.

52. Rouleau M, Patel A, Hendzel MJ, et al. PARP inhibition: PARP1 and beyond. *Nat Rev Cancer.* 2010;10:293–301.

53. Fong PC, Yap TA, Boss DS, et al. Poly(ADP-ribose) polymerase inhibition: Frequent durable responses in BRCA carrier ovarian cancer correlating with platinum-free interval. *J Clin Oncol.* 2010;28:2512–2519.

54. Audeh MW, Carmichael J, Penson RT, et al. Oral poly(ADP-ribose) polymerase inhibitor olaparib in patients with BRCA1 or BRCA2 mutations and recurrent ovarian cancer: A proof-of-concept trial. *Lancet.* 2010;376:245–251.

55. Gelmon KA, Tischkowitz M, Mackay H, et al. Olaparib in patients with recurrent high-grade serous or poorly differentiated ovarian carcinoma or triple-negative breast cancer: A phase 2, multicentre, open-label, non-randomized study. *Lancet Oncol.* 2011;12:852–861.

56. Ledermann J, Harter P, Gourley C, et al. Olaparib maintenance therapy in platinum-sensitive relapsed ovarian cancer. *N Engl J Med.* 2012;366:1382–1392.

57. Finch A, Beiner M, Lubinski J, et al. Salpingo-oophorectomy and the risk of ovarian, fallopian tube and peritoneal cancers in women with a BRCA1 or BRCA2 mutation. *JAMA.* 2006;296:185–192.

58. Kauff ND, Domcheck SM, Friebel TM, et al. Risk-reducing salpingo-oophorectomy for the prevention of BRCA1- and BRCA2-associated breast and gynecologic cancer: A multicenter, prospective study. *J Clin Oncol.* 2008;26:1331–1337.

59. Rebbeck TR, Kauff ND, Domcheck SM. Meta-analysis of risk reduction estimates associated with risk-reducing salpingo-oophorectomy in BRCA1 and BRCA2 mutation carriers. *J Natl Cancer Inst.* 2009;101:80–87.

60. Domcheck SM, Friebel TM, Singer CF, et al. Association of risk-reducing surgery in BRCA1 or BRCA2 mutation carriers with cancer risk and mortality. *JAMA.* 2010;304:967–975.

61. Rebbeck TR, Levin AM, Eisen A, et al. Breast cancer risk after bilateral prophylactic oophorectomy in BRCA1 mutation carriers. *J Natl Cancer Inst.* 1999;91:1475–1479.

62. Eisen A, Lubinski J, Klijn J, et al. Breast cancer risk following bilateral oophorectomy in BRCA1 and BRCA2 mutation carriers: An international case-control study. *J Clin Oncol.* 2005;23:7491–7496.

63. Powell CB, Kenley E, Chen L, et al. Risk-reducing salpingo-oophorectomy in BRCA mutation carriers: Role of serial sectioning in the detection of occult malignancy. *J Clin Oncol.* 2005;23:127–132.

64. Finch A, Shaw P, Rosen B, et al. Clinical and pathologic findings of prophylactic salpingo-oophorectomy in 159 BRCA1 and BRCA2 carriers. *Gynecol Oncol.* 2006;100:58–64.

65. Domchek SM, Friebel TM, Garber JE, et al. Occult ovarian cancers identified at risk-reducing salpingo-oophorectomy in a prospective cohort of BRCA1/2 mutation carriers. *Breast Cancer Res Treat.* 2010;124:195–203.

66. Movahedi-Lankarani S, Baker PM, Giks B, et al. Protocol for the examination of specimens from patients with carcinoma of the ovary. Available at: http://www.cap.org/apps/docs/committees/cancer/cancer_protocols/2009/Ovary_09protocol.pdf. Accessed on April 14, 2012.

67. Stirling D, Evans DGR, Pichert G, et al. Screening for familial ovarian cancer: Failure of current protocols to detect ovarian cancer at an early stage according to the International Federation of Gynecology and Obstetrics System. *J Clin Oncol.* 2005;23:5588–5596.

68. Narod SA, Risch H, Moslehi R, et al. Oral contraceptives and the risk of hereditary ovarian cancer. Hereditary Ovarian Cancer Clinical Study Group. *N Engl J Med.* 1998;39:424–428.

69. Iodice S, Barile M, Rotmensz N, et al. Oral contraceptive use and breast or ovarian cancer risk in BRCA1/2 carriers: A meta-analysis. *Eur J Cancer.* 2010;46:2275–2284.

70. Narod SA, Dube MP, Klijn J, et al. Oral contraceptives and the risk of breast cancer in BRCA1 and BRCA2 mutation carriers. *J Natl Cancer Inst.* 2002;94:1773–1779.

71. Milne RL, Knight JA, John EM, et al. Oral contraceptive use and risk of early-onset breast cancer in carriers and noncarriers of BRCA1 and BRCA2 mutations. *Cancer Epidemiol Biomarkers Prev.* 2005;14:350–356.

72. Haile RW, Thomas DC, McGuire V, et al. BRCA1 and BRCA2 mutation carriers, oral contraceptive use, and breast cancer before age 50. *Cancer Epidemiol Biomarkers Prev.* 2006;15:1863–1870.

73. Lee E, Ma H, McKean-Cowdin R, et al. Effect of reproductive factors and oral contraceptives on breast cancer risk in BRCA1/2 mutation carriers and noncarriers: Results from a population based study. *Cancer Epidemiol Biomarkers Prev.* 2008;17:3170–3178.

74. Kurian AW, Munoz DF, Rust P, et al. Online tool to guide decisions for BRCA1/2 mutation carriers. *J Clin Oncol.* 2012;30:497–506.

75. Watson P, Bützow R, Lynch HT, et al. The clinical features of ovarian cancer in hereditary nonpolyposis colorectal cancer. *Gynecol Oncol.* 2001;82:223–228.

76. Weissman SM, Bellcross C, Bittner CC, et al. Genetic counseling considerations in the evaluation of families for Lynch syndrome—a review. *J Genet Counsel.* 2011;20:5–19.

77. Palomaki GE, McClain MR, Melillo S, et al. EGAPP supplementary evidence review: DNA testing strategies aimed at reducing morbidity and mortality from Lynch syndrome. *Genet Med.* 2009;11:42–65.

78. Weissman SM, Burt R, Church J, et al. Identification of individuals at risk for Lynch syndrome using targeted evaluations and genetic testing: National Society of Genetic Counselors and the Collaborative Group of the Americans on Inherited Colorectal Cancer Joint Practice Guideline. *J Genet Counsel.* 2012;21:484–493.

79. Hendriks YM, Wagner A, Morreau H, et al. Cancer risk in hereditary nonpolyposis colorectal cancer due to MSH6 mutations: Impact on counseling and surveillance. *Gastroenterology.* 2004;127:17–25.

80. Senter L, Clendenning M, Sotamaa K, et al. The clinical phenotype of Lynch syndrome due to germline PMS2 mutations. *Gastroenterology.* 2008;135:419–428.

81. Vasen HF, Mecklin JP, Khan PM, et al. The International Collaborative Group on hereditary nonpolyposis colorectal cancer (ICG-HNPCC). *Dis Colon Rectum.* 1991;34:424–425.

82. Vasen HF, Watson P, Mecklin JP, et al. New clinical criteria for hereditary nonpolyposis colorectal cancer (HNPCC, Lynch syndrome) proposed by the International Collaborative group on HNPCC. *Gastroenterology.* 1999;116:1453–1456.

83. Hampel H, Frankel WL, Martin E, et al. Feasibility of screening for Lynch syndrome among patients with colorectal cancer. *J Clin Oncol.* 2008;26:5783–5788.

84. Barrow E, Alduaij W, Robinson L, et al. Colorectal cancer in HNPCC: Cumulative lifetime incidence, survival and tumour distribution. A report of 121 families with proven mutations. *Clin Genet.* 2008;74:233–242.

85. Watson P, Vasen HF, Mecklin JP, et al. The risk of extra-colonic, extra-endometrial cancer in the Lynch syndrome. *Int J Cancer.* 2008;123:444–449.

86. Pal T, Permuth-Wey J, Kumar A, et al. Systematic review and meta-analysis of ovarian cancers: Estimation of microsatellite-high frequency and characterization of mismatch repair deficient tumor histology. *Clin Cancer Res.* 2008;14:6847–6854.

87. Crijnen TE, Janssen-Heijnen ML, Gelderblom H, et al. Survival of patients with ovarian cancer due to a mismatch repair defect. *Fam Cancer.* 2005;4:301–305.

88. Jensen KC, Mariappan MR, Putcha GV, et al. Microsatellite instability and mismatch repair protein defects in ovarian epithelial neoplasms in patients 50 years of age and younger. *Am J Surg Pathol.* 2008;32:1029–1037.

89. Domanska K, Malander S, Måsbäck A, et al. Ovarian cancer at young age: The contribution of mismatch-repair defects in a population-based series of epithelial ovarian cancer before age 40. *Intl J Gynecol Cancer.* 2007;17:789–793.

90. NCCN Clinical Practice Guidelines in Oncology (NCCN Guidelines). Colorectal Cancer Screening. V2.2012. Available at: http://www.nccn.org/professionals/physician_gls/pdf/colorectal_screening. pdf. Accessed on April 30, 2012.

91. Allen BA, Terdiman JP. Hereditary polyposis syndromes and hereditary non-polyposis colorectal cancer. *Best Pract Res Clin Gastroenterol.* 2003;17:237–258.

92. Lindor NM, McMaster ML, Lindor CJ, et al. Concise handbook of familial cancer susceptibility syndromes—second edition. *J Natl Cancer Inst Monogr.* 2008:1–93.

93. Schreibman IR, Baker M, Amos C et al. The hamartomatous polyposis syndromes: A clinical and molecular review. *Am J Gastroenterol.* 2005;100:476–490.

94. Boardman LA. Heritable colorectal cancer syndromes: Recognition and preventive management. *Gastroenterol Clin North Am.* 2002;31:1107–1131.

95. McGarrity TJ, Kulin HE, Zaino RJ. Peutz–Jeghers syndrome. *Am J Gastroenterol.* 2000;95:596–604.

96. Beggs AD, Latchford AR, Vasen HF et al. Peutz–Jeghers syndrome: A systematic review and recommendations for management. *Gut.* 2010;59:975–986.

97. Giardello FM, Brensinger JD, Tersmette AC. Very high risk of cancer in familial Peutz–Jeghers syndrome. *Gastroenterology.* 2000;119:1447–1453.

98. van Lier MGF, Mathus-Vliegen FMH, Wagner A, et al. High cancer risk in Peutz–Jeghers syndrome: A systematic review and surveillance recommendations. *Am J Gastroenterol.* 2010;105:1258–1264.

99. Young RH, Welch WR, Dickersin GR, et al. Ovarian sex cord tumor with annular tubules: Review of 74 cases including 27 with Peutz–Jeghers syndrome and four with adenoma malignum of the cervix. *Cancer.* 1982;50:1384–1402.

100. Dozois RR, Kempers RD, Dahlin DC, et al. Ovarian tumors associated with the Peutz–Jeghers syndrome. *Ann Surg.* 1970;172:233–238.

101. Hemminki A, Markie D, Tomlinson I, et al. A serine/threonine kinase gene defective in Peutz–Jeghers syndrome. *Nature.* 1998;391:184–187.

102. Jenne DE, Reimann H, Nezu J, et al. Peutz–Jeghers syndrome is caused by mutations in a novel serine threonine kinase. *Nat Genet.* 1998;18:38–43.

103. Volikos E, Robinson J, Aittomäki K, et al. LKB1 exonic and whole gene deletions are a common cause of Peutz–Jeghers syndrome. *J Med Genet.* 2006;43:e18.

104. Salloch H, Reinacher-Schick A, Schulmann K, et al. Truncating mutations in Peutz–Jeghers syndrome are associated with more polyps, surgical interventions and cancers. *Int J Colorectal Dis.* 2010;25:97–107.

105. Amos CI, Keitheri-Cheteri MB, Sabripour M, et al. Genotype–phenotype correlations in Peutz–Jeghers. *J Med Genet.* 2004;41:327–333.

106. Mehenni H, Resta N, Guanti G, et al. Molecular and clinical characteristics in 46 families affected with Peutz–Jeghers syndrome. *Dig Dis Sci.* 2007;52:1924–1933.
107. Aretz S, Steinen D, Uhlhaas S, et al. High proportion of large genomic STK11 deletions in Peutz–Jeghers syndrome. *Human Mutat.* 2005;26:513–519.
108. Hearle N, Lucassen A, Wang R, et al. Mapping of a translocation breakpoint in a Peutz–Jeghers hamartoma to the putative PJS locus at 19q13.4 and mutation analysis of candidate genes in polyp and STK11-negative PJS cases. *Genes Chromosomes Cancer.* 2004;41:163–169.
109. Mehenni H, Gehrig C, Nezu J, et al. Loss of LKB1 kinase activity in Peutz–Jeghers syndrome, and evidence for allelic and locus heterogeneity. *Am J Hum Genet.* 1998;63:1641–1650.
110. Boardman LA, Couch FJ, Burgart LJ, et al. Genetic heterogeneity in Peutz–Jeghers syndrome. *Human Mutat.* 2000;16:23–30.
111. Vaz F, Hanenberg H, Schuster B, et al. Mutation of the RAD51C gene in a Fanconi anemia-like disorder. *Nat Genet.* 2010;42:406–409.
112. Meindl A, Hellebrand H, Wiek C, et al. Germline mutations in breast and ovarian cancer pedigrees establish RAD51C as a human cancer susceptibility gene. *Nat Genet.* 2010;42:410–414.
113. Vuorela P, Pylkäs K, Hartikainen JM, et al. Further evidence for the contribution of the RAD51C gene in hereditary breast and ovarian cancer susceptibility. *Breast Cancer Res Treat.* 2011;130:1003–1010.
114. Thompson ER, Boyle SE, Johnson J, et al. Analysis of RAD51C germline mutations in high-risk breast and ovarian cancer families and ovarian cancer patients. *Hum Mutat.* 2012;33:95–99.
115. Osorio A, Endt D, Fernández F. Predominance of pathogenic missense variants in the RAD51C gene occurring in breast and ovarian cancer families. *Hum Mol Genet.* 2012:1–10.
116. Pelttari LM, Heikkinen T, Thompson D, et al. RAD51C is a susceptibility gene for ovarian cancer. *Hum Mol Genet.* 2011;20:3278–3288.
117. Loveday C, Turnbull C, Ramsay E, et al. Germline mutations in RAD51D confer susceptibility to ovarian cancer. *Nat Genet.* 2011;43:879–882.
118. Osher DJ, De Leeneer K, Michils G, et al. Mutation analysis of RAD51D in non-BRCA1/2 ovarian and breast cancer families. *Br J Cancer.* 2012;106:1460–1463.

7 Genetic Testing by Cancer Site

Colon (Polyposis Syndromes)

Kory W. Jasperson

Hereditary colonic polyposis conditions account for less than 1% of all colorectal cancers (CRCs). Accurate classification of these conditions is imperative, given their distinct cancer risks, management strategies, and consequent risk to relatives. However, overlapping features and atypical or attenuated presentations make diagnosis difficult in some cases. Determining the histologic types of colorectal polyps identified is especially useful in guiding diagnostic strategies. Adenomatous polyps are the predominant lesion in familial adenomatous polyposis (FAP), attenuated FAP (AFAP), and *MUTYH* (MutY human homolog)-associated polyposis (MAP), whereas hamartomatous polyps are the primary gastrointestinal lesion in Peutz–Jeghers syndrome (PJS), juvenile polyposis syndrome (JPS), and Cowden syndrome (CS). Extracolonic features, which are highlighted for each syndrome in Tables 7.1 to 7.3, are also important clues in the diagnostic workup. Genetic testing is now available for these conditions and in most cases allows for a precise diagnosis.

ADENOMATOUS POLYPOSIS

FAP and AFAP

Of all of the colonic polyposis conditions, FAP is both the most common and the best characterized. FAP is caused by germline mutations in the adenomatous polyposis coli (*APC*) gene and is estimated to occur in about 1 in 10,000 individuals. With the classic presentation of FAP, hundreds to thousands of adenomatous polyps occur by the age of 20 to 40 years.[1] The attenuated or less severe colonic phenotype associated with AFAP may mimic sporadic colon polyps and cancer, or other known syndromes, such as MAP. This creates diagnostic difficulties when evaluating an individual with moderate adenomatous polyposis. Other conditions linked to germline *APC* mutations include Gardner syndrome (association of colonic polyposis and osteomas, epidermoid cysts, fibromas, and/or desmoid tumors) and Turcot syndrome (association of colonic polyposis and medulloblastomas).[2] However, it is now believed that the features associated with Gardner

TABLE 7.1	**Characteristic Features and Recommendations: Adenomatous Polyposis Conditions**	

Lifetime Cancer Risks	Management Recommendations	Nonmalignant Features
FAP (*APC*)		
Colorectum (100%)	Annual colonoscopy/ sigmoidoscopy by 10–12 y until colectomy	100s to 1,000s of colorectal adenomas
Duodenum (5%)	Upper endoscopy every 1–4 y by 25–30 y	Fundic gland polyposis
Stomach (≤1%)		Duodenal polyposis
Thyroid (1–2%)	Annual physical examination	CHRPE, epidermoid cysts, osteomas
Pancreas (1–2%)		Dental abnormalities
Hepatoblastoma (1–2%)		Desmoid tumors
Medulloblastoma (<1%)		
AFAP (*APC*)		
Colorectum (70%)	Colonoscopy every 1–2 y by 18–20 y	10–100 colonic adenomas (range, 0–100s)
Duodenum (5%)	Upper endoscopy every 1–4 y by 25–30 y	Fundic gland polyposis
Stomach (≤1%)		Duodenal polyposis
Thyroid (1–2%)	Annual physical examination	Other nonmalignant features are uncommon
Pancreas (1–2%)		
MAP (biallelic *MUTYH*)		
Colorectum (80%)	Colonoscopy every 3 y by 25–30 y	10–100 colonic adenomas (range, 0–100s)
Duodenum (4%)	Upper endoscopy every 3–5 y by 30–35 y	Multiple hyperplastic and sessile serrated polyps possible
		Duodenal adenomatous polyposis

Data derived from: NCCN clinical practice guidelines in oncology. Colorectal cancer screening; V1.2012. 2012. Available at: http://www.nccn.org. Accessed on April 3, 2012.

syndrome and Turcot syndrome are the result of variable expressivity of *APC* mutations as opposed to being distinct clinical entities.

Colon Phenotype

Although adenomatous polyps associated with FAP have a similar malignancy rate as those that develop in the general population, the sheer number of polyps present in FAP results in nearly a 100% lifetime risk of CRC in untreated individuals. In FAP, colorectal polyps begin to develop on average around the age of 16 years.[1] The mean age at CRC onset is 39 years, with 7% developing CRC by 21 years and 95% before the age of 50 years.[3]

In AFAP, the lifetime risk of CRC is approximately 70% with an average age at onset in the 50s.[4] The colonic phenotype of AFAP is quite variable, even within the same family. Colonoscopies in 120 mutation-positive individuals within the same family revealed that 37% had less than 10 adenomatous colon polyps (average age, 36 years; range, 16 to 67 years), 28% had 10 to 50 polyps (average age, 39 years; range, 21 to 76 years), and 35% had greater than 50 polyps (average age, 48 years; range, 27 to 49 years).[4] In addition, the total number of polyps per individual ranged from 0 to 470.[4]

Extracolonic Features

The most common extracolonic finding in individuals with FAP and AFAP is upper gastrointestinal tract polyps. Although the colonic phenotype in AFAP is less severe than in FAP, the upper gastrointestinal phenotype is comparable. Adenomatous polyps of the duodenum (20% to 100%) and periampullary region (at least 50%) are common.[5,6] The relative risk of duodenal or periampullary carcinoma in FAP is estimated to be 100 to 330 times greater than the general population, although the absolute risk is only around 5%.[5] The majority of FAP- and AFAP-associated small-bowel carcinomas arise in the duodenum.

Fundic gland polyps are found in most cases of FAP/AFAP and often number in the hundreds.[7] Unlike polyps in the colon or small bowel, fundic gland polyps are a type of hamartoma. They are typically small (1 to 5 mm), sessile, and usually asymptomatic and are located in the fundus and body of the stomach.[7] Adenomatous polyps of the stomach are occasionally found in FAP and AFAP.[8] Gastric cancers arising from fundic gland polyps have been reported in FAP, although most are believed to arise from adenomatous polyps.[8]

Individuals with FAP have an 800-fold increased risk for desmoid tumors (aggressive fibromatoses), with a lifetime risk of 10% to 30%.[9-11] Risk factors for desmoid tumors in FAP include family history of desmoid tumors, *APC* mutations 3′ to codon 1,399 (genotype–phenotype correlation), female sex, and previous abdominal surgery.[10] Although desmoid tumors do not metastasize, they can be locally invasive, aggressive, and difficult to treat, resulting in significant morbidity and the second leading cause of mortality in FAP.[12]

The phenotypic spectrum of germline *APC* mutations also includes other benign findings such as osteomas, epidermoid cysts, fibromas, dental abnormalities, and congenital hypertrophy of the retinal pigment epithelium (CHRPE). In addition, there are increased risks for other cancers including those of the pancreas, thyroid, bile duct, brain (typically medulloblastoma), and liver (specifically hepatoblastoma).[6]

Management

Without treatment, CRC is inevitable in FAP. However, with early screening and polypectomies, in addition to prophylactic colectomy after polyps become too difficult to manage endoscopically, most CRCs can be prevented in AFAP and FAP. In FAP, annual colonoscopies or flexible sigmoidoscopies are recommended starting around the age of 10 years.[13] In AFAP, screening begins in the late teenage years, and colonoscopies, rather than sigmoidoscopies, are necessary because of proximally located polyps.[13] Colectomy can sometimes be avoided in AFAP, which is not the case for individuals with FAP. After polyps become too numerous (usually >20 to 30 polyps) to manage endoscopically or when adenomas with advanced histology are identified, prophylactic colectomy is advised.[13] Proctocolectomy with ileal pouch anal anastomosis is the standard surgery in FAP, whereas total colectomy with ileorectal anastomosis is often the preferred approach with AFAP or in FAP cases with limited rectal involvement.[13,14] Continued screening of the remaining rectum or ileal pouch is still necessary.[13]

Recently, it has been shown that duodenal cancer detected through surveillance improves survival compared with individuals presenting because of symptoms.[15] The National Comprehensive Cancer Network (NCCN) currently recommends consideration of esophagogastroduodenoscopy (EGD) with side-viewing examination beginning around the age of 25 years for duodenal cancer surveillance.[13] The extent of duodenal polyps, as defined by the Spigelman staging criteria, is used to determine the EGD follow-up interval.[13] Additional considerations for management in individuals with germline *APC* mutations are outlined and updated annually by the NCCN (www.nccn.org).

Genetic Testing and Counseling

A clinical diagnosis of FAP is considered when at least 100 colorectal adenomatous polyps are detected by the second or third decade of life.[6] Genetic testing of *APC* is still recommended to clarify extracolonic cancer risks and to help determine FAP status in relatives. Genetic testing has also been shown to be cost-effective,[16] although it is unlikely to change colon management for cases with extensive adenomatous polyposis.

Given the phenotypic variability, a consensus as to what constitutes a diagnosis of AFAP has not been reached. The NCCN currently recommends that individuals with greater than 10 cumulative colorectal adenomas be referred for genetic counseling and consideration of genetic testing.[13] Identification of an *APC* mutation in these less severe polyp cases confirms a diagnosis of AFAP. It is also noteworthy that individuals with 100 or more adenomatous polyps may have AFAP if polyp development occurs at a later age (typically after 40 years).

Differentiating among FAP, AFAP, and other colonic polyposis conditions is not always straightforward. Family history consistent with an autosomal dominant mode of inheritance is suggestive of FAP/AFAP and increases the likelihood of finding an *APC* mutation.[6] However, 10% to 30% of probands with germline *APC* mutations are de novo (new mutation) cases, and consequently their parents are unaffected.[6,17] In addition, it is not uncommon for individuals with AFAP to have less than 10 cumulative adenomatous polyps.[4] In patients with fewer polyps, it is not clear whether genetic testing should be performed.[13] However, it is important that these individuals be closely followed up, and if multiple adenomas continue to develop, genetic testing should be reconsidered.

Unlike what is found in some of the other conditions described in this review, hyperplastic or hamartomatous colon polyps are not known to be associated with FAP/AFAP. Therefore, if multiple hyperplastic or hamartomatous colon polyps are found in an individual, genetic testing of *APC* is unlikely to be informative. Other features associated with *APC* mutations that may assist with making a diagnosis of AFAP or FAP include fundic gland polyposis, duodenal adenomatous polyps, osteomas, CHRPE, desmoid tumors, and hepatoblastoma.[6]

MUTYH-associated Polyposis

As the name implies, MAP is a colonic polyposis condition caused by germline mutations in the *MUTYH* gene. Contrary to the other conditions described in this review, MAP is inherited in an autosomal recessive pattern. Al-Tassan et al.[18] in 2002 were the first to describe a family with biallelic (homozygous or compound heterozygous) mutations in *MUTYH*, which is part of the base excision repair system. In this family, three siblings had CRC and/or multiple colorectal adenomas, but no detectable mutations in *APC*.[18] All three of the affected siblings were found to have compound heterozygous mutations in *MUTYH*, whereas the other four unaffected siblings did not.[18]

It is now widely accepted that MAP is associated with a significant increased risk for multiple colorectal adenomas and cancer. Whether monoallelic *MUTYH* carriers have a modest increase in risk of CRC is debatable.[19] Monoallelic mutations in *MUTYH* are found in 1% to 2% of the general population, whereas biallelic mutations account for less than 1% of all CRCs.[20]

Colonic Phenotype

There are a number of similarities between the colonic phenotype of MAP and AFAP, including the average number, proximal distribution, and young age at onset of adenomas and cancers.[4,19] *MUTYH*-associated polyposis is associated with a 28-fold increased risk of CRC, with a penetrance of 19% by the age of 50 years, 43% by 60 years, and 80% by 70 years.[19,21] Although the risk of CRC has been reported to be as high as 100%,[22] the actual penetrance is likely to be incomplete and similar to that of AFAP. The total number of polyps in MAP is also highly variable, with some individuals developing CRC without polyps, whereas others have more than 500 colorectal polyps.[23] Typically, affected individuals have between 10 and 100 polyps.[23]

Adenomas are the predominant polyp type seen not only in AFAP and FAP, but also in MAP. Unlike individuals with germline *APC* mutations, serrated polyps are common in MAP. Serrated polyps include hyperplastic polyps, sessile serrated polyps (also referred to as sessile serrated adenomas), and traditional serrated adenomas.[24] Boparai et al.[25] evaluated 17 individuals with MAP and found that almost one-half (47%) had hyperplastic and/or sessile serrated polyps. In addition, three met criteria for hyperplastic polyposis, now known as serrated polyposis. The World Health Organization diagnostic criteria for serrated polyposis include an individual with any of the following: (1) at least five serrated polyps proximal to the sigmoid colon with at least two larger than 10 mm; (2) greater than 20 serrated polyps of any size, but distributed through the colon; and (3) any number of serrated polyps proximal to the sigmoid colon in an individual with a first-degree relative with serrated polyposis.[24] Interestingly, Chow et al.[26] also identified biallelic *MUTYH* mutations in 1 (~3%) of 38 cases meeting hyperplastic polyposis/serrated polyposis criteria. Another family involving three brothers with biallelic *MUTYH* mutations has recently been reported, further highlighting this variability in phenotype. Their history included one with CRC at the age of 48 years but had no additional polyps, another was 38 years old and reportedly met criteria for serrated polyposis but had only two confirmed adenomas, and the other brother was 46 years old and had four hyperplastic polyps removed.[27] Currently, the etiology of serrated polyposis is largely unknown; however, there is growing evidence that the base excision repair pathway may be involved in a minority of these cases.

Boparai et al.[25] also compared the frequency of *K-ras* mutations and G:C to T:A transversions in hyperplastic or sessile serrated polyps in individuals with MAP to controls. In MAP, 51 (70%) of 73 serrated polyps had *K-ras* mutations, and 48 (94%) of these 51 had G:C to T:A transversions, whereas in the control group, only 7 (17%) of 41 serrated polyps had *K-ras* mutations, and 2 (29%) of 7 had G:C to T:A transversions.[25] These findings support an association between MAP and serrated polyps.

Extracolonic Features

A number of extracolonic findings have been reported in individuals with MAP.[23] However, it is still unclear whether most of these manifestations are chance occurrences or due to an underlying defective *MUTYH*. In a study of 276 individuals with MAP, only two developed duodenal cancer.[22] However, compared with the general population, the risk of duodenal cancer was significantly elevated, with a standard incidence ratio of 129 and an estimated lifetime risk of 4%.[22] Although the lifetime risk of duodenal cancer is similar between MAP and FAP/AFAP (4% and 5%), gastric and duodenal polyps are far less common in MAP. Of 150 individuals with MAP who underwent an EGD, 11% had gastric polyps, whereas 17% had duodenal polyps.[22]

Extraintestinal malignancies have also been reported in MAP,[22] although the data supporting an association are conflicting.[28,29] Desmoid tumors, thyroid and brain cancer, CHRPE, osteomas, and epidermoid cysts are rarely seen in MAP.[23]

Genetic Counseling and Testing

Since the first reported family with biallelic *MUTYH* mutations was described in 2002, more than 500 individuals with MAP have been confirmed.[23] As was the case with this first MAP family, genetic testing strategies to evaluate for *MUTYH* are typically targeted toward individuals with multiple colorectal adenomas. However, there are many other factors that can influence genetic testing approaches for *MUTYH* and *APC* mutations. Family history; age at polyp onset; types, location, and total number of polyps; CRC history (including age at onset and location); ethnicity; and extracolonic features are just some of the factors that influence genetic testing strategies and detection rates. The purpose of this review was not to present every scenario and strategy for *MUTYH* and *APC* genetic testing, but instead to outline some key concepts and considerations when multiple adenomas are detected.

Given the inheritance pattern of MAP, it is uncommon for more than one generation to be affected; however, a family history of CRC in more than one generation does not exclude MAP. Consanguinity (sharing a common ancestor) is seen in some MAP families and is an important element to evaluate for when taking a history. Siblings of affected individuals have a one (25%) in four chances of having MAP, whereas parents and children are obligate carriers. Therefore, when there is clear evidence of recessive inheritance in a family (>1 sibling affected in a family, but no one else), genetic testing should start with *MUTYH*. *APC* should still be evaluated in these families if no *MUTYH* mutations are identified, as germline mosaicism can result in more than one affected sibling with FAP and unaffected parents.[30] To clarify risk to offspring, spouses of individuals with MAP should also be offered *MUTYH* genetic testing. This strategy has been shown to be cost-effective.[31]

Generally, germline *APC* mutations are more common than biallelic *MUTYH* mutations; therefore, unless there is clear evidence for recessive inheritance in a family, *APC* genetic testing typically precedes *MUTYH* analysis. There are two common mutations in *MUTYH* that are found in the majority of affected individuals: Y179C and G396D (previously known as Y165C and G382D). These hotspot mutations were found in the original MAP family.[18] According to Nielsen et al.,[23] a review up to 2009 revealed more than 100 distinct *MUTYH* mutations. In individuals with Northern European ancestry and MAP, at least one of the two hotspot mutations are found in 90% of cases.[23,32] Testing specifically for the hotspot mutations, followed by full *MUTYH* sequencing only if one of these mutations is found, is often performed. In other populations, the scope of *MUTYH* mutations is less well understood, and therefore, full gene sequencing of *MUTYH* is often performed in individuals of non-Northern European ancestry.

Similar to *APC*, genetic testing of *MUTYH* is considered when greater than 10 adenomas are documented.[13,23] The detection rates of biallelic *MUTYH* mutations in individuals with 10 to 100 and 100 to 1,000 polyps are 28% and 14%, respectively.[23] Given the growing evidence that hyperplastic and sessile serrated polyps are associated with MAP, these polyps should also be included in the total polyp count when considering when to test someone for *MUTYH* mutations. Individuals with FAP/AFAP are not known to develop numerous serrated polyps; therefore, genetic testing of *APC* in someone with multiple serrated polyps is unlikely to be informative. The

NCCN guidelines do not currently recommend genetic testing of *MUTYH* in individuals with multiple serrated polyps and no adenomas.[13]

It is not unusual for individuals with MAP or AFAP to present with early-onset CRC and few to no polyps.[4,33] However, a consensus as to whether genetic testing of *APC* or *MUTYH* should be performed in these cases has not yet been reached.[13,23]

Management

Colonoscopy screening starting at around the age of 25 years is recommended for individuals with MAP.[13] The frequency of screening depends on polyp burden. As is the case with AFAP and FAP, colectomy is advised when polyps become endoscopically uncontrollable. EGDs should be considered in the 30s and, if duodenal adenomas are found, managed the same as in AFAP and FAP.[13] Currently, the evidence does not support increased CRC screening in monoallelic *MUTYH* carriers.

HAMARTOMATOUS POLYPOSIS

Peutz–Jeghers Syndrome

PJS is an autosomal dominant condition caused by mutations in the *STK11/LKB1* gene. It is estimated to occur in 1 in 50,000 to 200,000 births.[34] The two most characteristic manifestations of PJS are the distinct gastrointestinal-type hamartomas, called Peutz–Jeghers polyps, and the mucocutaneous melanin pigmentation. Both of these features are included in the diagnostic criteria for PJS (Table 7.2). Although it is not 100% penetrant and can fade with time, mucocutaneous hyperpigmentation in PJS typically presents in childhood. By the age of 20 years, 50% of individuals present with small-bowel obstruction, intussusception, and/or bleeding due to small-bowel polyps.[35] The polyps in PJS can also number in the hundreds and are most often found in the small intestine, followed by the colon and the stomach.[34]

The cancer risks associated with PJS are more significant after the age of 30 years, although earlier-onset malignancies do occur. In the largest study to date of 419 individuals with PJS, the risk of developing any cancer was 2% by the age of 20 years, 5% by 30 years, 17% by 40 years, 31% by 50 years, 60% by 60 years, and 85% by 70 years.[36] Gastrointestinal tract cancers had the highest cumulative risk. The specific cancer risks associated with PJS are outlined in Table 7.3.

Juvenile Polyposis Syndrome

JPS is an autosomal dominant condition caused by germline mutations in *SMAD4* or *BMPR1A* genes, with an incidence of 0.6 to 1 in 100,000 and a de novo rate of 25% to 50%.[37,38] Juvenile polyps are the hallmark lesion in JPS.[38] They are most commonly found in the colorectum and can number in the hundreds, although carpeting of polyps is not usually seen in JPS like it is in FAP.[38] Of note, solitary juvenile polyps can occur in children without JPS (Table 7.2). Hematochezia is the most common presenting symptom, and similar to PJS, intussusception and obstruction are common.

TABLE 7.2	Testing and Diagnostic Criteria for PJS, JPS, and CS

PJS

A clinical diagnosis of PJS is considered when any of the following are met:
(1) ≥3 histologically confirmed Peutz–Jeghers polyps
(2) Any number of Peutz–Jeghers polyps and a family history of PJS
(3) Characteristic, prominent, mucocutaneous pigmentation and a family history of PJS
(4) ≥1 Peutz–Jeghers polyp and characteristic, prominent, mucocutaneous pigmentation

JPS

A clinical diagnosis of JPS is considered when any of the following are met:
(1) 3–5 Juvenile polyps of the colorectum
(2) Juvenile polyps throughout the gastrointestinal tract
(3) ≥1 Juvenile polyp in an individual with a family history of JPS

CS[a]

Genetic testing for CS is considered in individuals meeting any of the following criteria:

(1) Adult onset Lhermitte–Duclos disease
(2) Autism spectrum disorder and macrocephaly
(3) ≥2 major criteria (one must be macrocephaly)
(4) ≥3 major criteria without macrocephaly
(5) Bannayan–Riley–Ruvalcaba syndrome
(6) One major and ≥3 minor criteria
(7) ≥2 biopsy-proven trichilemmomas
(8) ≥4 minor criteria

Major Criteria	Minor Criteria
Multiple gastrointestinal (GI) hamartomas/ ganglioneuromas	A single GI hamartoma/ ganglioneuroma
Nonmedullary thyroid cancer	Thyroid adenoma or multinodular goiter
Breast cancer	Fibrocystic disease of the breast
Endometrial cancer	Mental retardation (i.e., IQ ≤ 75)
Mucocutaneous lesions	Autism spectrum disorder
One biopsy proven trichilemmoma	Fibromas
Multiple palmoplantar keratoses	Renal cell carcinoma
Multiple cutaneous facial papules	Uterine fibroids
Macular pigmentation of glans penis	Lipomas
Multifocal/extensive oral mucosal papillomatosis	
Macrocephaly (megalocephaly) (at least 97th percentile)	

[a]Data derived from: NCCN guidelines genetic/familial high-risk assessment: Breast and ovarian cancer, V.1.2012. Available at: http://www.nccn.org.

TABLE 7.3	Characteristic Features and Recommendations: PJS and JPS	

Lifetime Cancer Risks	Management Recommendations	Nonmalignant Features
PJS (*STK11*)		
Breast (54%)	Annual mammogram and breast magnetic resonance imaging by age 25 y	Mucocutaneous pigmentation
Colon (39%)	Colonoscopy every 2–3 y by age 25 y	
Pancreas (11–36%)	CA-19-9 and magnetic resonance cholangiopancreatography and/or endoscopic ultrasound every 1–2 y	Peutz–Jeghers polyps
Stomach (29%)	Upper endoscopy by 25–30 y; consider small-bowel visualization (CT enterography, small-bowel enteroclysis) by 8–10 y	
Small bowel (13%)		
Ovary[a] (21%)	Annual pelvic examination and Pap smear	
Uterine/cervix[b] (11%)		
Lung (15%)	No specific recommendations	
Testicle[c] (<1%)	Annual testicular examination	
JPS (*SMAD4* and *BMPR1A*)		
Colon (40–50%)	Colonoscopy by age 15 y repeating annually if polyps are present and every 2–3 y if no polyps	Juvenile polyps Features of HHT
Stomach (21% if gastric polyps are present)	Upper endoscopy by age 15 y repeating annually if polyps are present and every 2–3 y if no polyps	Congenital defects

[a] Sex cord tumor with annular tubules.
[b] Adenoma malignum.
[c] Sertoli cell tumor.
HHT, hereditary hemorrhagic telangiectasia.
Data derived from: NCCN clinical practice guidelines in oncology. Colorectal cancer screening; V1.2012. 2012. Available at: http://www.nccn.org. Accessed on April 3, 2012.

The highest risk of cancer (Table 7.3) in JPS is CRC. Gastric cancers typically occur only in the setting of gastric polyposis, which is more commonly present in individuals with mutations in *SMAD4* than in *BMPR1A*.[37] JPS occurring in infancy (also known as juvenile polyposis of infancy) is often fatal, but rare. Hereditary hemorrhagic telangiectasia symptoms, such as arteriovenous malformations, telangiectasia, and epistaxis, occur in some individuals with mutations in *SMAD4*, but not *BMPR1A*.[37]

Cowden Syndrome

CS, which is part of the PTEN hamartoma tumor syndrome, occurs in about 1 in 200,000 to 1 in 250,000 individuals and is caused by germline mutations in the *PTEN* gene.[39] It is a multisystem disorder associated with characteristic mucocutaneous features, macrocephaly, and a variety of cancers and gastrointestinal manifestations.[39] Although other malignancies may be seen in CS, the primary cancers associated with CS include breast (25% to 50%), nonmedullary thyroid (3% to 10%), and endometrial (5% to 10%).[39] A recent study estimated that the lifetime risk for these cancers in *PTEN* mutation carriers was 85%, 35%, and 28%, respectively.[40] However, these risks are likely overestimates, as Tan et al.[40] failed to accurately account for ascertainment bias in their study.

Gastrointestinal polyps are one of the most common features in CS.[41] Polyps develop throughout the gastrointestinal tract, from the esophagus to the rectum, and numerous polyps or diffuse polyposis can be seen.[41] Multiple, white flat plaques in the esophagus, called glycogenic acanthosis, also occur in the setting of CS. In a large study of 127 individuals with *PTEN* mutations, 39 underwent at least 1 EGD, and 8 (~23%) had glycogenic acanthosis, 26 (~67%) had duodenal and/or gastric polyps, and only 2 (5%) had fundic gland polyps.[41] Of the 67 individuals who underwent at least 1 colonoscopy, 62 (~93%) had colonic polyps, and 16 met criteria for hyperplastic polyposis.[41] Although hamartomas predominate, a variety of other colon polyps also develop, including adenomatous, hyperplastic, sessile serrated, ganglioneuromatous, inflammatory, lymphoid, and lipomatous. Of all of the mutation carriers in this large study, nine (7%) were diagnosed with CRC.[41]

PJS, JPS, AND CS: GENETIC COUNSELING AND TESTING

Hamartomatous polyps consist of an overgrowth of cells native to the tissue in which they occur. They are rare, account for a minority of all colon polyps, and can be a red flag for an underlying cancer predisposition syndrome. When hamartomatous polyps are found in an individual, the differential diagnosis depends, in part, on the histologic type, total number, and age at onset of the polyps. Hamartomas can often be misdiagnosed as other polyp types, and therefore, review by a gastrointestinal pathologist should be considered.[42] When hamartomatous colonic polyps are identified, EGD and a thorough physical examination may identify extracolonic manifestations leading to a precise diagnosis. A detailed family history is also imperative. Diagnostic criteria for JPS and PJS are summarized in Table 7.2. Guidelines for genetic testing of CS, which are quite extensive and include a number of extraintestinal features, are also included in Table 7.2. Given the complexity of genetic testing for CS, the NCCN updates their guidelines annually.[43] Management considerations are reviewed for PJS and JPS in Table 7.3 and are also updated annually by the NCCN.[13]

CONCLUSIONS

There are numerous presentations that may warrant genetic testing for hereditary colonic polyposis conditions. Simplified guidelines for referral for genetic counseling include individuals with any of the following: (1) greater than 10 colonic adenomas, (2) three or more hamartomatous polyps, or (3) at least one Peutz–Jeghers polyp. Other manifestations in these individuals may help target genetic testing to a specific condition. Once the genetic cause has been identified in an affected individual, predictive testing in at-risk relatives is critical. Family members who test negative can be spared the increased surveillance and risk-reducing procedures that are warranted for family members who test positive. It is important that health care providers involved in the care of patients with hereditary colonic polyposis conditions stay updated with management guidelines as recommendations are constantly evolving.

REFERENCES

1. Petersen GM, Slack J, Nakamura Y. Screening guidelines and premorbid diagnosis of familial adenomatous polyposis using linkage. *Gastroenterology.* 1991;100:1658–1664.
2. Foulkes WD. A tale of four syndromes: Familial adenomatous polyposis, Gardner syndrome, attenuated APC and Turcot syndrome. *QJM.* 1995;88:853–863.
3. Jasperson KW, Tuohy TM, Neklason DW, et al. Hereditary and familial colon cancer. *Gastroenterology.* 2010;138:2044–2058.
4. Burt RW, Leppert MF, Slattery ML, et al. Genetic testing and phenotype in a large kindred with attenuated familial adenomatous polyposis. *Gastroenterology.* 2004;127:444–451.
5. Gallagher MC, Phillips RK, Bulow S. Surveillance and management of upper gastrointestinal disease in familial adenomatous polyposis. *Fam Cancer.* 2006;5:263–273.
6. Jasperson KW, Burt RW. APC-associated polyposis conditions. In: Pagon RA, Bird TD, Dolan CR, et al., eds. *Gene Reviews.* Seattle, WA: University of Washington. 1993.
7. Burt RW. Gastric fundic gland polyps. *Gastroenterology.* 2003;125:1462–1469.
8. Garrean S, Hering J, Saied A, et al. Gastric adenocarcinoma arising from fundic gland polyps in a patient with familial adenomatous polyposis syndrome. *Am Surg.* 2008;74:79–83.
9. Nieuwenhuis MH, Casparie M, Mathus-Vliegen LM, et al. A nation-wide study comparing sporadic and familial adenomatous polyposis-related desmoid-type fibromatoses. *Int J Cancer.* 2011;129:256–261.
10. Nieuwenhuis MH, Lefevre JH, Bulow S, et al. Family history, surgery, and APC mutation are risk factors for desmoid tumors in familial adenomatous polyposis: An international cohort study. *Dis Colon Rectum.* 2011;54:1229–1234.
11. Sinha A, Tekkis PP, Gibbons DC, et al. Risk factors predicting desmoid occurrence in patients with familial adenomatous polyposis: A meta-analysis. *Colorectal Dis.* 2011;13:1222–1229.
12. Nieuwenhuis MH, Mathus-Vliegen EM, Baeten CG, et al. Evaluation of management of desmoid tumours associated with familial adenomatous polyposis in Dutch patients. *Br J Cancer.* 2011;104:37–42.
13. NCCN clinical practice guidelines in oncology. Colorectal cancer screening; V1.2012. 2012. Available at: http://www.nccn.org. Accessed on April 3, 2012.
14. Guillem JG, Wood WC, Moley JF, et al. ASCO/SSO review of current role of risk-reducing surgery in common hereditary cancer syndromes. *J Clin Oncol.* 2006;24:4642–4660.
15. Bulow S, Christensen IJ, Hojen H, et al. Duodenal surveillance improves the prognosis after duodenal cancer in familial adenomatous polyposis. *Colorectal Dis.* 2011;14:947–952. doi: 10.1111/j.1463-1318.2011.02844.x.

16. Cromwell DM, Moore RD, Brensinger JD, et al. Cost analysis of alternative approaches to colorectal screening in familial adenomatous polyposis. *Gastroenterology*. 1998;114:893–901.

17. Hes FJ, Nielsen M, Bik EC, et al. Somatic APC mosaicism: An underestimated cause of polyposis coli. *Gut*. 2008;57:71–76.

18. Al-Tassan N, Chmiel NH, Maynard J, et al. Inherited variants of MYH associated with somatic G:C–>T:A mutations in colorectal tumors. *Nat Genet*. 2002;30:227–232.

19. Lubbe SJ, Di Bernardo MC, Chandler IP, et al. Clinical implications of the colorectal cancer risk associated with MUTYH mutation. *J Clin Oncol*. 2009;27:3975–3980.

20. Cleary SP, Cotterchio M, Jenkins MA, et al. Germline MutY human homologue mutations and colorectal cancer: A multisite case-control study. *Gastroenterology*. 2009;136:1251–1260.

21. Jenkins MA, Croitoru ME, Monga N, et al. Risk of colorectal cancer in monoallelic and biallelic carriers of MYH mutations: A population-based case-family study. *Cancer Epidemiol Biomarkers Prev*. 2006;15:312–314.

22. Vogt S, Jones N, Christian D, et al. Expanded extracolonic tumor spectrum in MUTYH-associated polyposis. *Gastroenterology*. 2009;137:1976–1985, e1–e10.

23. Nielsen M, Morreau H, Vasen HF, et al. MUTYH-associated polyposis (MAP). *Crit Rev Oncol Hematol*. 2011;79:1–16.

24. Snover DC, Ahnen DJ, Burt RW, et al. Serrated polyps of the colon and rectum and serrated polyposis. In: Bosman FT, Carneiro F, Hruban RH, et al, eds. *WHO Classification of Tumours of the Digestive System*. 4th ed. Lyon, France: IARC; 2010:160–165.

25. Boparai KS, Dekker E, Van Eeden S, et al. Hyperplastic polyps and sessile serrated adenomas as a phenotypic expression of MYH-associated polyposis. *Gastroenterology*. 2008;135:2014–2018.

26. Chow E, Lipton L, Lynch E, et al. Hyperplastic polyposis syndrome: Phenotypic presentations and the role of MBD4 and MYH. *Gastroenterology*. 2006;131:30–39.

27. Zorcolo L, Fantola G, Balestrino L, et al. MUTYH-associated colon disease: Adenomatous polyposis is only one of the possible phenotypes. A family report and literature review. *Tumori*. 2011;97:676–680.

28. Out AA, Wasielewski M, Huijts PE, et al. MUTYH gene variants and breast cancer in a Dutch case-control study. *Breast Cancer Res Treat*. 2012;134:219–227. doi: 10.1007/s10549-012-1965-0.

29. Santonocito C, Paradisi A, Capizzi R, et al. Common genetic variants of MUTYH are not associated with cutaneous malignant melanoma: Application of molecular screening by means of high-resolution melting technique in a pilot case-control study. *Int J Biol Markers*. 2011;26:37–42.

30. Schwab AL, Tuohy TM, Condie M, et al. Gonadal mosaicism and familial adenomatous polyposis. *Fam Cancer*. 2008;7:173–177.

31. Nielsen M, Hes FJ, Vasen HF, et al. Cost-utility analysis of genetic screening in families of patients with germline MUTYH mutations. *BMC Med Genet*. 2007;8:42.

32. Goodenberger M, Lindor NM. Lynch syndrome and MYH-associated polyposis: Review and testing strategy. *J Clin Gastroenterol*. 2011;45:488–500.

33. Wang L, Baudhuin LM, Boardman LA, et al. MYH mutations in patients with attenuated and classic polyposis and with young-onset colorectal cancer without polyps. *Gastroenterology*. 2004;127:9–16.

34. Offerhaus GJA, Billaud M, Gruber SB. Peutz–Jeghers syndrome. In: Bosman FT, Carneiro F, Hruban RH, et al., eds. *WHO Classification of Tumours of the Digestive System*. 4th ed. Lyon, France: IARC; 2010:168–170.

35. Latchford AR, Phillips RK. Gastrointestinal polyps and cancer in Peutz–Jeghers syndrome: Clinical aspects. *Fam Cancer*. 2011;10:455–461.

36. Hearle N, Schumacher V, Menko FH, et al. Frequency and spectrum of cancers in the Peutz–Jeghers syndrome. *Clin Cancer Res*. 2006;12:3209–3215.

37. Gammon A, Jasperson K, Kohlmann W, et al. Hamartomatous polyposis syndromes. *Best Pract Res Clin Gastroenterol*. 2009;23:219–231.

38. Offerhaus GJ, Howe JR. Juvenile polyposis. In: Bosman FT, Carneiro F, Hruban RH, et al., eds. *WHO Classification of Tumours of the Digestive System*. 4th ed. Lyon, France: IARC; 2010:166–167.

39. Pilarski R. Cowden syndrome: A critical review of the clinical literature. *J Genet Couns*. 2009;18:13–27.

40. Tan MH, Mester JL, Ngeow J, et al. Lifetime cancer risks in individuals with germline PTEN mutations. *Clin Cancer Res.* 2012;18:400–407.
41. Heald B, Mester J, Rybicki L, et al. Frequent gastrointestinal polyps and colorectal adenocarcinomas in a prospective series of PTEN mutation carriers. *Gastroenterology.* 2010;139:1927–1933.
42. Sweet K, Willis J, Zhou XP, et al. Molecular classification of patients with unexplained hamartomatous and hyperplastic polyposis. *JAMA.* 2005;294:2465–2473.

8 Genetic Testing by Cancer Site

Colon (Nonpolyposis Syndromes)

Leigha Senter

Approximately 5% to 10% of colorectal cancers (CRCs) are hereditary and are often categorized by the presence or absence of polyposis as a predominant feature. Lynch syndrome (LS), also sometimes referred to as hereditary nonpolyposis CRC, is the most common form of hereditary CRC, accounting for approximately 2.2%[1] of population-based CRC diagnosed in the United States. LS also accounts for 2.3%[2] of all newly diagnosed endometrial cancers (ECs), and individuals with LS also have an increased risk of developing other cancers, including cancers of the ovary, stomach, small bowel, urothelium, and biliary tract.[3] Given these increased cancer risks, cancer screening recommendations for individuals with LS differ significantly from general population screening recommendations with a goal of reducing cancer risk and burden to the extent possible.

Mutations in 1 of 4 mismatch repair genes (*MLH1*, *MSH2*, *MSH6*, and *PMS2*) cause LS, and clinical genetic testing is available for all of them. Unlike most other hereditary cancer syndromes, though, clinical testing for LS typically begins with microsatellite instability (MSI) testing and/or immunohistochemical (IHC) staining of tumor tissue before germline genetic testing. This difference in testing approach, although not always possible, allows for targeted genetic analysis and, in most cases, reduced cost. Here, we review key considerations in genetic counseling for LS.

CANCER RISKS

CRC and EC are the two most common LS-associated malignancies, and there have been several calculations of lifetime cancer risks reported in the literature. Differences in ascertainment and testing approaches have led not only to wealth of data but also to a wide range of risk estimates for consideration by clinicians and patients. Consistently, studies have found that the lifetime CRC risk for men with LS is higher than the risk for women with LS. The lifetime CRC for males is 27% to 92%, whereas the risk for females is 22% to 68%.[4,5] The most recent large study of carriers of *MLH1*, *MSH2*, and *MSH6* mutations estimated lifetime CRC risks for males and

125

females to be 38% and 31%, respectively.[6] The average age at CRC diagnosis tends to be younger in LS (estimated 45 to 59 years) than that in the general population.[6,7] The lifetime risk of EC for women with LS based on recent data is estimated to be 33% to 39%.[6,8] Individuals with LS who have already been diagnosed with CRC also have an increased risk (10-year risk of 16%) of developing a second primary CRC.[9]

In addition to sex differences in LS-associated cancer risks, there appear to be some differences in gene-specific–associated cancer risks, as well. *MLH1* and *MSH2* seem to be associated with a higher overall cancer risk than risks associated with *MSH6* or *PMS2*.[10,11] Variable expression of phenotype both within and among families with LS is common. Therefore, as a general rule, management of families with LS (discussed later) should always take into account the family history.

Malignancies of the ovary, stomach, small bowel, urothelium, and biliary tract are also seen with greater frequency in individuals with LS when compared with the general population. Although cumulative risk estimates of these less common tumor types have been published, they are usually based on fewer cases than studies focused on CRC and EC, and have typically shown a lifetime cancer risk of less than 10%.[3] There have also been reports of LS-associated pancreatic and breast cancers, but the data have been inconsistent. A recent prospective study showed an increased risk of developing both tumor types when comparing carriers of *MMR* gene mutations to their unaffected relatives.[12] Additional data are necessary, however, to determine whether screening recommendations should change based on these reported risks.

Some individuals with LS also have a predisposition to developing sebaceous lesions and keratoacanthomas of the skin. When an individual has one of these lesions in addition to a visceral organ malignancy, they have a variant of LS called Muir–Torre syndrome.[13] Some recent studies suggest that these skin lesions are more common in LS than originally thought and that sebaceous tumors of the skin should be considered part of the typical LS spectrum.[14]

Another variant of LS characterized by the presence of glioblastomas is called Turcot syndrome. Turcot syndrome is more commonly caused by mutations in the *APC* gene but has been described in individuals with MMR deficiency, as well.[15]

CLINICAL CLASSIFICATION: AMSTERDAM CRITERIA AND BETHESDA GUIDELINES

In 1991, the International Collaborative Group on Hereditary Non-Polyposis CRC wrote the Amsterdam I criteria[16] and revised them in 1999 (Amsterdam II criteria)[17] to clinically classify families as having LS (Table 8.1). The Amsterdam criteria rely heavily on extensive family history and do not take into account the full spectrum of possible LS-associated tumors. The less stringent Bethesda guidelines (written in 1997 and revised in 2004)[18,19] (Table 8.2) were written to include these less common LS-associated tumors as well as pathologic features that are common in LS-associated CRCs. Unlike the Amsterdam criteria, which were meant to diagnose LS based on familial criteria, the Bethesda guidelines were meant to determine who should have

TABLE 8.1	**Revised Amsterdam Criteria**

≥3 relatives with colorectal, endometrial, small bowel, ureter, and/or renal pelvis cancer and
1 of these relatives is a first-degree relative[a] of the other 2 and
≥2 successive generations are affected and
At least 1 diagnosis is at the age of <50 y
Familial adenomatous polyposis is excluded
Tumors should be verified pathologically/histologically

[a]First-degree relative: Parent, sibling, or child.

From: Vasen HF, Watson P, Mecklin JP, et al. New clinical criteria for hereditary nonpolyposis colorectal cancer (HNPCC, Lynch syndrome) proposed by the International Collaborative group on HNPCC. *Gastroenterology*. 1999;116:1453–1456.

tumor screening for LS and relied less on family history. It has been repeatedly shown, however, that these clinical classification systems do not reliably predict LS in all patient populations, particularly those outside the cancer genetics clinics dedicated to high-risk patients.[1,20]

TABLE 8.2	**Revised Bethesda Guidelines**

Individuals with CRC should be tested for MSI if they have any of the following:
- CRC at the age of <50 y
- Synchronous CRC (>1 CRC at the same time) or metachronous CRC (>1 CRC diagnosed at different times) or other LS-associated tumors[a]
- CRC with MSI-H histology (tumor-infiltrating lymphocytes, Crohn-like lymphocytic reaction, mucinous or signet-ring differentiation, medullary growth pattern) in a patient aged <60 y
- CRC or LS-associated tumor[a] diagnosed at the age of <50 y in FDR
- CRC or LS-associated tumor[a] in 2 FDR and/or SDR at any age

[a]CRC, EC, stomach, small bowel, ovary, pancreas, ureter and renal pelvis, biliary tract, brain tumor, sebaceous adenomas, keratoacanthomas.

FDR, first-degree relative (parent, sibling, child); SDR, second-degree relative (grandparent, aunt, uncle, grandchild).

From: Umar A, Boland CR, Terdiman JP, et al. Revised Bethesda guidelines for hereditary nonpolyposis colorectal cancer (Lynch syndrome) and microsatellite instability. *J Natl Cancer Inst*. 2004;96:261–268.

TUMOR SCREENING

Microsatellites are pieces of DNA sequence where a single nucleotide or group of nucleotides is repeated multiple times. In general, the number of repeated nucleotide sequences should remain the same within a person's cells, but when this number of repeats differs in one or two alleles, MSI is present.[21] In the case of LS, five microsatellite markers are used as the standard with which to measure MSI, and a tumor is considered to have a high level of MSI (MSI-H) if at least 40% of the markers are unstable.[22] Nearly all LS-associated tumors display MSI, but the presence of MSI is not diagnostic of LS, given that approximately 10% to 15% of all CRCs, in general, also display MSI.[23,24] MSI testing, however, can be used as a screening test to help identify individuals for whom germline genetic testing for mutations in *MLH1*, *MSH2*, *MSH6*, and/or *PMS2* is indicated. A clinical diagnosis of LS can be made if a person has an MSI-H CRC and meets the Amsterdam II criteria (Table 8.1).

Immunohistochemistry can be used to determine the presence or absence of MMR proteins in a tumor specimen and is another available screening test for LS. The absence of one or more MMR proteins in tumor tissue indicates dysfunction of the corresponding *MMR* gene, but additional analyses are required to determine if the dysfunction is germline or somatic in nature. The benefit of performing IHC staining over MSI testing is that results from IHC staining can direct the approach to genetic testing. For instance, if a patient has CRC that demonstrates absence of MSH2 and MSH6 proteins, testing for MSH2 with procession to testing for MSH6 if the MSH2 test results are negative is recommended. In the context of this IHC result, it is generally not necessary to test for mutations in *MLH1* and/or *PMS2*. Strategies for genetic testing based on IHC results are included in Table 8.3.[25,26] In comparing

TABLE 8.3	Genetic Testing Strategies Based on IHC Pattern
Absence MLH1 and PMS2	*MLH1* methylation and/or *BRAF* testing[a] OR *MLH1* germline testing[b] • If negative, consider *PMS2* germline testing[20]
Absence PMS2 only	*PMS2* germline testing • If negative consider *MLH1* germline testing[21]
Absence MSH2 and MSH6	*MSH2* germline testing • If negative, *TACSTD1* deletion testing • If negative, *MSH6* germline testing
Absence MSH6 only	*MSH6* germline testing • If negative, consider *MSH2* germline testing

[a]If personal/family history highly suggestive of LS, it is appropriate to forgo *MLH1* methylation/*BRAF* testing.
[b]Unless otherwise noted, "germline testing" here refers to sequencing/large rearrangement testing.

tumor screening strategies, using MSI and IHC staining together will identify the majority of LS cases. Since the sensitivity of either test is not 100%, using either test alone will leave 5% to 10% of LS cases undetected.[27,28]

Epigenetic events unrelated to LS can cause a tumor to demonstrate MSI and absence of MLH1 and PMS2 proteins upon IHC staining. These results can often be attributed to hypermethylation of the *MLH1* promoter and/or a somatic *BRAF* mutation (V600E). Several studies have shown that the V600E *BRAF* mutations are not associated with LS, and there have been very few exceptions.[11,29] Both of these tests can be performed on CRC tissue to help determine whether germline genetic testing should be pursued, further streamlining the genetic testing process but should be interpreted in the context of clinical familial presentation because sensitivities and specificities for these tests are not 100%. It is important to note that it is possible but rare to have inherited *MLH1* promoter hypermethylation.[30]

Similar approaches to screening EC with MSI and/or IHC staining are appropriate. However, because somatic *BRAF* mutations are uncommon in ECs, *BRAF* testing is not an appropriate test for ECs that are MSI-H and/or MLH1 and PMS2 protein deficient.[31] There are less data to support MSI and/or IHC testing using other LS-associated tumor tissue, but many reports suggest that it is at least feasible in the absence of additional testing options.[32]

In 2009, the Evaluation of Genomic Application in Practice and Prevention Working Group recommended that individuals with newly diagnosed CRC be offered genetic testing for LS. Although the Evaluation of Genomic Application in Practice and Prevention working group did not specify the best approach for genetic testing, performing tumor analysis with IHC staining allows for more targeted genetic testing and was considered to be an acceptable strategy.[33] In addition, multiple reports have shown that tumor screening with IHC staining is a cost-effective strategy for identifying LS in the CRC patient population.[34,35] Ladabaum et al.[35] compared the differences among multiple testing strategies with regard to effect of life years, cancer morbidity and mortality, and cost. They concluded that IHC staining with inclusion of *BRAF* gene testing if MLH1 protein was absent was the preferred method of identifying LS among CRC patients.[35] Effectiveness of screening for LS in these reports has been dependent on the ability to test family members of the initially diagnosed LS patient, so genetic counseling and dissemination of information to relatives of probands are crucial for effective diagnosis and prevention of cancer.

GENETIC TESTING

In many situations, as mentioned above, tumor screening tests are performed before germline genetic testing, but there are situations where this is not possible or desired (e.g., sufficient tumor tissue is unavailable, or all individuals affected with cancer in a family are deceased). In the absence of IHC results to direct genetic testing, germline testing is typically done in a stepwise fashion beginning with *MLH1* and *MSH2*, which account for 32% and 38% of mutations, respectively.[9] If no mutations are identified, testing for mutations in *MSH6* and *PMS2* is indicated. Mutations in these 2 genes are less common and account for 14% and 15% of LS, respectively.[9] It is important for testing to include sequencing as well as analysis of deletions and duplications because all mutation types have been reported in the *MMR* genes.

Recently, deletions in *TACSTD1* (also known as *EPCAM*), which is not an *MMR* gene, have been reported to cause inactivation of *MSH2* and lack of expression of MSH2 protein when IHC staining is performed. Therefore, testing for deletions in *TACSTD1* is indicated when MSH2 protein is absent on IHC staining, but no germline *MSHS2* mutation has been identified.[36]

GENETIC COUNSELING FOR LS

Inherited in an autosomal dominant manner, first-degree relatives of individuals with LS have a 50% chance of having inherited the syndrome, as well, making communication of these risks to family members of patients with LS very important. Data have shown that compliance with the screening recommendations reviewed below is effective in reducing the risk of dying of cancer in individuals with LS, and this should be communicated to at-risk families. A large study of *MMR* mutation carriers in Finland found that despite the increased risks of CRC and EC, cancer mortality was not increased when individuals followed the intensive screening protocol and/or opted to have prophylactic surgery.[37]

MANAGEMENT OF LS

Individuals with LS require personalized management planning with the goal of reducing their cancer risks. Although many groups have put forth screening recommendations in the literature, the LS surveillance and screening recommendations from the National Comprehensive Cancer Network, which are updated annually, are used commonly in clinical practice. Based on these current recommendations, individuals with LS should have colonoscopy every 1 to 2 years beginning at the age of 20 to 25 years or 2 to 5 years earlier than the youngest CRC in the family if diagnosed before the age of 25 years (colonoscopy may be recommended to start at the age of 30 years in families with *MSH6* and *PMS2* mutations if the CRC age at onset in the family is not younger than the age of 30 years given the reduced penetrance with these genes). Given that there is no clear evidence to support screening for endometrial and/or ovarian cancers, women with LS are recommended to consider prophylactic hysterectomy and bilateral salpingo-oophorectomy upon completion of childbearing. Some clinicians may find endometrial sampling, transvaginal ultrasound, and CA-125 serum screening to be helpful; however, these tools should be used at their discretion. To screen for gastric and small-bowel cancers, individuals with LS should consider esophagogastroduodenoscopy with extended duodenoscopy and capsule endoscopy every 2 to 3 years beginning at the age of 30 to 35 years. Annual urinalysis beginning at the age of 25 to 30 years can be used to screen for urothelial cancers, and an annual physical examination to assess for symptoms of central nervous system tumors is reasonable.[38]

A 2011 study by Burn et al.[39] showed through a randomized trial with postintervention double-blind follow-up that daily use of 600 mg of aspirin for a minimum of

25 months reduced the risk of CRC by almost 60% in individuals with LS. Like other studies of aspirin use on cancer risk, cumulative use seemed to make a difference in the study as reduced risk became evident over time. The optimum dose and duration of use of aspirin in individuals with LS still need to be established, but based on this evidence, many clinicians are considering aspirin therapy as chemoprevention in this population.

ACKNOWLEDGMENT

The author thanks Kory Jasperson for his review of the manuscript.

REFERENCES

1. Hampel H, Frankel WL, Martin E, et al. Screening for the Lynch syndrome (hereditary nonpolyposis colorectal cancer). *N Engl J Med.* 2005;352:1851–1860.
2. Hampel H, Panescu J, Lockman J, et al. Comment on: Screening for Lynch syndrome (hereditary nonpolyposis colorectal cancer) among endometrial cancer patients. *Cancer Res.* 2007;67:9603.
3. Barrow E, Robinson L, Alduaij W, et al. Cumulative lifetime incidence of extracolonic cancers in Lynch syndrome: A report of 121 families with proven mutations. *Clin Genet.* 2009;75:141–149.
4. Vasen HF, Wijnen JT, Menko FH, et al. Cancer risk in families with hereditary nonpolyposis colorectal cancer diagnosed by mutation analysis. *Gastroenterology.* 1996;110:1020–1027.
5. Quehenberger F, Vasen HF, van Houwelingen HC. Risk of colorectal and endometrial cancer for carriers of mutations of the hMLH1 and hMSH2 gene: Correction for ascertainment. *J Med Genet.* 2005;42:491–496.
6. Bonadona V, Bonaiti B, Olschwang S, et al. Cancer risks associated with germline mutations in MLH1, MSH2, and MSH6 genes in Lynch syndrome. *JAMA.* 2011;305:2304–2310.
7. Hampel H, Stephens JA, Pukkala E, et al. Cancer risk in hereditary nonpolyposis colorectal cancer syndrome: Later age of onset. *Gastroenterology.* 2005;129:415–421.
8. Stoffel E, Mukherjee B, Raymond VM, et al. Calculation of risk of colorectal and endometrial cancer among patients with Lynch syndrome. *Gastroenterology.* 2009;137:1621–1627.
9. Palomaki GE, McClain MR, Melillo S, et al. EGAPP supplementary evidence review: DNA testing strategies aimed at reducing morbidity and mortality from Lynch syndrome. *Genet Med.* 2009;11:42–65.
10. Baglietto L, Lindor NM, Dowty JG, et al. Risks of Lynch syndrome cancers for MSH6 mutation carriers. *J Natl Cancer Inst.* 2010;102:193–201.
11. Senter L, Clendenning M, Sotamaa K, et al. The clinical phenotype of Lynch syndrome due to germline PMS2 mutations. *Gastroenterology.* 2008;135:419–428.
12. Win AK, Young JP, Lindor NM, et al. Colorectal and other cancer risks for carriers and noncarriers from families with a DNA mismatch repair gene mutation: A prospective cohort study. *J Clin Oncol.* 2012;30:958–964.
13. Lynch HT, Lynch PM, Pester J, et al. The cancer family syndrome. Rare cutaneous phenotypic linkage of Torre's syndrome. *Arch Intern Med.* 1981;141:607–611.
14. South CD, Hampel H, Comeras I, et al. The frequency of Muir-Torre syndrome among Lynch syndrome families. *J Natl Cancer Inst.* 2008;100:277–281.
15. Hamilton SR, Liu B, Parsons RE, et al. The molecular basis of Turcot's syndrome. *N Engl J Med.* 1995;332:839–847.
16. Vasen HF, Mecklin JP, Khan PM, et al. The International Collaborative Group on Hereditary Non-Polyposis Colorectal Cancer (ICG-HNPCC). *Dis Colon Rectum.* 1991;34:424–425.
17. Vasen HF, Watson P, Mecklin JP, et al. New clinical criteria for hereditary nonpolyposis colorectal cancer (HNPCC, Lynch syndrome) proposed by the International Collaborative group on HNPCC. *Gastroenterology.* 1999;116:1453–1456.

18. Rodriguez-Bigas MA, Boland CR, Hamilton SR, et al. A National Cancer Institute Workshop on Hereditary Nonpolyposis Colorectal Cancer Syndrome: Meeting highlights and Bethesda guidelines. *J Natl Cancer Inst.* 1997;89:1758–1762.

19. Umar A, Boland CR, Terdiman JP, et al. Revised Bethesda guidelines for hereditary nonpolyposis colorectal cancer (Lynch syndrome) and microsatellite instability. *J Natl Cancer Inst.* 2004;96:261–268.

20. Morrison J, Bronner M, Leach BH, et al. Lynch syndrome screening in newly diagnosed colorectal cancer in general pathology practice: From the revised Bethesda guidelines to a universal approach. *Scand J Gastroenterol.* 2012;46:1340–1348.

21. de la Chapelle A, Hampel H. Clinical relevance of microsatellite instability in colorectal cancer. *J Clin Oncol.* 2010;28:3380–3387.

22. Boland CR, Thibodeau SN, Hamilton SR, et al. A National Cancer Institute Workshop on Microsatellite Instability for cancer detection and familial predisposition: Development of international criteria for the determination of microsatellite instability in colorectal cancer. *Cancer Res.* 1998;58:5248–5257.

23. Hampel H, Frankel WL, Martin E, et al. Feasibility of screening for Lynch syndrome among patients with colorectal cancer. *J Clin Oncol.* 2008;26:5783–5788.

24. Samowitz WS, Curtin K, Lin HH, et al. The colon cancer burden of genetically defined hereditary nonpolyposis colon cancer. *Gastroenterology.* 2001;121:830–838.

25. Niessen RC, Kleibeuker JH, Westers H, et al. PMS2 involvement in patients suspected of Lynch syndrome. *Genes Chromosomes Cancer.* 2009;48:322–329.

26. Zighelboim I, Powell MA, Babb SA, et al. Epitope-positive truncating MLH1 mutation and loss of PMS2: Implications for IHC-directed genetic testing for Lynch syndrome. *Fam Cancer.* 2009;8:501–504.

27. Lindor NM, Burgart LJ, Leontovich O, et al. Immunohistochemistry versus microsatellite instability testing in phenotyping colorectal tumors. *J Clin Oncol.* 2002;20:1043–1048.

28. Ruszkiewicz A, Bennett G, Moore J, et al. Correlation of mismatch repair genes immunohistochemistry and microsatellite instability status in HNPCC-associated tumours. *Pathology.* 2002;34:541–547.

29. Loughrey MB, Waring PM, Tan A, et al. Incorporation of somatic BRAF mutation testing into an algorithm for the investigation of hereditary non-polyposis colorectal cancer. *Fam Cancer.* 2007;6:301–310.

30. Hitchins MP, Ward RL. Constitutional (germline) MLH1 epimutation as an aetiological mechanism for hereditary non-polyposis colorectal cancer. *J Med Genet.* 2009;46:793–802.

31. Mutch DG, Powell MA, Mallon MA, et al. RAS/RAF mutation and defective DNA mismatch repair in endometrial cancers. *Am J Obstet Gynecol.* 2004;190:935–942.

32. Weissman SM, Bellcross C, Bittner CC, et al. Genetic counseling considerations in the evaluation of families for Lynch syndrome—a review. *J Genet Couns.* 2011;20:5–19.

33. Recommendations from the EGAPP Working Group: Genetic testing strategies in newly diagnosed individuals with colorectal cancer aimed at reducing morbidity and mortality from Lynch syndrome in relatives. *Genet Med.* 2009;11:35–41.

34. Mvundura M, Grosse SD, Hampel H, et al. The cost-effectiveness of genetic testing strategies for Lynch syndrome among newly diagnosed patients with colorectal cancer. *Genet Med.* 2010;12:93–104.

35. Ladabaum U, Wang G, Terdiman J, et al. Strategies to identify the Lynch syndrome among patients with colorectal cancer: A cost-effectiveness analysis. *Ann Intern Med.* 2011;155:69–79.

36. Niessen RC, Hofstra RM, Westers H, et al. Germline hypermethylation of MLH1 and EPCAM deletions are a frequent cause of Lynch syndrome. *Genes Chromosomes Cancer.* 2009;48:737–744.

37. Jarvinen HJ, Renkonen-Sinisalo L, Aktan-Collan K, et al. Ten years after mutation testing for Lynch syndrome: Cancer incidence and outcome in mutation-positive and mutation-negative family members. *J Clin Oncol.* 2009;27:4793–4797.

38. NCCN. NCCN Guidelines Version 1.2012: Colorectal Cancer Screening. NCCN Guidelines for Detection, Prevention, and Risk Reduction [v.1.2012]. 2012.

39. Burn J, Gerdes AM, Macrae F, et al. Long-term effect of aspirin on cancer risk in carriers of hereditary colorectal cancer: An analysis from the CAPP2 randomised controlled trial. *Lancet.* 2011;378:2081–2087.

9

Genetic Testing by Cancer Site

Uterus

Molly S. Daniels

terine cancer is the most common invasive gynecologic cancer in the United States.[1] The median age at diagnosis of uterine cancer in the general population is 60 years.[1] The average woman's lifetime risk of developing uterine cancer is approximately 2.6%.[2] The vast majority of uterine cancers are endometrial in origin. Five percent or less of uterine cancers are nonendometrial; examples include endometrial stromal sarcoma and uterine leiomyosarcoma.[3]

Endometrial cancers can be further subdivided into type I and type II. Type I endometrial cancers are endometrioid in histology and account for more than 75% of endometrial cancers. Type II endometrial cancers include all nonendometrioid histologies, such as uterine papillary serous carcinoma (UPSC), clear cell carcinoma, and carcinosarcoma (also called malignant mixed Müllerian tumor).[4] Type II endometrial cancers are generally diagnosed at later stages and have a poorer prognosis than type I endometrial cancers.[5]

Type I endometrial cancers, in particular, are associated with personal medical history risk factors, likely due to their impact on the amount of estrogen to which the endometrium is exposed. Other than long-term use of unopposed estrogen (which is no longer prescribed for women with an intact uterus because of the associated endometrial cancer risk) and hereditary cancer predisposition (which will be discussed below), the biggest risk factor for endometrial cancer is obesity. Obese women have up to a sixfold risk of endometrial cancer when compared with women at ideal body weight.[6] Other risk factors include nulliparity, early age at menarche, late age at menopause, and tamoxifen use.[6] Use of combination oral contraceptives decreases risk of endometrial cancer in the general population, with a relative risk of 0.6.[1]

This review also discusses uterine leiomyomas, commonly referred to as uterine fibroids. Uterine leiomyomas are benign smooth muscle tumors that are common in the general population. A US study found that more than 80% of black women and almost 70% of white women develop uterine leiomyomas, although not all were symptomatic.[7] Symptoms of uterine leiomyomas can include pelvic pain, infertility, pregnancy complications, and menometrorrhagia.[7]

LYNCH SYNDROME, ALSO KNOWN AS HEREDITARY NONPOLYPOSIS COLORECTAL CANCER SYNDROME

Since Lynch syndrome has been extensively described elsewhere in this book, this section focuses on Lynch syndrome–associated endometrial cancer. Lynch syndrome is an autosomal dominant hereditary cancer predisposition syndrome characterized by significantly increased risks of colorectal, endometrial, and other cancers. Mutations in the DNA mismatch repair genes *MLH1*, *MSH2*, *MSH6*, *PMS2*, and *EPCAM* (via disruption of *MSH2* expression) have been associated with Lynch syndrome.

Two to three percent of women with endometrial cancer have Lynch syndrome.[8,9] Average age at diagnosis of endometrial cancer for women with Lynch syndrome is in the 40s to 50s in many[8–10] (but not all[11]) studies, younger than the general population. The likelihood of Lynch syndrome is increased in women with endometrial cancer; diagnosed at younger than 50 years,[12,13] who have also had colorectal cancer,[14] with lower body mass index,[12] with lower uterine segment tumors,[15] or with family history of colorectal and/or endometrial cancers.[16,17] Models to assess risk of Lynch syndrome based on personal and family history are available.[16,17] The identification of Lynch syndrome in the endometrial cancer patient allows her to take steps to reduce her colorectal cancer risk and also allows family members to benefit from predictive genetic testing and subsequent targeted cancer risk reduction strategies.

The optimal way to screen endometrial cancer patients for Lynch syndrome is an area of active discussion. Historically, endometrial cancer patients with personal and/or family histories suggestive of Lynch syndrome have been referred for cancer genetic risk assessment. More recently, some institutions have undertaken universal screening of all endometrial cancer patients by immunohistochemistry (IHC) and/or microsatellite instability (MSI) analysis of the endometrial tumor.[18] The advantage to this approach is that it has the potential to detect all Lynch syndrome–associated endometrial cancers, some of which occur in the absence of a known family history and would be missed by any strategy that screens patients by family history.[8,9] Limitations to the universal screening approach include high cost per mutation identified[19] and lower than expected uptake of genetic counseling and genetic testing among endometrial cancer patients identified via universal screening.[18]

By whatever method endometrial cancer patients are selected for Lynch syndrome evaluation, the recommended first step in genetic testing is tumor studies: IHC for the mismatch repair proteins and/or MSI analysis.[20,21] Nearly all Lynch syndrome–associated endometrial cancers will demonstrate high MSI (MSI-H) and/or IHC loss of one or more mismatch repair proteins, and the IHC results often allow genetic testing to be targeted to one Lynch syndrome gene.[20] *MLH1* promoter hypermethylation analysis is recommended as a follow-up study when an endometrial tumor is MSI-H, and IHC shows loss of *MLH1* and *PMS2*, because 15% to 20% of sporadic endometrial cancers exhibit *MLH1* promoter hypermethylation.[22] Whereas sporadic MSI-H colorectal cancers often have somatic *BRAF* mutations, sporadic MSI-H endometrial cancers usually do not,[23] and therefore, *BRAF* mutation analysis is not recommended for distinguishing sporadic MSI-H endometrial cancers from Lynch syndrome–associated endometrial cancers. Lynch syndrome is confirmed by the finding of a germline mutation in a mismatch repair gene through molecular genetic testing, and family members can subsequently undergo predictive genetic testing. Currently, molecular genetic testing is not always able to identify a pathogenic Lynch syndrome mutation when tumor studies are suggestive of Lynch syndrome; possible explanations in these cases include limited genetic test sensitivity for the known mismatch repair genes, other as yet unidentified Lynch syndrome genes, and as yet unidentified other epigenetic causes for the tumor phenotype. Given that Lynch syndrome has not been ruled out in a patient with suggestive tumor studies and negative genetic test results, consideration should be given to following Lynch syndrome management guidelines in these cases.[20,21]

The lifetime risk of endometrial cancer for women with Lynch syndrome has been recently reported as 33% to 40%.[10,24] Endometrial cancer risk may vary by gene, with risks highest for women with *MLH1*, *MSH2*, and *MSH6* mutations. Lower endometrial cancer risks have been reported for women with *PMS2* mutations (15% lifetime risk[25]) or *EPCAM* mutations (up to 12% lifetime risk[26,27]). Lynch syndrome–associated endometrial cancers can be both type I (endometrioid) and type II (nonendometrioid); nonendometrioid histologies observed in women with Lynch syndrome include clear cell carcinoma, UPSC, and malignant mixed Müllerian tumor (carcinosarcoma).[28]

Given the high risk of endometrial cancer for women with Lynch syndrome, both cancer screening and risk reduction options should be considered. Patient education regarding endometrial cancer symptoms (such as abnormal vaginal bleeding) and the importance of reporting them promptly are also important.[21] In terms of risk reduction, hysterectomy (plus bilateral salpingo-oophorectomy [BSO], because ovarian cancer risk is also elevated) is clearly effective in preventing endometrial cancer[29] and can be considered if childbearing is completed and/or after menopause.[21,30,31] If a woman with Lynch syndrome is undergoing surgery for colon cancer, concomitant hysterectomy/BSO can be considered.[30,31] Risk-reducing hysterectomy/BSO has not been demonstrated to reduce mortality in women with Lynch syndrome. Oral contraceptives reduce risk of endometrial and ovarian cancer in the general population[1]; their efficacy in women with Lynch syndrome has not been determined. There is no proven benefit to endometrial cancer screening in women with Lynch syndrome; screening guidelines are based on expert opinion. Transvaginal ultrasound alone does not appear to be an effective screening test in this population[32,33]; endometrial biopsy plus transvaginal ultrasound may be more effective.[34] The National Comprehensive Cancer Network currently recommends considering annual endometrial biopsy as an option.[21]

PTEN HAMARTOMA TUMOR SYNDROME (ALSO KNOWN AS COWDEN SYNDROME, BANNAYAN–RUVALCABA–RILEY SYNDROME)

Since PTEN hamartoma tumor syndrome (PHTS) has also been extensively described elsewhere in this book, this section focuses on uterine manifestations of PHTS. PHTS is a rare autosomal dominant syndrome defined by the presence of a pathogenic *PTEN* mutation. PHTS can manifest in many organ systems, with phenotypic effects ranging from autism[35,36] to increased cancer risk[37,38] to characteristic mucocutaneous lesions.[39]

Uterine leiomyomas have been described as a common finding in women with PHTS,[40] and uterine leiomyomas are included as a minor diagnostic criterion of PHTS.[39] However, given the high prevalence of uterine leiomyomas in the general population,[7] it is not clear whether the prevalence is actually elevated in PHTS.[38,41] Uterine leiomyomas are a nonspecific finding and should not by themselves be considered particularly suggestive of PHTS.[38,41]

Endometrial cancer has been reported to occur at increased frequency in women with PHTS.[37,41] Reported ages at endometrial cancer diagnosis have been mostly in the 30s to 50s.[39,42] Endometrial cancer has been reported in adolescence in PHTS.[43] Endometrial cancer has been observed in 12 (17%) of 69[41] and 25 (16%) of 158[39] of adult women who were referred for *PTEN* genetic testing and tested positive. Data regarding lifetime risk of endometrial cancer in PHTS are sparse; studies to date have focused on probands and are thus subject to significant ascertainment bias. Therefore, a recent estimate of lifetime endometrial cancer risk in PHTS of 28%[37] is likely a significant overestimation. PHTS appears to account for a very small proportion of unselected endometrial cancers; a study by Black et al.[44] found no germline *PTEN* mutations in a series of 240 endometrial cancer patients.

In light of the limited data regarding lifetime risk of endometrial cancer for women with PHTS, the National Comprehensive Cancer Network does not currently recommend a specific endometrial cancer screening strategy beyond educating women to respond promptly to symptoms and considering enrollment in a clinical trial to determine effectiveness and necessity of screening.[45] Others have suggested that women with PHTS undergo annual endometrial biopsy and/or transvaginal ultrasound.[37,40] To date, there is no proven benefit to these screening strategies in the context of PHTS. Based on the lack of efficacy of transvaginal ultrasound as an endometrial cancer screening test for women with Lynch syndrome discussed above, if screening is undertaken, ultrasound may not be the ideal modality. The National Comprehensive Cancer Network also notes that risk-reducing hysterectomy can be discussed as an option on a case-by-case basis.[45]

HEREDITARY LEIOMYOMATOSIS AND RENAL CELL CARCINOMA

Hereditary leiomyomatosis and renal cell carcinoma (HLRCC) (OMIM 150800) is characterized by increased risk of type 2 papillary renal cell carcinoma, cutaneous leiomyomas, and uterine leiomyomas. The fumarate hydratase (*FH*) gene is the only gene that has been associated with HLRCC. HLRCC exhibits autosomal dominant inheritance. Both point mutations and large rearrangements of the *FH* gene have been reported in individuals with HLRCC.[46] If germline mutations in both copies of the *FH* gene are present, this causes the severe autosomal recessive condition fumarase deficiency (OMIM 606812), which is characterized by encephalopathy and psychomotor retardation, and is frequently lethal in infancy or childhood.

The uterine leiomyomas seen in the context of HLRCC tend to occur at younger ages than in the general population, with a mean age at diagnosis around 30 years.[47,48] Women with HLRCC frequently report complications from uterine leiomyomas, including symptoms of menorrhagia, pelvic pain, and reduced fertility,[49] and are more likely than women with uterine leiomyomas who do not have HLRCC to have had treatment, including hysterectomy.[48] In a study of North Americans with HLRCC, 98% of women had uterine leiomyomas, and 89% had undergone hysterectomy, often before the age of 30 years.[47]

Uterine leiomyosarcoma has been reported in Finnish women with HLRCC, but a recent review notes that only one clinically malignant uterine leiomyosarcoma has been confirmed in a patient with an *FH* germline mutation.[50] Therefore, to what extent the risk of uterine leiomyosarcoma may be elevated over that in the general population is not yet clear. It also appears that germline *FH* mutations are not common in women with isolated uterine leiomyosarcoma; a series of 67 uterine leiomyosarcomas diagnosed in Finland were tested for *FH* mutations, and only one patient was found to have a *FH* missense sequence variant, which was present in both tumor and normal tissue but is of uncertain significance.[51]

The presence of multiple cutaneous leiomyomas should prompt consideration of HLRCC; studies of patients with multiple cutaneous leiomyomas have found *FH* mutations in 80% to 89%.[47,49,52] Cutaneous leiomyomas vary in appearance; biopsy is required for diagnosis.[49] Pain and paresthesias associated with cutaneous leiomyomas are frequently reported.[47] Ages at onset were reported to be from 10 to 47 years, with mean age at onset of 25 years.[47] The absence of cutaneous leiomyomas does not exclude the possibility of HLRCC; some patients with HLRCC showed no evidence of cutaneous leiomyoma after detailed skin examination.[47,53] Rarely, cutaneous leiomyosarcoma has been reported with HLRCC.[47,53]

The type 2 papillary renal cell carcinomas associated with HLRCC are usually unilateral and unifocal but nonetheless appear to be aggressive in that they can already be metastatic when the primary tumor is still small (<1 cm).[50] Penetrance of renal cell carcinoma in HLRCC has been reported as approximately 20%.[52] Age at diagnosis of renal cell carcinoma has been reported as early as 11 years[54] and 16 years,[49] with average age at diagnosis in the 40s.[47,52] Other types of kidney cancer have also been reported in patients with HLRCC, including collecting duct carcinoma, oncocytoma, clear cell renal cell carcinoma, and Wilms tumor.[50]

Given the relative rarity of HLRCC (estimated approximately 180 families identified worldwide[50]), guidelines for screening and management are still evolving and are based on expert opinion only. Pediatric kidney cancers have been reported in HLRCC but appear to be rare; thus, there is some debate regarding at what age predictive genetic should be offered as well as at what age screening should begin. Proposed kidney cancer screening recommendations have included magnetic resonance imaging, computed tomography, or positron emission tomography–computed tomography; annual or biannual; and beginning at age 18 to 20 or as early as the age of 5 years (perhaps particularly if pediatric kidney cancer has occurred in a family member).[50] Ultrasound may not be effective at detecting HLRCC-associated kidney cancers and is not recommended.[47] The aggressive nature of the type 2 papillary renal cell carcinomas also makes designing an effective screening program challenging, and there is not yet evidence that instituting screening favorably impacts morbidity or mortality for patients with HLRCC.

UTERINE CANCER AND OTHER HEREDITARY CANCER SYNDROMES

UPSC is histologically similar to ovarian serous carcinoma[5] and has been observed in Ashkenazi Jewish women with *BRCA1/BRCA2* mutations who also had personal and/or family histories of breast and/or ovarian cancer.[55] However, other studies of consecutive series of Jewish endometrial cancer patients found a *BRCA*-positive rate that is similar to that of the general Jewish population.[56,57] It therefore seems unlikely that a personal history of endometrial cancer, UPSC or otherwise, increases the likelihood for a woman to have a germline *BRCA1/BRCA2* mutation.

Patients with hereditary retinoblastoma are at increased risk to develop a variety of second malignancies. A recent study found that women with hereditary retinoblastoma are at significantly increased risk for uterine leiomyosarcoma in particular.[58]

CONCLUSIONS

Approximately 2% to 3% of endometrial cancers are attributable to Lynch syndrome. Early age at diagnosis, low body mass index, and personal and/or family history of Lynch syndrome–associated cancers increase the likelihood for an endometrial cancer patient to have Lynch syndrome, but not all Lynch syndrome–associated endometrial cancers occur in the presence of these risk factors. MSI and IHC analyses are the recommended first step in Lynch syndrome evaluation. The identification of Lynch syndrome in the endometrial cancer patient allows her to take steps to reduce her colorectal cancer risk and also allows family members to benefit from predictive genetic testing and subsequent targeted cancer risk reduction strategies. Unaffected women with Lynch syndrome are at significantly increased risk to develop endometrial cancer and should be educated regarding signs and symptoms of endometrial cancer and should be offered screening and prevention options.

The proportion of endometrial cancer attributable to PHTS (Cowden syndrome) is not precisely known but appears to be less than 1%. The risk for endometrial cancer is likely elevated in women with PHTS, but the magnitude of this risk is not well defined at this time. Women with PHTS should be educated regarding signs and symptoms of endometrial cancer. Endometrial cancer screening and surgical risk reduction can be considered for women with PHTS.

Symptomatic uterine leiomyomas are more common in those with HLRCC than in the general population, with a tendency toward earlier age at diagnosis. Multiple cutaneous leiomyomas are a characteristic finding in HLRCC. Uterine leiomyosarcoma has occurred in the context of HLRCC, but whether and to what extent this risk exceeds that in the general population remains to be determined. Individuals with HLRCC are at increased risk to develop an aggressive subtype of kidney cancer, and therefore, should consider periodic kidney cancer screening.

REFERENCES

1. National Cancer Institute. Endometrial cancer prevention (PDQ). Available at: http://www.cancer.gov/cancertopics/pdq/prevention/endometrial/
2. National Cancer Institute. SEER stat fact sheets: Corpus and uterus, NOS. Available at: http://seer.cancer.gov/statfacts/html/corp.html#risk. Accessed on April 16, 2012.
3. National Cancer Institute. Uterine sarcoma. Available at: http://www.cancer.gov/cancertopics/types/uterinesarcoma. Accessed on April 16, 2012.
4. Broaddus R. Pathology of Lynch syndrome–associated gynecological cancers. In: Lu KH, ed. *Hereditary Gynecologic Cancer: Risk, Prevention, and Management.* New York: Informa Healthcare;2008.
5. Mendivil A, Schuler KM, Gehrig PA. Non-endometrioid adenocarcinoma of the uterine corpus: A review of selected histological subtypes. *Cancer Control.* 2009;16:46–52.
6. Buchanan EM, Weinstein LC, Hillson C. Endometrial cancer. *Am Fam Physician.* 2009;80:1075–1080.
7. Day Baird D, Dunson DB, Hill MC, et al. High cumulative incidence of uterine leiomyoma in black and white women: Ultrasound evidence. *Am J Obstet Gynecol.* 2003;188:100–107.
8. Hampel H, Frankel W, Panescu J, et al. Screening for Lynch syndrome (hereditary nonpolyposis colorectal cancer) among endometrial cancer patients. *Cancer Res.* 2006;66:7810–7817.
9. Hampel H, Panescu J, Lockman J, et al. Comment on: Screening for Lynch syndrome (hereditary nonpolyposis colorectal cancer) among endometrial cancer patients. *Cancer Res.* 2007;67:9603.
10. Stoffel E, Mukherjee B, Raymond VM, et al. Calculation of risk of colorectal and endometrial cancer among patients with Lynch syndrome. *Gastroenterology.* 2009;137:1621–1627.
11. Hampel H, Stephens JA, Pukkala E, et al. Cancer risk in hereditary nonpolyposis colorectal cancer syndrome: Later age of onset. *Gastroenterology.* 2005;129:415–421.
12. Lu KH, Schorge JO, Rodabaugh KJ, et al. Prospective determination of prevalence of Lynch syndrome in young women with endometrial cancer. *J Clin Oncol.* 2007;25:5158–5164.
13. Berends MJ, Wu Y, Sijmons RH, et al. Toward new strategies to select young endometrial cancer patients for mismatch repair gene mutation analysis. *J Clin Oncol.* 2003;21:4364–4370.
14. Millar AL, Pal T, Madlensky L, et al. Mismatch repair gene defects contribute to the genetic basis of double primary cancers of the colorectum and endometrium. *Hum Mol Genet.* 1999;8:823–829.
15. Westin SN, Lacour RA, Urbauer DL, et al. Carcinoma of the lower uterine segment: A newly described association with Lynch syndrome. *J Clin Oncol.* 2008;26:5965–5971.
16. Balmana J, Stockwell DH, Steyerberg EW, et al. Prediction of MLH1 and MSH2 mutations in Lynch syndrome. *JAMA.* 2006;296:1469–1478.
17. Chen S, Wang W, Lee S, et al. Prediction of germline mutations and cancer risk in the Lynch syndrome. *JAMA.* 2006;296:1479–1487.
18. Backes FJ, Leon ME, Ivanov I, et al. Prospective evaluation of DNA mismatch repair protein expression in primary endometrial cancer. *Gynecol Oncol.* 2009;114:486–490.
19. Kwon JS, Scott JL, Gilks CB, et al. Testing women with endometrial cancer to detect Lynch syndrome. *J Clin Oncol.* 2011;29:2247–2252.
20. Weissman SM, Bellcross C, Bittner CC, et al. Genetic counseling considerations in the evaluation of families for Lynch syndrome—a review. *J Genet Couns.* 2011;20:5–19.
21. National Comprehensive Cancer Network. Colorectal cancer screening, V1.2012. Available at: http://www.nccn.org/professionals/physician_gls/pdf/colorectal_screening.pdf. Accessed on April 16, 2012.
22. Esteller M, Levine R, Baylin SB, et al. MLH1 promoter hypermethylation is associated with the microsatellite instability phenotype in sporadic endometrial carcinomas. *Oncogene.* 1998;17:2413–2417.

23. Kawaguchi M, Yanokura M, Banno K, et al. Analysis of a correlation between the BRAF V600E mutation and abnormal DNA mismatch repair in patients with sporadic endometrial cancer. *Int J Oncol.* 2009;34:1541–1547.

24. Bonadona V, Bonaiti B, Olschwang S, et al. Cancer risks associated with germline mutations in MLH1, MSH2, and MSH6 genes in Lynch syndrome. *JAMA.* 2011;305:2304–2310.

25. Senter L, Clendenning M, Sotamaa K, et al. The clinical phenotype of Lynch syndrome due to germline PMS2 mutations. *Gastroenterology.* 2008;135:419–428.

26. Kempers MJ, Kuiper RP, Ockeloen CW, et al. Risk of colorectal and endometrial cancers in EPCAM deletion-positive Lynch syndrome: A cohort study. *Lancet Oncol.* 2011;12:49–55.

27. Lynch HT, Riegert-Johnson DL, Snyder C, et al. Lynch syndrome–associated extracolonic tumors are rare in two extended families with the same EPCAM deletion. *Am J Gastroenterol.* 2011;106:1829–1836.

28. Broaddus RR, Lynch HT, Chen LM, et al. Pathologic features of endometrial carcinoma associated with HNPCC: A comparison with sporadic endometrial carcinoma. *Cancer.* 2006;106:87–94.

29. Schmeler KM, Lynch HT, Chen LM, et al. Prophylactic surgery to reduce the risk of gynecologic cancers in the Lynch syndrome. *N Engl J Med.* 2006;354:261–269.

30. Lindor NM, Petersen GM, Hadley DW, et al. Recommendations for the care of individuals with an inherited predisposition to Lynch syndrome: A systematic review. *JAMA.* 2006;296:1507–1517.

31. Vasen HF, Moslein G, Alonso A, et al. Guidelines for the clinical management of Lynch syndrome (hereditary non-polyposis cancer). *J Med Genet.* 2007;44:353–362.

32. Rijcken FE, Mourits MJ, Kleibeuker JH, et al. Gynecologic screening in hereditary nonpolyposis colorectal cancer. *Gynecol Oncol.* 2003;91:74–80.

33. Dove-Edwin I, Boks D, Goff S, et al. The outcome of endometrial carcinoma surveillance by ultrasound scan in women at risk of hereditary nonpolyposis colorectal carcinoma and familial colorectal carcinoma. *Cancer.* 2002;94:1708–1712.

34. Renkonen-Sinisalo L, Butzow R, Leminen A, et al. Surveillance for endometrial cancer in hereditary nonpolyposis colorectal cancer syndrome. *J Int Cancer.* 2007;120:821–824.

35. Butler MG, Dasouki MJ, Zhou XP, et al. Subset of individuals with autism spectrum disorders and extreme macrocephaly associated with germline PTEN tumour suppressor gene mutations. *J Med Genet.* 2005;42:318–321.

36. Varga EA, Pastore M, Prior T, et al. The prevalence of PTEN mutations in a clinical pediatric cohort with autism spectrum disorders, developmental delay, and macrocephaly. *Genet Med.* 2009;11:111–117.

37. Tan MH, Mester JL, Ngeow J, et al. Lifetime cancer risks in individuals with germline PTEN mutations. *Clin Cancer Res.* 2012;18:400–407.

38. Pilarski R. Cowden syndrome: A critical review of the clinical literature. *J Genet Couns.* 2009;18:13–27.

39. Tan MH, Mester J, Peterson C, et al. A clinical scoring system for selection of patients for PTEN mutation testing is proposed on the basis of a prospective study of 3042 probands. *Am J Hum Genet.* 2011;88:42–56.

40. Eng C. PTEN hamartoma tumor syndrome (PHTS). In: Pagon RA, Bird TD, Dolan CR, et al., eds. *Gene Reviews.* Seattle, WA: University of Washington, Seattle. 1993.

41. Pilarski R, Stephens JA, Noss R, et al. Predicting PTEN mutations: An evaluation of Cowden syndrome and Bannayan–Riley–Ruvalcaba syndrome clinical features. *J Med Genet.* 2011;48:505–512.

42. Starink TM, van der Veen JP, Arwert F, et al. The Cowden syndrome: A clinical and genetic study in 21 patients. *Clin Genet.* 1986;29:222–233.

43. Schmeler KM, Daniels MS, Brandt AC, et al. Endometrial cancer in an adolescent: A possible manifestation of Cowden syndrome. *Obstet Gynecol.* 2009;114(2 pt 2):477–479.

44. Black D, Bogomolniy F, Robson ME, et al. Evaluation of germline PTEN mutations in endometrial cancer patients. *Gynecol Oncol.* 2005;96:21–24.

45. National Comprehensive Cancer Network. Genetic/familial high-risk assessment: breast and ovarian. V1.2011. Available at: www.nccn.org. Accessed on April 7, 2011.

46. Bayley JP, Launonen V, Tomlinson IP. The FH mutation database: An online database of fumarate hydratase mutations involved in the MCUL (HLRCC) tumor syndrome and congenital fumarase deficiency. *BMC Med Genet.* 2008;9:20.

47. Toro JR, Nickerson ML, Wei MH, et al. Mutations in the fumarate hydratase gene cause hereditary leiomyomatosis and renal cell cancer in families in North America. *Am J Hum Genet.* 2003;73:95–106.

48. Stewart L, Glenn GM, Stratton P, et al. Association of germline mutations in the fumarate hydratase gene and uterine fibroids in women with hereditary leiomyomatosis and renal cell cancer. *Arch Dermatol.* 2008;144:1584–1592.

49. Alam NA, Barclay E, Rowan AJ, et al. Clinical features of multiple cutaneous and uterine leiomyomatosis: An underdiagnosed tumor syndrome. *Arch Dermatol.* 2005;141:199–206.

50. Lehtonen HJ. Hereditary leiomyomatosis and renal cell cancer: Update on clinical and molecular characteristics. *Fam Cancer.* 2011;10:397–411.

51. Ylisaukko-oja SK, Kiuru M, Lehtonen HJ, et al. Analysis of fumarate hydratase mutations in a population-based series of early onset uterine leiomyosarcoma patients. *Int J Cancer.* 2006;119:283–287.

52. Gardie B, Remenieras A, Kattygnarath D, et al. Novel FH mutations in families with hereditary leiomyomatosis and renal cell cancer (HLRCC) and patients with isolated type 2 papillary renal cell carcinoma. *J Med Genet.* 2011;48:226–234.

53. Wei MH, Toure O, Glenn GM, et al. Novel mutations in FH and expansion of the spectrum of phenotypes expressed in families with hereditary leiomyomatosis and renal cell cancer. *J Med Genet.* 2006;43:18–27.

54. Alrashdi I, Levine S, Paterson J, et al. Hereditary leiomyomatosis and renal cell carcinoma: Very early diagnosis of renal cancer in a paediatric patient. *Fam Cancer.* 2010;9:239–243.

55. Lavie O, Hornreich G, Ben-Arie A, et al. BRCA germline mutations in Jewish women with uterine serous papillary carcinoma. *Gynecol Oncol.* 2004;92:521–524.

56. Barak F, Milgram R, Laitman Y, et al. The rate of the predominant Jewish mutations in the BRCA1, BRCA2, MSH2 and MSH6 genes in unselected Jewish endometrial cancer patients. *Gynecol Oncol.* 2010;119:511–515.

57. Levine DA, Lin O, Barakat RR, et al. Risk of endometrial carcinoma associated with BRCA mutation. *Gynecol Oncol.* 2001;80:395–398.

58. Francis JH, Kleinerman RA, Seddon JM, et al. Increased risk of secondary uterine leiomyosarcoma in hereditary retinoblastoma. *Gynecol Oncol.* 2012;124:254–259.

10 Genetic Testing by Cancer Site
Urinary Tract

Gayun Chan-Smutko

Cancers of the urinary tract include renal cell carcinoma (RCC) and transitional cell, or urothelial carcinoma (UC). About 64,770 cases of invasive cancer of the kidney and renal pelvis, 74,510 cases of urinary bladder cancer, and 2,860 cases of cancer of the ureter and other urinary organs are expected to be diagnosed in men and women in the United States in 2012.[1] The lifetime risk of cancer of the kidney and renal pelvis is 1.6%, with an average age at diagnosis (based on statistics from 2005 to 2009) of 64 years.[2] A family history of RCC is associated with a 2.2- to 2.8-fold increased risk for developing RCC.[3] Most cases of RCC are sporadic, and approximately 4% are due to a hereditary susceptibility.

RCC is a heterogeneous disease, which has been divided into the following subtypes based on the World Health Organization 2004 classification system: Clear cell (80%), papillary types 1 and 2 (10%), chromophobe (5%), collecting duct (1%), and RCC unclassified (4% to 6%). Additional rarer types that collectively account for less than 2% of RCCs have been described as well.[4] The molecular pathways driving tumorigenesis in hereditary syndromes such as von Hippel–Lindau (VHL) disease, Birt–Hogg–Dubé (BHD) syndrome, hereditary leiomyomatosis and renal cell carcinoma, and hereditary papillary renal cell carcinoma (HPRCC) have provided greater insight into the molecular mechanisms behind the four major subtypes of RCC. This understanding has led to targeted therapies aimed at specific molecular pathways such as the hypoxia-inducible factor (HIF) pathway. This review is devoted primarily to the discussion of renal neoplasms in the adult population and their associated hereditary syndromes (Table 10.1). Genetic testing for susceptibility to urothelial cancers of the upper urinary tract is also presented.

GENETIC SUSCEPTIBILITY TO RCC
von Hippel–Lindau Disease

VHL disease is an autosomal dominant condition that affects approximately 1 in 36,000 live births worldwide. The VHL gene is located on the short arm of

TABLE

10.1

Genetic Susceptibility to RCC

Syndrome	Acronym	Gene(s)	Phenotype	RCC Type	Genetic Testing Sensitivity
von Hippel–Lindau	VHL	*VHL*	Hemangioblastoma (cerebellum, spine, retina), pheochromocytoma, papillary cystadenoma (pancreas, epididymis, adnexal organs, endolymphatic sac pancreatic NET, and cysts)	Clear cell	Nearly 100%[a]
Birt–Hogg–Dubé syndrome	BHD	Folliculin, *FLCN*	Fibrofolliculoma, trichodiscoma, acrochordon, lung cysts, spontaneous pneumothorax	50% Chromophobe/ oncocytic hybrid, 34% chromophobe, 9% clear cell, 5% oncocytoma, 2% papillary	~88%[20]
Hereditary leiomyomatosis and RCC	HLRCC	*FH*	Cutaneous leiomyoma, uterine leiomyoma	Papillary type 2	~93%[25]
Hereditary papillary RCC	HPRCC	*MET*	No additional features	Papillary type 1	Not well established as families are rare
Hereditary paraganglioma/ pheochromocytoma	HPGL	*SDHB*, possibly *SDHD* and *SDHC*	Pheochromocytoma and paraganglioma	Not well defined, but clear cell and papillary types reported.	Unknown in families with RCC and no paraganglioma or pheochromocytoma

[a]Stolle C, Glenn G, Zbar B, et al. Improved detection of germline mutations in the von Hippel–Lindau disease tumor suppressor gene. *Hum Mutat.* 1998;12:417–423.

TABLE
10.2

VHL Genotype/Phenotype Correlations

VHL Phenotype	Pheo	RCC	HB	Predominant Mutation Type
Type 1	Rare or absent	High	High	Large deletions, nonsense, frameshift
Type 2A	High	Rare	High	Missense
Type 2B	High	High	High	Missense
Type 2C (uncommon)	High	Absent	Absent	Missense

Note: The majority of type 1 mutations are partial or complete deletions and protein truncating (nonsense and frameshift), whereas 96% of type 2 mutations are missense. Missense mutations that disrupt amino acid residues on the surface of the VHL protein confer a higher pheo risk than missense mutations that disrupt protein structure.

Pheo, pheochromocytoma; HB, hemangioblastoma.

From: Maher ER, Webster AR, Richards FM, et al. Phenotypic expression in von Hippel–Lindau disease: Correlations with germline VHL gene mutations. *J Med Genet*. 1996;33:328–332; and Ong KR, Woodward ER, Killick P, et al. Genotype–phenotype correlations in von Hippel–Lindau disease. *Hum Mutat*. 2007;28:143–149.

chromosome 3 (3p25) and is the only known susceptibility locus associated with the condition. It is a well-studied tumor suppressor gene that demonstrates loss of heterozygosity in RCCs of patients with VHL disease and sporadic clear cell RCC as well.

VHL disease is a multisystem condition, and an affected individual is at risk to develop any of the following lesions: (1) hemangioblastoma of the cerebellum, spine, or retina; (2) papillary cystadenoma of the epididymis, the adnexal organs, or the endolymphatic sac; (3) adrenal pheochromocytoma and occasionally extra-adrenal paraganglioma; (4) pancreatic cysts, serous cystadenomas, and neuroendocrine tumors (NETs); and (5) multiple and/or bilateral RCC and cysts.

Although the penetrance of VHL disease is 100%, where individuals will develop at least one associated lesion by their sixth decade of life, the expressivity is highly variable even among individuals sharing the same gene mutation. The disease is phenotypically categorized into type 1 and type 2 based on risk for developing pheochromocytoma, with the latter further divided into three subtypes (2A, 2B, and 2C) based on risk for developing RCC. The genotype/phenotype correlations within each type are described in Table 10.2.

Renal Lesions

RCCs of patients with VHL disease are of exclusively clear cell histology. The lifetime risk for developing RCC is 25% to 45%, and when renal cysts are included, the risk rises to 60%.[5] Renal cysts and RCCs develop at an earlier age in patients with VHL in comparison to sporadic counterparts, with an average age of 39 years (range, 16 to 67 years).[5] Cystic lesions are typically asymptomatic; however, complex cysts must be monitored closely with computed tomography (CT) or magnetic resonance imaging as they will harbor a visibly solid RCC component. RCC will often arise from noncystic parenchyma as well.

Nonrenal Clinical Features

With the exception of RCC and pancreatic NETs, the malignancy risk with VHL-associated tumors is very low. Renal lesions and hemangioblastoma of the cerebellum, spine, or retina are common presenting lesions in VHL. The risk for developing a single hemangioblastoma of the spine, cerebellum, and brainstem is 60% to 80%, and the average age is 33 years (range, 9 to 73 years),[5] although most patients can develop multiple lesions at any point in their lifetime. Patients may remain completely asymptomatic especially during periods of no growth or slow growth. Surgical resection is delayed until onset of symptoms.

Retinal hemangioblastomas (retinal angiomas) are usually multifocal and bilateral. These hypervascular tumors can lead to retinal detachment and vision loss. Retinal hemangioblastomas have been observed in 25% to 60% of patients with an average age of 25 years (range, 1 to 67 years). Approximately 5% of lesions are seen younger than 10 years, making genetic testing of at-risk children essential as affected children should undergo annual retinal examinations beginning at birth. Pheochromocytoma has also been observed in young children and can present as a hypertensive crisis. The average age at presentation is 30 years (range, 5 to 58 years), and the risk is 10% to 20%.[5]

Pancreatic manifestations include multiple simple cysts and serous cystadenomas (47% and 11%, respectively), which follow a benign course and are almost always asymptomatic in patients. Pancreatic NETs are less common (15%); however, approximately 2% undergo malignant transformation.[6] A NET tends to be indolent and is seldom the initial presenting lesion; however, close monitoring is indicated for timing of surgical resection.

A less common manifestation of VHL is a papillary cystadenoma of the endolymphatic sac, or inner ear, which is extremely rare in the general population but more prevalent in VHL disease (~11%). Papillary cystadenomas may also arise in the epididymis in men and less commonly in the adnexal organs in women.

VHL Molecular Genetics

The *VHL* gene was cloned by Latif et al.[7] in 1993 and is the most well studied of the familial RCC syndromes. Loss of *VHL* function has been demonstrated to cause RCC formation in VHL disease as well as in the majority of sporadic clear cell RCCs.[8,9] The *VHL* gene encodes the pVHL protein, which in normoxic conditions forms a complex with elongin B, elongin C, Cullin 2, and Rbx1. The VHL complex targets HIF-1α and HIF-2α for ubiquitin-mediated degradation. The HIF-1α and HIF-2α

genes, along with HIF-3α, encode the α subunit of the HIF heterodimer. In hypoxic conditions, the VHL complex does not interact with HIF-1α and HIF-2α, leading to an accumulation of these subunits and downstream transcription of HIF-dependent genes. Loss of VHL protein function in renal tumors simulates low tissue oxygen levels, or "pseudohypoxia" where HIF-1α and HIF-2α accumulate, causing upregulation of many genes involved in tumorigenesis such as vascular endothelial growth factor (proangiogenesis), epidermal growth factor receptor (cell proliferation and survival), and glucose transporter 1 (regulation of glucose uptake).

VHL Genetic Testing

Genetic testing of the VHL gene is available on a clinical basis and involves full-gene sequencing and large gene rearrangement analysis. When both methods are used, the mutation detection rate is nearly 100% in patients with a clinical diagnosis of VHL.[10] Approximately 80% of patients have a parent with VHL, and ~20% represent de novo cases where neither parent carries the mutation. Genetic testing is recommended for a proband with a personal and family history of VHL, as the identification of causative mutations aids in determining disease subtype (Table 10.2). Disease subtype information along with a careful, detailed family history aids in guiding screening and surveillance of VHL patients. In simplex cases, where a patient has two or more VHL-associated lesions and a negative family history, genetic testing is recommended to establish a diagnosis. When a mutation is identified in a proband, at-risk family members should be offered predictive testing. Since young children with VHL are known to be at risk for retinal lesions and pheochromocytoma, genetic testing should be offered anytime after birth.

Birt–Hogg–Dubé Syndrome

In 1977, Drs. Birt, Hogg, and Dubé first described a multigenerational kindred showing autosomal dominant transmission of fibrofolliculomas with trichodiscomas and acrochordons.[11] The phenotype was later expanded beyond dermatologic manifestations to include lung cysts and pneumothorax, and renal tumors.[12] The number of families with BHD syndrome described in the literature to date is small, and therefore, the exact incidence is unknown. Inherited mutations in the folliculin (*FLCN*) gene are associated with BHD syndrome.

Renal Lesions

An individual with BHD syndrome is at increased risk of developing multiple and bilateral renal tumors, frequently of more than one histologic type even within the same renal unit, and at younger ages compared with the general population. The lifetime risk is in the range of 27% to 45%,[13,14] and the wide range may be a reflection of ascertainment bias introduced when families are recruited predominantly through dermatology clinics versus urology. The most common tumor pathology found in patients is a hybrid oncocytic RCC, which contains a mixture of oncocytic and chromophobe cells. Furthermore, radical nephrectomy specimens of patients have demonstrated oncocytosis where tiny nodules of cells similar to the larger hybrid tumors are diffusely scattered throughout the renal parenchyma. A retrospective study by Pavlovich et al.[15] examined 130 tumor specimens from 30 patients (25 males, 5 females) in 19 different BHD families. The authors found that hybrid oncocytic (50%) and chromophobe (34%) were the more common histologic findings, followed by clear cell (9%), benign oncocytoma (5%), and papillary (2%). The average age at first tumor was 50.7 years, and patients averaged 5.3 tumors each (range, 1 to 28). Other studies reporting histologic subtypes of BHD syndrome–related renal tumors have similar findings.

Nonrenal Manifestations

Skin findings associated with BHD syndrome are benign and consist of fibrofolliculoma, trichodiscoma (which are histologically and clinically indistinguishable from angiofibroma), perifollicular fibroma, and acrochordons. Fibrofolliculoma is highly specific for BHD syndrome, whereas trichodiscomas and acrochordons are not. Onset for skin lesions is typically at older than 25 years, and a dermatologic diagnosis of BHD syndrome can be made on the basis of the presence of five or more facial or truncal papules with at least one histologically confirmed fibrofolliculoma.

Approximately 83% to 89% of patients with BHD syndrome will have multiple pulmonary cysts[14,16,17] identified upon chest CT. The lifetime risk of spontaneous pneumothorax is 24% to 32%,[14,18] and the majority of patients have their first event by age 50 years. The presence of lung cysts is strongly associated with risk of pneumothorax,[17] but the mechanism behind this is not known. A possible association between BHD syndrome and parotid oncocytoma has also been reported in a small number of cases.[14]

FLCN Molecular Genetics

The *FLCN* gene is located on chromosome 17p11.2 and was cloned by Nickerson et al.[12] in 2002. The gene has 14 exons and encodes the protein folliculin. The role of *FLCN* and tumorigenesis has not been fully established, but animal studies and loss of heterozygosity studies in renal tumors provide some evidence that it is a tumor suppressor gene. Folliculin binds with folliculin-interacting proteins (FNIP1 and FNIP2) and then binds AMP-activated protein kinase, which is part of the cellular energy and nutrient sensing system. AMP-activated protein kinase also helps regulates mTOR activity (mTORC1 and mTORC2). Studies of renal tumors from heterozygous BHD knockout mice and renal tumors from patients with BHD syndrome show mTOR activation. Therapeutic agents inhibiting mTOR activity in sporadic chromophobe tumors are currently under investigation and may have implications for patients with BHD syndrome–related renal tumors.[19]

The mutation detection rate for *FLCN* clinical testing is approximately 89%, and nearly all of the mutations described to date have been truncating point mutations (frameshift and nonsense). Splice-site mutations have also been reported in a small number of BHD families, and one missense mutation in a patient with bilateral renal tumors has been reported as well.[20] A mutational hotspot in a polycytosine tract in exon 11 has been suggested.[14]

Hereditary Papillary RCC

HPRCC is inherited in an autosomal dominant manner with reduced penetrance where patients with HPRCC are at risk of developing multiple and/or bilateral papillary RCCs at a young age. The phenotype is limited to the risk of papillary RCC alone, particularly papillary type 1, although the distinction between type 1 and type 2 is not always made on initial pathology review.

Germline mutations in the *c-met* or *MET* proto-oncogene on chromosome 7q31.2 have been associated with HPRCC.[21] This is a comparatively uncommon condition, and few families with a *MET* mutation have been reported to date. Missense mutations found in HPRCC families occur in exons 16, 17, 18, and 19 of the *MET* proto-oncogene, which encodes the tyrosine kinase domain of the protein product. These mutations have been shown to be activating or gain-of-function mutations, unlike most hereditary cancer susceptibility syndromes, which are associated with loss-of-function mutations in tumor suppressor genes. Papillary tumors obtained from patients with HPRCC typically show duplication of chromosome 7, as do their sporadic counterparts.[22] Furthermore, HPRCC-associated tumors show nonrandom duplication of the chromosome 7 copy harboring the mutation *MET* allele,[22,23] suggesting that overexpression of *MET* may lead to cellular proliferation, although the exact mechanism has not yet been elucidated.

Analysis by Lindor et al.[24] of 59 apparently sporadic patients with papillary type 1 tumors including 13 cases with multifocal or bilateral disease found no germline mutations in *MET*. This suggests differing etiology in sporadic versus papillary type 1 cancers. The rarity of the disease and low likelihood of identifying mutation carriers in isolated cases poses a challenge for genetic counseling of these patients. In the setting of a positive family history, *MET* genetic testing should be offered to patients with papillary type 1 RCC. A negative genetic test result; however, does not exclude the possibility of a hereditary susceptibility.

Hereditary Leiomyomatosis and RCC

Susceptibility to papillary type 2 RCC has been associated with hereditary leiomyomatosis and RCC (HLRCC) syndrome demonstrating autosomal dominant transmission. Most individuals with HLRCC-associated renal lesions present with unilateral, solitary tumors; however, bilateral and multifocal disease has also been observed.[25] The tumors tend to be highly aggressive with poor prognosis, which has implications for screening and early detection in at-risk patients. Although papillary type 2 is the predominant histology, collecting duct RCC and mixed cystic, papillary, and tubulopapillary RCC have also been reported. The incidence of RCC in individuals with HLRCC is approximately 25% to 40%.[25,26]

Cutaneous leiomyomatosis and uterine leiomyomatosis are additional features of the disease. Leiomyomas of the skin appear as firm skin-colored to light brown papules and can be distributed anywhere along the trunk, extremities, head, or neck. Uterine leiomyomas (fibroids) are common in the general population; however, HLRCC-associated burden tends to be greater in women with HLRCC. Compared with the general population, the average age at onset is younger where many women become symptomatic before the age of 30 years, significantly impacting their child-bearing years. The fibroids tend to be multiple (ranging from 1 to 15 in 1 series of 22 women from 16 families studied) and large (1 to 8 cm), often requiring myomectomy or hysterectomy for treatment.[25] Not all individuals with HLRCC will have cutaneous manifestations, although it is worthwhile to note that the presence of cutaneous leiomyomas has a strong concordance with uterine leiomyoma. A very small number of cases have been reported of cutaneous and uterine leiomyosarcoma in HLRCC families.

The fumarate hydratase gene, or *FH*, is the only gene associated with the disease to date. Fumarate hydratase functions in the Krebs cycle to convert fumarate to malate. Alteration of the *FH* gene results in accumulation of fumarate, which inhibits HIF-α prolyl hydroxylase enzymes (HPH). HIF-α is hydroxylated by HPH in normoxic conditions, but when HPH is inhibited, HIF-α levels rise, leading to increased transcription of downstream genes involved in tumorigenesis.[19]

Hereditary Paraganglioma and Pheochromocytoma Associated with SDHB

Several genes have been implicated in hereditary paraganglioma with and without pheochromocytoma, such as the succinate dehydrogenase complex genes (*SDHB*, *SDHD*, and *SDHC*), as well as *TMEM127*, *SDHAF2*, *VHL*, *MEN2*, and others. The reader is referred to the "Genetic Testing: Endocrine Tumors" this book for a detailed discussion of these genes.

Earlier reports of families with mutations in *SDHB* also noted renal tumors in a minority of these families with a paraganglioma/pheochromocytoma phenotype.[27] Different renal tumor histologic findings have been reported including clear cell, chromophobe, carcinoma not classifiable, papillary type 2, or oncocytoma.[27-31] Gill et al.[32] examined five renal tumors from four families with an *SDHB* mutation and suggest that *SDHB*-associated renal tumors share common morphologic features such as bubbly eosinophilic cytoplasm with intracytoplasmic inclusions and indistinct cell borders.

Genetic testing of *SDHB* should be considered in patients presenting with early-onset and/or multifocal/bilateral RCC and a family history of paraganglioma or pheochromocytoma. Testing can also be considered in familial RCC especially in multigeneration and early-onset families, although there are not enough data at this time to suggest whether many *SDHB* carriers will be identified in the absence of known paraganglioma or pheochromocytoma. Ricketts et al.[29] studied a cohort of 68 patients with RCC and no evidence of syndromic

RCC susceptibility and identified three *SDHB* mutation carriers (4.4%). One had a personal history of RCC at 24 years and a positive family history; two had a history of bilateral disease, one at the age of 30 years and the other at the age of 38 years; none of the three cases had a personal or family history of paraganglioma or pheochromocytoma.[29]

GENETIC SUSCEPTIBILITY TO UROTHELIAL CANCERS
Hereditary Nonpolyposis Colorectal Cancer or Lynch Syndrome

Hereditary nonpolyposis colorectal cancer or Lynch syndrome is an inherited syndrome characterized by and increased risk for carcinoma of the colon, uterus, stomach, ovary, pancreas, and upper urinary tract. Inherited mutations in the DNA mismatch repair genes (*MLH1*, *MSH2*, *MSH6*, and *PMS2*) are associated with the syndrome. A detailed discussion of Lynch syndrome and genetic testing can be found in "Genetic Testing: Colon Nonpolyposis" section of this book.

Upper urinary tract cancers are the third most common cancer in Lynch syndrome with a 5% to 6% lifetime risk. The associated cancers are mainly UCs of the ureter and renal pelvis with a relative-risk of 22 times higher than that of the general population and a median age at onset of 56 years, or 10 to 15 years earlier.[33] Upper urinary UC may be the initial presenting feature in some patients from Lynch families. Most of the reported cases are in families with *MSH2* mutations, but have been observed in smaller number of *MLH1* and *MSH6* families as well. Bladder UC has been reported in patients with Lynch syndrome, with some studies reporting a relative risk similar or slightly higher to that of the general population.[34] In a cohort of Dutch families with Lynch syndrome, the relative risk of bladder cancer compared with the Dutch population was higher: 4.2 for men and 2.5 for women. *MSH2* mutation carriers in this cohort showed an even higher risk of 7 for men and 5.8 for women.[35]

Upper urinary tract cancers may be an underrecognized entity in Lynch syndrome, particularly in the urology specialty setting. Patients with UC of the ureter and renal pelvis may warrant a referral to genetics for risk assessment when presenting at young ages and/or synchronous or metachronous disease. Family history positivity for upper urinary tract cancers and other Lynch-associated tumors should be an indication for referral as well.

INDICATIONS FOR GENETIC TESTING

One or more of the indicators listed below should prompt a referral for evaluating a patient for genetic susceptibility to RCC. Possible entry points for the patient include a diagnosis of RCC, pheochromocytoma or paraganglioma, spontaneous pneumothorax, bilateral cystic kidneys, cystic pancreas, or suspicious cutaneous lesions. A proposed guide to making a differential diagnosis is depicted in Figure 10.1.

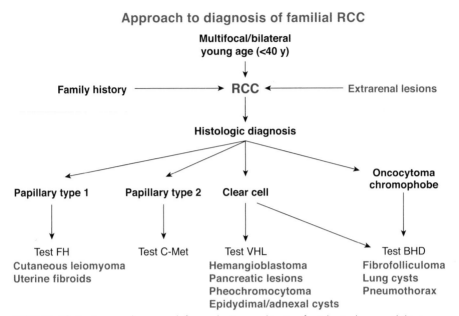

FIGURE 10.1. Proposed approach for evaluation and testing for inherited susceptibility to RCC. Family history, age at onset, extrarenal lesions, and renal histology guide testing.

- Syndromic features: A thorough medical history and physical examination may provide supporting evidence of syndromic features. Review of available radiology examinations is warranted. Patients with suspicious cutaneous lesions should be referred to dermatology for biopsy and histologic confirmation.
- Personal diagnosis of RCC: Even in the absence of known family history, early-onset (<40 years) and/or presence of multifocal or bilateral lesions warrants referral.
- Family history: Obtaining and reviewing pathology reports on renal tumors from family members are essential. Patients should be queried for a positive family history of related tumors such as pheochromocytoma, skin findings, and colon cancer.

GENETIC TESTING AND COUNSELING

Genetic testing for *VHL, FLCN, MET, FH,* and *SDHB* is clinically available for approximately $1,000 to $1,200 per gene, although the per-gene cost is anticipated to decrease as the cost of sequencing technologies decreases and more multigene panels are offered. Lynch syndrome testing is also available; however, it is a genetically heterogeneous disease, and tumor screening with microsatellite instability analysis and immunohistochemistry of the DNA mismatch repair genes can help guide germline testing (see "Colon Nonpolyposis" section of this book).

A summary of the mutation detection rates for each gene can be found in Table 10.1. Testing sensitivity is predictably highest in syndromic cases with uncommon tumors that are highly specific for the syndrome such as hemangioblastoma (VHL) and fibrofolliculoma (BHD). Genetic testing is still warranted in less suspicious cases as a positive test result in a patient (i.e., germline mutation) prompts close monitoring in a rational, targeted manner. This includes screening for new renal tumors and nonrenal manifestations such as pheochromocytoma and paraganglioma. High-risk, aggressive papillary type 2 tumors are associated with HLRCC and warrant prompt intervention. Early detection and monitoring of nonpapillary type 2 renal lesions provide the patient and physician with information on disease burden, tumor size, and doubling time. Since patients with hereditary conditions such as VHL are at high risk of developing multiple RCC over their lifetime, close surveillance provides necessary clinical information for timing surgical intervention and increases the likelihood that nephron-sparing approaches can be used.

When a deleterious mutation is identified, at-risk family members should be offered predictive genetic testing. Genetic counseling regarding the natural history of the condition, the risk of carrying the mutation, age-appropriate screening, and the limitations of genetic testing is essential. In the case of BHD, HPRCC, and HLRCC, there is no consensus for a minimum age at which genetic testing should be considered. Timing of testing of asymptomatic relatives may be guided by ages at onset within the family. Each first-degree relative of a mutation carrier has an empiric risk of 50%. A negative test effectively rules out the disease and spares the individual from unnecessary imaging and screening. A positive test prompts close monitoring, such as regular imaging of the kidneys with CT or magnetic resonance imaging. With respect to limitations, it is important for patients to understand that a positive test result does not predict which tumors they will develop over their lifetime, age at onset of tumors, or severity of their disease. VHL disease represents an exception where genetic testing should be offered anytime after a child is born. When a child tests negative for the familial VHL mutation, he/she is spared unnecessary screening; a child who carries the mutation must begin annual retinal examinations within the first year of life, with additional imaging examinations of the abdomen and brain around the onset of puberty. Multiple cases of retinal hemangioblastomas (angioma) in young children have been reported, and the morbidity of undiagnosed retinal tumors is high. Similarly, childhood-onset pheochromocytoma is also known to be associated with VHL and hereditary paraganglioma/pheochromocytoma syndromes.

Predictive testing of minors in their teenage years should be treated with a greater sensitivity to the minor's intellectual and emotional capacity. Some parents include their child on the decision to test, depending on the age and emotional maturity of their child. This helps maintain trust between the child and the parent, and lays a foundation for greater comprehension of the test result and the implications, whether the results are positive or negative. In the setting of genetic predisposition counseling, the concept of risk and the struggle to cope with risk information is a tenuous position for any adult patient. This is no less stressful for a teenager and his/her parents demanding elevated sensitivity and awareness from the provider and genetic counselor caring for the family.

Not including an older child in the testing decision is also the parents' prerogative; however, the health care provider or genetic counselor working with the family should help parents consider the potential ramifications of initiating testing without the child's knowledge. Questions to consider include when and how they would disclose the results to their child in an age-appropriate way. When we consider a teenaged minor who is intellectually capable of giving assent for genetic testing, the process of obtaining the minor's assent involves the health care professional who together with the parents provides age-appropriate information about the genetic disease, what is involved in carrying out the test, and how results will be disclosed. Parents may wish to test their teenage minor without his/her knowledge primarily because they are hoping for a "good news" scenario of a negative test result where both the teen and the parents can be worry-free. When parents request testing for their teenager without his/her knowledge, the provider should help parents anticipate that they may be putting their child's trust in them (and their child's trust in the medical community) at risk, particularly, if it results in a positive diagnosis.

The role of the genetic counselor and health care provider is to support the patient and family with a focus on improving their understanding of their disease and on helping the family find a common language with which to communicate their fears, concerns, and needs. Families often benefit from participating in multidisciplinary practices staffed by a combination of medical oncology, advanced practice nursing, genetic counseling, urosurgery, and other practitioners.[36] These disease specialty clinics are geared toward meeting the medical and informational needs of the patient and family, which are expected to evolve with age and with major life transitions.

SUMMARY

The genetic basis of heritable susceptibility to cancers of the urinary tract is a complex problem composed of many different genes and molecular pathways. Careful inspection of family medical history, tumor histology, and physical findings such as cutaneous lesions provide the opportunity for a stepwise approach to genetic risk assessment of the cancer patient. Genetic testing of cancer susceptibility genes has downstream implications for surveillance and treatment of disease, and identification of causative mutations provides valuable information for patients and their at-risk family members. Genetic counseling of patients and their family members allows for enhanced understanding of the disease and treatment.

REFERENCES

1. Siegel R, Naishadham D, Jemal A. Cancer statistics. *CA Cancer J Clin.* 2012;62:10–29.
2. National Cancer Institute. Available at: http://seer.cancer.gov/statfacts/html/kidrp.html#risk. Accessed on May 2, 2012.
3. Clague J, Lin J, Cassidy A, et al. Family history and risk of renal cell carcinoma: Results from a case-control study and systematic meta-analysis. *Cancer Epidemiol Biomarkers Prev.* 2009;18:801–807.
4. Deng FM, Melamed J. Histologic variants of renal cell carcinoma: Does tumor type influence outcome? *Urol Clin North Am.* 2012;39:119–132.

5. Lonser RR, Glenn GM, Walther M, et al. von Hippel–Lindau disease. *Lancet.* 2003;361:2059–2067.
6. Charlesworth M, Verbeke CS, Falk GA, et al. Pancreatic lesions in von Hippel–Lindau disease? A systematic review and meta-synthesis of the literature. *J Gastrointest Surg.* 2012;16:1422–1428.
7. Latif F, Tory K, Gnarra J, et al. Identification of the von Hippel–Lindau disease tumor suppressor gene. *Science.* 1993;260:1317–1320.
8. Gnarra JR, Tory K, Weng Y, et al. Mutations of the VHL tumour suppressor gene in renal carcinoma. *Nat Genet.* 1994;7:85–90.
9. Shuin T, Kondo K, Torigoe S, et al. Frequent somatic mutations and loss of heterozygosity of the von Hippel–Lindau tumor suppressor gene in primary human renal cell carcinomas. *Cancer Res.* 1994;54:2852–2855.
10. Schimke RN, Collins DL, Stolle CA. *von Hippel–Lindau Syndrome.* 1993.
11. Birt AR, Hogg GR, Dube WJ. Hereditary multiple fibrofolliculomas with trichodiscomas and acrochordons. *Arch Dermatol.* 1977;113:1674–1677.
12. Nickerson ML, Warren MB, Toro JR, et al. Mutations in a novel gene lead to kidney tumors, lung wall defects, and benign tumors of the hair follicle in patients with the Birt–Hogg–Dube syndrome. *Cancer Cell.* 2002;2:157–164.
13. Pavlovich CP, Grubb RL 3rd, Hurley K, et al. Evaluation and management of renal tumors in the Birt–Hogg–Dube syndrome. *J Urol.* 2005;173:1482–1486.
14. Schmidt LS, Nickerson ML, Warren MB, et al. Germline BHD-mutation spectrum and phenotype analysis of a large cohort of families with Birt–Hogg–Dube syndrome. *Am J Hum Genet.* 2005;76:1023–1033.
15. Pavlovich CP, Walther MM, Eyler RA, et al. Renal tumors in the Birt–Hogg–Dube syndrome. *Am J Surg Pathol.* 2002;26:1542–1552.
16. Zbar B, Alvord WG, Glenn G, et al. Risk of renal and colonic neoplasms and spontaneous pneumothorax in the Birt–Hogg–Dube syndrome. *Cancer Epidemiol Biomarkers Prev.* 2002;11:393–400.
17. Toro JR, Pautler SE, Stewart L, et al. Lung cysts, spontaneous pneumothorax, and genetic associations in 89 families with Birt–Hogg–Dube syndrome. *Am J Respir Crit Care Med.* 2007;175:1044–1053.
18. Houweling AC, Gijezen LM, Jonker MA, et al. Renal cancer and pneumothorax risk in Birt–Hogg–Dube syndrome; an analysis of 115 FLCN mutation carriers from 35 BHD families. *Br J Cancer.* 2011;105:1912–1919.
19. Singer EA, Bratslavsky G, Middelton L, et al. Impact of genetics on the diagnosis and treatment of renal cancer. *Curr Urol Rep.* 2011;12:47–55.
20. Toro JR, Wei MH, Glenn GM, et al. BHD mutations, clinical and molecular genetic investigations of Birt–Hogg–Dube syndrome: A new series of 50 families and a review of published reports. *J Med Genet.* 2008;45:321–331.
21. Schmidt L, Duh FM, Chen F, et al. Germline and somatic mutations in the tyrosine kinase domain of the MET proto-oncogene in papillary renal carcinomas. *Nat Genet.* 1997;16:68–73.
22. Fischer J, Palmedo G, von Knobloch R, et al. Duplication and overexpression of the mutant allele of the MET proto-oncogene in multiple hereditary papillary renal cell tumours. *Oncogene.* 1998;17:733–739.
23. Zhuang Z, Park WS, Pack S, et al. Trisomy 7–harbouring non-random duplication of the mutant MET allele in hereditary papillary renal carcinomas. *Nat Genet.* 1998;20:66–69.
24. Lindor NM, Dechet CB, Greene MH, et al. Papillary renal cell carcinoma: Analysis of germline mutations in the MET proto-oncogene in a clinic-based population. *Genet Test.* 2001;5:101–106.
25. Wei MH, Toure O, Glenn GM, et al. Novel mutations in FH and expansion of the spectrum of phenotypes expressed in families with hereditary leiomyomatosis and renal cell cancer. *J Med Genet.* 2006;43:18–27.
26. Gardie B, Remenieras A, Kattygnarath D, et al. Novel FH mutations in families with hereditary leiomyomatosis and renal cell cancer (HLRCC) and patients with isolated type 2 papillary renal cell carcinoma. *J Med Genet.* 2011;48:226–234.
27. Vanharanta S, Buchta M, McWhinney SR, et al. Early-onset renal cell carcinoma as a novel extraparaganglial component of SDHB-associated heritable paraganglioma. *Am J Hum Genet.* 2004;74:153–159.
28. Henderson A, Douglas F, Perros P, et al. SDHB-associated renal oncocytoma suggests a broadening of the renal phenotype in hereditary paragangliomatosis. *Fam Cancer.* 2009;8:257–260.
29. Ricketts C, Woodward ER, Killick P, et al. Germline SDHB mutations and familial renal cell carcinoma. *J Natl Cancer Inst.* 2008;100:1260–1262.

30. Ricketts CJ, Forman JR, Rattenberry E, et al. Tumor risks and genotype–phenotype–proteotype analysis in 358 patients with germline mutations in SDHB and SDHD. *Hum Mutat.* 2010;31:41–51.

31. Srirangalingam U, Walker L, Khoo B, et al. Clinical manifestations of familial paraganglioma and pheochromocytomas in succinate dehydrogenase B (SDH-B) gene mutation carriers. *Clin Endocrinol (Oxf).* 2008;69:587–596.

32. Gill AJ, Pachter NS, Chou A, et al. Renal tumors associated with germline SDHB mutation show distinctive morphology. *Am J Surg Pathol.* 2011;35:1578–1585.

33. Rouprêt M, Yates DR, Comperat E, et al. Upper urinary tract urothelial cell carcinomas and other urological malignancies involved in the hereditary nonpolyposis colorectal cancer (Lynch syndrome) tumor spectrum. *Eur Urol.* 2008;54:1226–1236.

34. Crockett DG, Wagner DG, Holmäng S, et al. Upper urinary tract carcinoma in Lynch syndrome cases. *J Urol.* 2011;185:1627–1630.

35. van der Post RS, Kiemeney LA, Ligtenberg MJ, et al. Risk of urothelial bladder cancer in Lynch syndrome is increased, in particular among MSH2 mutation carriers. *J Med Genet.* 2010;47:464–470.

36. A list of VHL specialty clinics in the United States and other countries. Available at: www.vhl.org.

11 Genetic Testing by Cancer Site

Pancreas

Jennifer E. Axilbund and Elizabeth A. Wiley

I t is estimated that 5% to 10% of pancreatic cancer (adenocarcinoma) is familial,[1,2] and individuals with a family history of pancreatic cancer are at greater risk of developing pancreatic cancer, themselves.[3] Although there is evidence of a major pancreatic cancer susceptibility gene,[4] it remains elusive. Therefore, the majority of families with multiple cases of pancreatic cancer do not have an identifiable causative gene or syndrome, making risk assessment and counseling challenging. However, a subset of pancreatic cancer is attributable to known inherited cancer predisposition syndromes (Table 11.1).

BRCA2

The *BRCA2* gene is associated with hereditary breast and ovarian cancer syndrome, and often presents as premenopausal breast cancer, ovarian cancer, and/or male breast cancer. The Breast Cancer Linkage Consortium[5] reported a 3.5-fold (95% confidence interval [CI], 1.9 to 6.6) increased risk of pancreatic cancer in *BRCA2* gene mutation carriers. Subsequent studies in the United Kingdom and the Netherlands showed a relative risk of 4.1 and 5.9, respectively.[6,7] In a US-based study, 10.9% (17/156) of families with a *BRCA2* mutation reported a family history of pancreatic cancer. The median ages at diagnosis for males and females were 67 and 59 years, respectively, which differed statistically from the SEER (Surveillance, Epidemiology and End Results) database (70 years old for males and 74 years old for females; $P = 0.011$).[8] Although genotype–phenotype data remain sparse, the *BRCA2* K3326X variant was found in 5.6% (8/144) of familial pancreatic cancer patients compared with 1.2% (3/250) of those with sporadic pancreatic cancer (odds ratio [OR], 4.84; 95% CI, 1.27 to 18.55; $P < 0.01$).[9]

Approximately, 17% of pancreatic cancer patients who have at least two additional relatives with pancreatic cancer carry deleterious mutations in the *BRCA2* gene.[10] Estimates for the prevalence of *BRCA2* mutations with two first-degree relatives with pancreatic cancer are 6% to 12%,[11,12] and *BRCA2* mutations also explain a portion of

157

TABLE 11.1	Inherited Cancer Predisposition Syndromes that Increase the Risk for Pancreatic Cancer		
Syndrome	**Gene(s)**	**Risk of PC**	**Predominant Features**
Hereditary breast and ovarian cancer	*BRCA1*	RR, 2.26–3	Malignancies: Breast (particularly premenopausal), ovary, male breast, prostate
	BRCA2	RR, 3.5–5.9	Malignancies: Breast (particularly premenopausal), ovary, male breast, prostate, melanoma (cutaneous and ocular)
Familial atypical multiple mole and melanoma	*CDKN2A*	RR, 7.4–47.8	Malignancies: Melanoma (often multiple and early onset)
			Other: Dysplastic nevi
Hereditary pancreatitis	*PRSS1*	SIR, 57	Other: Chronic pancreatitis
Hereditary nonpolyposis colorectal cancer (Lynch syndrome)	*MLH1*	SIR, 0–8.6	Malignancies: Colorectum, endometrium, ovary, stomach, small bowel, urinary tract (ureter, renal pelvis), biliary, brain (glioblastoma), skin (sebaceous)
	MSH2		
	MSH6		
	PMS2		
	EPCAM		
PJS	*STK11*	SIR, 132	Malignancies: Colorectum, small bowel, stomach, breast, gynecologic
			Other: Melanin pigmentation (mucocutaneous), small-bowel intussusception

SIR, standardized incidence ratio; RR, relative risk.

apparently sporadic pancreatic cancers.[13] However, prevalence varies between populations. Six (4.1%) of one hundred forty-five Ashkenazi Jews with pancreatic cancer were found to have a deleterious *BRCA2* mutation when compared with cancer-free controls (OR, 3.85; 95% CI, 2.1 to 10.8; $P = 0.007$), although no differences were noted in age at diagnosis or clinical pathologic features.[14] An earlier, smaller study found a deleterious *BRCA2* mutation in 3 (13%) of 23 Ashkenazi Jews with pancreatic cancer, unselected for family history.[15] Among Ashkenazi Jewish probands with breast cancer who reported a family history of pancreatic cancer, 7.6% (16/211) had a *BRCA2* mutation.[16] By comparison, no *BRCA2* mutations were found in studies of pancreatic cancer in Korea or Italy.[17,18]

BRCA1

Similar to *BRCA2*, mutations in *BRCA1* are associated with markedly increased risk for premenopausal breast cancer and ovarian cancer. The Breast Cancer Linkage Consortium reported a 2.26-fold (95% CI, 1.26 to 4.06) increased risk of pancreatic cancer in families with a *BRCA1* mutation,[19] and Brose et al.[20] estimated a threefold higher lifetime risk. However, more recently, Moran et al.[6] in the United Kingdom found no elevation in pancreatic cancer risk in 268 families with a known *BRCA1* mutation. A US-based study reported that 11% (24/219) of their families with a *BRCA1* mutation had at least one individual with pancreatic cancer, with median ages at diagnosis of 59 years for males and 68 years for females. Again, this was significantly younger than reported in the SEER database ($P = 0.0014$).[8] Molecularly, Al-Sukhni et al.[21] evaluated pancreatic tumors from seven known *BRCA1* mutation carriers and found loss of heterozygosity of *BRCA1* in five (71%), with confirmed loss of the wild-type allele in three of the five compared with only one (11%) of nine sporadic controls. This suggests that *BRCA1* germline mutations do, in fact, predispose to pancreatic cancers in at least some individuals.

Familial breast cancer registries in the United States and Israel have evaluated the mutation status of families that reported pancreatic cancer in addition to breast cancer and ovarian cancer. In the US study of 19 families with breast, ovarian, and pancreatic cancer, 15 carried a deleterious mutation in *BRCA1* and 4 in BRCA2,[22] whereas the Israeli study reported an equal number of *BRCA1* and *BRCA2* families.[23]

Another study, specifically of Ashkenazi Jewish families, reported a *BRCA1* mutation in 7% of probands with breast cancer who also had a family history of pancreatic cancer,[16] which was, again, equal to the prevalence of *BRCA2* mutations. Thus, within the Ashkenazi Jewish population, *BRCA1* and *BRCA2* mutations may contribute more equally to risk in families with both breast and pancreatic cancer. However, these studies all examined cohorts of families selected because of clustering of breast and/or ovarian cancer with pancreatic cancer. When families were selected on the basis of familial pancreatic cancer, alone, *BRCA1* mutations were less prevalent. Zero of sixty-six families with three or more cases of pancreatic cancer had a deleterious *BRCA1* mutation, including those who also reported a family history of breast and/or ovarian cancer.[24] Evaluation of Ashkenazi Jewish patients ascertained on the basis of pancreatic cancer, alone, showed a 1.3% (2/145) prevalence of *BRCA1* mutations.[14] Therefore, *BRCA1* may explain a small subset of families showing a clustering of pancreatic cancer with breast and/or ovarian cancer, but is unlikely to explain most families with site-specific pancreatic cancer.

PALB2

PALB2 (partner and localizer of BRCA2) was recognized as the FANCN gene in 2007, and biallelic mutation carriers develop Fanconi anemia.[25,26] Monoallelic mutation carriers were shown to be at increased risk for breast cancer (relative risk [RR], 2.3; 95% CI, 1.4 to 3.9).[27] Prevalence of PALB2 mutations among familial breast cancer cases is low across ethnicities; PALB2 mutations are relatively nonexistent in breast cancers in the Irish and Icelandic populations and are found in approximately 1% of Italians, US African Americans, Chinese, and Spanish breast cancer families, and in 2% of young South African breast cancer patients.[28–35] Analysis of 1,144 US familial breast cancer cases found a PALB2 mutation in 3.4% (33/972) of non-Ashkenazi Jews and none (0/172) of Ashkenazi Jews. The estimated risk for breast cancer was 2.3-fold by the age of 55 years (95% CI, 1.5 to 4.2) and 3.4-fold by the age of 85 years (95% CI, 2.4 to 5.9). There was also a fourfold risk for male breast cancer ($P = 0.0003$) and a sixfold risk for pancreatic cancer ($P = 0.002$).[36] Among French Canadian women with bilateral breast cancer, a PALB2 mutation was found in 0.9% (5/559) compared with none of 565 women with unilateral breast cancer ($P = 0.04$), and first-degree relatives of PALB2 mutation carriers had a 5.3-fold risk for breast cancer (95% CI, 1.8 to 13.2).[37]

PALB2 founder mutations have been identified in several populations, including the c.2323 C > T (Q775X) mutation in French Canadians.[38] Another example is the Finnish founder mutation c.1592delT. This mutation was found in 2.7% (3/113) of familial breast and/or breast/ovarian cancer families compared with 0.2% (6/2,501) of controls (OR, 11.3; 95% CI, 1.8 to 57.8; $P = 0.005$).[39] One percent (18/1,918) of breast cancer cases, unselected for family history, also had this founder mutation. The hazard ratio for breast cancer was estimated at 6.1 (95% CI, 2.2 to 17.2; $P = 0.01$), with a penetrance of 40% by the age of 70 years.[40]

PALB2 has not been shown to be a significant contributor to familial clustering of other cancers, including melanoma, ovarian cancer, and prostate cancer,[41–43] but has been identified in familial pancreatic cancer kindreds. Specifically, Jones et al.[44] identified a PALB2 mutation in a familial pancreatic cancer proband, and subsequently found PALB2 mutations in 3 of 96 additional families, suggesting that 3% to 4% of familial pancreatic cancer may be attributed to this gene. Other populations have found lower mutation frequencies, ranging from absent in Dutch (0/31) to 3.7% (3/81) in Germans.[45,46] When ascertained on the basis of co-occurrence of breast and pancreatic cancer in the same individual or family, prevalence varied, again, from absent in Dutch (0/45) and US-based studies (0/77) to 4.8% (3/62) in Italians.[42,47,48]

CDKN2A

The p16 transcript of the CDKN2A gene is an important cell cycle regulator. Germline mutations in the CDKN2A gene predispose to multiple early-onset melanomas. Somatic CDKN2A mutations are also frequently identified in pancreatic adenocarcinomas and precursor lesions, indicating a role for this gene in pancreatic cancer development and progression.[49–51]

The risk of pancreatic cancer with *CDKN2A* mutations varies based on genotype. In a study of 22 families with the Dutch founder mutation, p16-Leiden, which is a 19-base-pair deletion in exon 2, the relative risk of pancreatic cancer was 47.8 (95% CI, 28.4 to 74.7).[52] The age-related risks have been shown to be less than 1%, 4%, 5%, 12%, and 17% by ages 40, 50, 60, 70, and 75 years, respectively.[53] Regarding other mutations, the Genes, Environment and Melanoma Study assessed relative risks for nonmelanoma cancers in 429 first-degree relatives of 65 melanoma patients with a *CDKN2A* mutation. Five pancreatic cancers were reported compared with 41 pancreatic cancers among 23,452 first-degree relatives of 3,537 noncarriers, for a relative risk of 7.4 (95% CI, 2.3 to 18.7; $P = 0.002$).[54] A US-based study estimated penetrance to be 58% by the age of 80 years (95% CI, 8% to 86%) and noted a hazard ratio of 25.8 ($P = 2.1 \times 10^{-13}$) in those who ever smoked cigarettes.[55]

Mutation prevalence in pancreatic cancer families varies by population. In an Italian study, 5.7% of 225 consecutive patients with pancreatic cancer had an identified *CDKN2A* mutation.[56] The predominant mutations were the E27X and G101W founder mutations, although others were also represented. Five (31%) of sixteen patients classified as having familial pancreatic cancer carried *CDKN2A* mutations, leading the authors to conclude that this gene may account for a sizeable subset of Italian familial pancreatic families. By comparison, no *CDKN2A* mutations were found in 51 Polish pancreatic cancer patients diagnosed at younger than 50 years.[57] Similarly, analysis of 94 German pancreatic cancer patients, who had at least one other first-degree relative with pancreatic cancer, revealed no *CDKN2A* mutations.[58] However, two of five families with at least one pancreatic cancer and at least one melanoma had an identified mutation.[59] Similarly, a Canadian study found a *CDKN2A* mutation in 2 of 14 families with both pancreatic cancer and melanoma.[60] Finally, a US-based study found 9 *CDKN2A* mutations in an unselected series of 1,537 pancreatic cancer cases (0.6%). The prevalence increased to 3.3% and 5.3% for those who reported a first-degree relative with pancreatic cancer or melanoma, respectively.[55] Thus, in the majority of populations, co-occurrence of melanoma appears to be a significant indicator of an underlying *CDKN2A* mutation.

Hereditary Nonpolyposis Colorectal Cancer

Hereditary nonpolyposis colorectal cancer (HNPCC), also referred to as Lynch syndrome, is the most common form of hereditary colon cancer, and it accounts for 2% to 5% of colorectal cancers. In addition to a high lifetime risk for colorectal cancer, affected individuals are at increased risk for multiple other cancers. HNPCC results from mutations in mismatch repair (MMR) genes, and colon cancers that arise in Lynch syndrome typically demonstrate microsatellite instability (MSI). Four percent of all pancreatic adenocarcinomas demonstrate MSI.[61] Yamamoto et al.[62] assessed tumor characteristics in three *MLH1* mutation carriers with both colon and pancreatic cancer, and found that both tumor types had similar properties, including high MSI, loss of MLH1 protein expression, wild-type K-RAS and p53, and poor differentiation. These findings support an inherited basis for the development of both types of cancer.[62]

Pancreatic cancer has been described in HNPCC kindreds as early as 1985, although data regarding risk of pancreatic cancer in HNPCC have varied.[63-68] Barrow et al.[64] studied 121 families with known MMR mutations; 2 of 282 extracolonic cancers were pancreatic, leading to a 0.4% cumulative lifetime risk for pancreatic cancer (95% CI, 0% to 0.8%). By comparison, Geary et al.[65] studied 130 families with MMR mutations and found 22 cases of pancreatic cancer, half of which were in confirmed or in obligate carriers. Pancreatic cancer in these families was seven times more common than expected, and the familial relative risk was 3.8 ($P = 0.02$). In addition, these tumors were 15 times more common in individuals younger than 60 years, suggesting an earlier average age at diagnosis as compared with the general population.[65] Another US-based study of HNPCC families found the lifetime risk for pancreatic cancer to be 1.31% by the age of 50 years (95% CI, 0.31% to 2.32%) and 3.68% by the age of 70 years (95% CI, 1.45% to 5.88%). These risks are higher than those from the SEER data of 0.04% and 0.52% at ages 50 and 70 years, respectively.[66]

Regarding the prevalence of HNPCC in pancreatic cancer, Gargiulo et al.[69] assessed 135 pancreatic cancer patients. Nineteen of these patients had a family history that was suggestive of HNPCC, and of the 11 patients whose DNA was available for analysis, only one deleterious MMR mutation was found. Thus, MMR mutations presumably account for only a small proportion of pancreatic cancer patients.

Hereditary Pancreatitis

Hereditary pancreatitis (HP) is a rare form of chronic pancreatitis. Several genes have been linked to chronic pancreatitis, including *SPINK1*, *CTFR*, and *CTRC*, but the *PRSS1* gene on chromosome 7q35 accounts for the majority of hereditary cases. *PRSS1* mutations are inherited in an autosomal dominant fashion and have an 80% penetrance for pancreatitis. Affected individuals begin experiencing symptoms of pancreatic pain and acute pancreatitis early in life. Several studies have shown an increase in pancreatic cancer risk associated with HP, and cumulative lifetime risk estimates range from 18.8% to 53.5%.[70-72] Lowenfels et al.[71] observed an increased risk associated with paternal inheritance. Tobacco use in patients with HP has been shown to increase the risk for pancreatic cancer twofold (95% CI, 0.7 to 6.1), pancreatic and HP patients who smoke developed cancer 20 years earlier than did their nonsmoking counterparts.[73]

Peutz–Jeghers Syndrome

Peutz–Jeghers syndrome (PJS) is an autosomal dominant condition characterized by mucocutaneous pigmentation and hamartomatous polyps of the gastrointestinal tract. PJS is caused by mutations on the *STK11* (*LKB1*) gene. The lifetime risk to develop any cancer has been estimated to be as high as 93%,[74] with no sex difference in cancer risk noted.[74,75] Risk for pancreatic cancer in PJS is estimated to be 8% to 36% by the age of 70 years.[74-76] Grützmann et al.[77] analyzed 39 individuals with familial pancreatic cancer, and none were found to carry mutations in *STK11*. In 2011, Schneider et al.[58] confirmed these findings in their study of 94 familial pancreatic

TABLE 11.2	Risk of Pancreatic Cancer in Familial Pancreatic Cancer Kindreds Based on Number of Affected First-degree Relatives (FDRs)

Number of Affected FDRs	SIR (95% CI)
1	4.5 (0.54–16.3)
2	6.4 (1.8–16.4)
3	32 (10.4–74.7)

cancer kindreds. Therefore, although *STK11* mutations confer a high lifetime risk for pancreatic cancer in individuals with PJS, germline *STK11* mutations are not thought to account for hereditary pancreatic cancer.

Empiric Risk Counseling and Management

Having a first-degree relative with apparently sporadic pancreatic cancer has a moderate effect on risk (OR, 1.76; 95% CI, 1.19 to 2.61).[78] In familial pancreatic cancer kindreds (defined as a family with a pair of affected first-degree relatives), the risk of pancreatic cancer increases with the number of affected first-degree relatives[3] (Table 11.2.) These findings suggest that high-penetrance genes may be causing the clustering of pancreatic cancer in families with two or three pancreatic cancer cases. Thus, individuals with multiple affected first-degree relatives are at appreciably increased risk for pancreatic cancer and may be candidates for increased surveillance.

Ideally, high-risk patients would be able to undergo noninvasive, inexpensive pancreatic cancer screening; however, to date, a highly sensitive and specific method for pancreas surveillance has not been recognized. Screening of high-risk patients with endoscopic ultrasound, magnetic resonance imaging, and/or magnetic resonance cholangiopancreatogram has been shown to be effective at identifying early neoplasms, both benign and malignant.[79–82] However, it is unknown if these methods actually prevent pancreatic cancer or improve overall survival by detecting presymptomatic disease. In addition, there is great interest in developing a biomarker for premalignant or early-stage disease, although none, including CA-19-9, has been proven effective.[83] Thus, whenever possible, it is recommended that high-risk patients undergo pancreatic screening through a research study.

REFERENCES

1. Lynch HT, Smyrk T, Kern SE, et al. Familial pancreatic cancer: A review. *Semin Oncol.* 1996;23:251–275.
2. Klein AP, Hruban RH, Brune KA, et al. Familial pancreatic cancer. *Cancer J.* 2001;7:266–273.
3. Klein AP, Brune KA, Petersen GM, et al. Prospective risk of pancreatic cancer in familial pancreatic cancer kindreds. *Cancer Res.* 2004;64:2634–2638.
4. Klein AP, Beaty TH, Bailey-Wilson JE, et al. Evidence for a major gene influencing risk of pancreatic cancer. *Genet Epidemiol.* 2002;23:133–149.

5. The Breast Cancer Linkage Consortium. Cancer risks in BRCA2 mutation carriers. *J Natl Cancer Inst.* 1999;91:1310–1316.

6. Moran A, O'Hara C, Khan S, et al. Risk of cancer other than breast or ovarian in individuals with BRCA1 and BRCA2 mutations. *Fam Cancer.* 2012;11:235–242.

7. van Asperen CJ, Brohet RM, Meijers-Heijboer EJ, et al. Cancer risks in BRCA2 families: Estimates for sites other than breast and ovary. *J Med Genet.* 2005;42:711–719.

8. Kim DH, Crawford B, Ziegler J, et al. Prevalence and characteristics of pancreatic cancer in families with BRCA1 and BRCA2 mutations. *Fam Cancer.* 2009;8:153–158.

9. Martin ST, Matsubayashi H, Rogers CD, et al. Increased prevalence of the BRCA2 polymorphic stop codon K3326X among individuals with familial pancreatic cancer. *Oncogene.* 2005;24:3652–3656.

10. Murphy KM, Brune KA, Griffin C, et al. Evaluation of candidate genes MAP2K4, MADH4, ACVR1B, and BRCA2 in familial pancreatic cancer: Deleterious BRCA2 mutations in 17%. *Cancer Res.* 2002;62:3789–3793.

11. Hahn SA, Greenhalf B, Ellis I, et al. BRCA2 germline mutations in familial pancreatic carcinoma. *J Natl Cancer Inst.* 2003;95:214–221.

12. Couch FJ, Johnson MR, Rabe KG, et al. The prevalence of BRCA2 mutations in familial pancreatic cancer. *Cancer Epidemiol Biomarkers Prev.* 2007;16:342–346.

13. Goggins M, Schutte M, Lu J, et al. Germline BRCA2 gene mutations in patients with apparently sporadic pancreatic carcinomas. *Cancer Res.* 1996;56:5360–5364.

14. Ferrone CR, Levine DA, Tang LH, et al. BRCA germline mutations in Jewish patients with pancreatic adenocarcinoma. *J Clin Oncol.* 2009;27:433–438.

15. Figer A, Irmin L, Geva R, et al. The rate of the 6174delT founder Jewish mutation in BRCA2 in patients with non-colonic gastrointestinal tract tumours in Israel. *Br J Cancer.* 2001;84:478–481.

16. Stadler ZK, Salo-Mullen E, Patil SM, et al. Prevalence of BRCA1 and BRCA2 mutations in Ashkenazi Jewish families with breast and pancreatic cancer. *Cancer.* 2012;118:493–499.

17. Cho JH, Bang S, Park SW, et al. BRCA2 mutations as a universal risk factor for pancreatic cancer has a limited role in Korean ethnic group. *Pancreas.* 2008;36:337–340.

18. Ghiorzo P, Pensotti V, Fornarini G, et al. Contribution of germline mutations in the BRCA and PALB2 genes to pancreatic cancer in Italy. *Fam Cancer.* 2012;11:41–47.

19. Thompson D, Easton DF. Cancer incidence in BRCA1 mutation carriers. *J Natl Cancer Inst.* 2002;94:1358–1365.

20. Brose MS, Rebbeck TR, Calzone KA, et al. Cancer risk estimates for BRCA1 mutation carriers identified in a risk evaluation program. *J Natl Cancer Inst.* 2002;94:1365–1372.

21. Al-Sukhni W, Rothenmund H, Borgida AE, et al. Germline BRCA1 mutations predispose to pancreatic adenocarcinoma. *Hum Genet.* 2008;124:271–278.

22. Lynch HT, Deters CA, Snyder CL, et al. BRCA1 and pancreatic cancer: Pedigree findings and their causal relationships. *Cancer Genet Cytogenet.* 2005;158:119–125.

23. Danes BS, Lynch HT. A familial aggregation of pancreatic cancer. An in vitro study. *JAMA.* 1982;247:2798–2802.

24. Axilbund JE, Argani P, Kamiyama M, et al. Absence of germline BRCA1 mutations in familial pancreatic cancer patients. *Cancer Biol Ther.* 2009;8:131–135.

25. Reid S, Schindler D, Hanenberg H, et al. Biallelic mutations in PALB2 cause Fanconi anemia subtype FA-N and predispose to childhood cancer. *Nat Genet.* 2007;39:162–164.

26. Xia B, Dorsman JC, Ameziane N, et al. Fanconi anemia is associated with a defect in the BRCA2 partner PALB2. *Nat Genet.* 2007;39:159–161.

27. Rahman N, Seal S, Thompson D, et al. PALB2, which encodes a BRCA2-interacting protein, is a breast cancer susceptibility gene. *Nat Genet.* 2007;39:165–167.

28. McInerney NM, Miller N, Rowan A, et al. Evaluation of variants in the CHEK2, BRIP1 and PALB2 genes in an Irish breast cancer cohort. *Breast Cancer Res Treat.* 2010;121:203–210.

29. Gunnarsson H, Arason A, Gillanders EM, et al. Evidence against PALB2 involvement in Icelandic breast cancer susceptibility. *J Negat Results Biomed.* 2008;7:5.

30. Papi L, Putignano AL, Congregati C, et al. A PALB2 germline mutation associated with hereditary breast cancer in Italy. *Fam Cancer.* 2010;9:181–185.

31. Ding YC, Steele L, Chu LH, et al. Germline mutations in PALB2 in African-American breast cancer cases. *Breast Cancer Res Treat.* 2011;126:227–230.

32. Zheng Y, Zhang J, Niu Q, et al. Novel germline PALB2 truncating mutations in African American breast cancer patients. *Cancer*. 2012;118:1362–1370.

33. Cao AY, Huang J, Hu Z, et al. The prevalence of PALB2 germline mutations in BRCA1/BRCA2 negative Chinese women with early onset breast cancer or affected relatives. *Breast Cancer Res Treat*. 2009;114:457–462.

34. Blanco A, de la Hoya M, Balmaæa J, et al. Detection of a large rearrangement in PALB2 in Spanish breast cancer families with male breast cancer. *Breast Cancer Res Treat*. 2012;132:307–315.

35. Sluiter M, Mew S, van Rensburg EJ. PALB2 sequence variants in young South African breast cancer patients. *Fam Cancer*. 2009;8:347–353.

36. Casadei S, Norquist BM, Walsh T, et al. Contribution of inherited mutations in the BRCA2-interacting protein PALB2 to familial breast cancer. *Cancer Res*. 2011;71:2222–2229.

37. Tischkowitz M, Capanu M, Sabbaghian N, et al. Rare germline mutations in PALB2 and breast cancer risk: A population-based study. *Hum Mutat*. 2012;33:674–680.

38. Foulkes WD, Ghadirian P, Akbari MR, et al. Identification of a novel truncating PALB2 mutation and analysis of its contribution to early-onset breast cancer in French-Canadian women. *Breast Cancer Res*. 2007;9:R83.

39. Erkko H, Xia B, Nikkilä J, et al. A recurrent mutation in PALB2 in Finnish cancer families. *Nature*. 2007;446:316–319.

40. Erkko H, Dowty JG, Nikkilä J, et al. Penetrance analysis of the PALB2c.1592delT founder mutation. *Clin Cancer Res*. 2008;14:4667–4671.

41. Sabbaghian N, Kyle R, Hao A, et al. Mutation analysis of the PALB2 cancer predisposition gene in familial melanoma. *Fam Cancer*. 2011;10:315–317.

42. Adank MA, van Mil SE, Gille JJ, et al. PALB2 analysis in BRCA2-like families. *Breast Cancer Res Treat*. 2011;127:357–362.

43. Tischkowitz M, Sabbaghian N, Ray AM, et al. Analysis of the gene coding for the BRCA2-interacting protein PALB2 in hereditary prostate cancer. *Prostate*. 2008;68:675–678.

44. Jones S, Hruban RH, Kamiyama M, et al. Exomic sequencing identifies PALB2 as a pancreatic cancer susceptibility gene. *Science*. 2009;324:217.

45. Harinck F, Kluijt I, van Mil SE, et al. Routine testing for PALB2 mutations in familial pancreatic cancer families and breast cancer families with pancreatic cancer is not indicated. *Eur J Hum Genet*. 2012;20:577–579.

46. Slater EP, Langer P, Niemczyk E, et al. PALB2 mutations in European familial pancreatic cancer families. *Clin Genet*. 2010;78:490–494.

47. Stadler ZK, Salo-Mullen E, Sabbaghian N, et al. Germline PALB2 mutation analysis in breast-pancreas cancer families. *J Med Genet*. 2011;48:523–525.

48. Peterlongo P, Catucci I, Pasquini G, et al. PALB2 germline mutations in familial breast cancer cases with personal and family history of pancreatic cancer. *Breast Cancer Res Treat*. 2011;126:825–828.

49. Kanda M, Matthaei H, Wu J, et al. Presence of somatic mutations in most early-stage pancreatic intraepithelial neoplasia. *Gastroenterology*. 2012;142:730–733.

50. Remmers N, Bailey JM, Mohr AM, et al. Molecular pathology of early pancreatic cancer. *Cancer Biomark*. 2011;9:421–440.

51. Bartsch D, Shevlin DW, Tung WS, et al. Frequent mutations of CDKN2 in primary pancreatic adenocarcinomas. *Genes Chromosomes Cancer*. 1995;14:189–195.

52. de Snoo FA, Bishop DT, Bergman W, et al. Increased risk of cancer other than melanoma in CDKN2A founder mutation (p16-Leiden)-positive melanoma families. *Clin Cancer Res*. 2008;14:7151–7157.

53. Vasen HF, Gruis NA, Frants RR, et al. Risk of developing pancreatic cancer in families with familial atypical multiple mole melanoma associated with a specific 19 deletion of p16 (p16-Leiden). *Int J Cancer*. 2000;87:809–811.

54. Mukherjee B, Delancey JO, Raskin L, et al. Risk of non-melanoma cancers in first-degree relatives of CDKN2A mutation carriers. *J Natl Cancer Inst*. 2012;104:953–856.

55. McWilliams RR, Wieben ED, Rabe KG, et al. Prevalence of CDKN2A mutations in pancreatic cancer patients: Implications for genetic counseling. *Eur J Hum Genet*. 2011;19:472–478.

56. Ghiorzo P, Fornarini G, Sciallero S, et al. CDKN2A is the main susceptibility gene in Italian pancreatic cancer families. *J Med Genet*. 2012;49:164–170.

57. Debniak T, van de Wetering T, Scott R, et al. Low prevalence of CDKN2A/ARF mutations among early-onset cancers of breast, pancreas and malignant melanoma in Poland. *Eur J Cancer Prev*. 2008;17:389–391.

58. Schneider R, Slater EP, Sina M, et al. German national case collection for familial pancreatic cancer (FaPaCa): Ten years experience. *Fam Cancer*. 2011;10:323–330.

59. Bartsch DK, Sina-Frey M, Lang S, et al. CDKN2A germline mutations in familial pancreatic cancer. *Ann Surg*. 2002;236:730–737.

60. Lal G, Liu L, Hogg D, et al. Patients with both pancreatic adenocarcinoma and melanoma may harbor germline CDKN2A mutations. *Genes Chromosomes Cancer*. 2000;27:358–361.

61. Goggins M, Offerhaus GJ, Hilgers W, et al. Pancreatic adenocarcinomas with DNA replication errors (RER⁺) are associated with wild-type K-ras and characteristic histopathology. Poor differentiation, a syncytial growth pattern, and pushing borders suggest RER⁺. *Am J Pathol*. 1998;152:1501–1507.

62. Yamamoto H, Itoh F, Nakamura H, et al. Genetic and clinical features of human pancreatic ductal adenocarcinomas with widespread microsatellite instability. *Cancer Res*. 2001;61:3136–3144.

63. Lynch HT, Voorhees GJ, Lanspa SJ, et al. Pancreatic carcinoma and hereditary nonpolyposis colorectal cancer: A family study. *Br J Cancer*. 1985;52:271–273.

64. Barrow E, Robinson L, Alduaij W, et al. Cumulative lifetime incidence of extracolonic cancers in Lynch syndrome: A report of 121 families with proven mutations. *Clin Genet*. 2009;75:141–149.

65. Geary J, Sasieni P, Houlston R, et al. Gene-related cancer spectrum in families with hereditary non-polyposis colorectal cancer (HNPCC). *Fam Cancer*. 2008;7:163–172.

66. Kastrinos F, Mukherjee B, Tayob N, et al. Risk of pancreatic cancer in families with Lynch syndrome. *JAMA*. 2009;302:1790–1795.

67. Aarnio M, Sankila R, Pukkala E, et al. Cancer risk in mutation carriers of DNA-mismatch-repair genes. *Int J Cancer*. 1999;81:214–218.

68. Vasen HF, Offerhaus GJ, den Hartog Jager FH, et al. The tumor spectrum in hereditary non-polyposis colorectal cancer: A study of 24 kindreds in the Netherlands. *Int J Cancer*. 1990;46:31–34.

69. Gargiulo S, Torrini M, Ollila S, et al. Germline MLH1 and MSH2 mutations in Italian pancreatic cancer patients with suspected Lynch syndrome. *Fam Cancer*. 2009;8:547–553.

70. Howes N, Lerch MM, Greenhalf W, et al. Clinical and genetic characteristics of hereditary pancreatitis in Europe. *Clin Gastroenterol Hepatol*. 2004;2:252–261.

71. Lowenfels AB, Maisonneuve P, DiMagno EP, et al. Hereditary pancreatitis and the risk of pancreatic cancer. International Hereditary Pancreatitis Study Group. *J Natl Cancer Inst*. 1997;89:442–446.

72. Rebours V, Boutron-Ruault MC, Schnee MF, et al. Risk of pancreatic adenocarcinoma in patients with hereditary pancreatitis: A national exhaustive series. *Am J Gastroenterol*. 2008;103:111–119.

73. Lowenfels AB, Maisonneuve P, Whitcomb DC, et al. Cigarette smoking as a risk factor for pancreatic cancer in patients with hereditary pancreatitis. *JAMA*. 2001;286:169–170.

74. Giardiello FM, Brensinger JD, Tersmette AC, et al. Very high risk of cancer in familial Peutz–Jeghers syndrome. *Gastroenterology*. 2000;119:1447–1453.

75. Lim W, Olschwang S, Keller JJ, et al. Relative frequency and morphology of cancers in STK11 mutation carriers. *Gastroenterology*. 2004; 126:1788–1794.

76. Hearle N, Schumacher V, Menko FH, et al. Frequency and spectrum of cancers in the Peutz–Jeghers syndrome. *Clin Cancer Res*. 2006;12:3209–3215.

77. Grützmann R, McFaul C, Bartsch DK, et al. No evidence for germline mutations of the LKB1/STK11 gene in familial pancreatic carcinoma. *Cancer Lett*. 2004;214:63–68.

78. Jacobs EJ, Chanock SJ, Fuchs CS, et al. Family history of cancer and risk of pancreatic cancer: A pooled analysis from the Pancreatic Cancer Cohort Consortium (PanScan). *Int J Cancer*. 2010;127:1421–1428.

79. Canto MI, Hruban RH, Fishman EK, et al. Frequent detection of pancreatic lesions in asymptomatic high-risk individuals. *Gastroenterology*. 2012;142:796–804.

80. Ludwig E, Olson SH, Bayuga S, et al. Feasibility and yield of screening in relatives from familial pancreatic cancer families. *Am J Gastroenterol*. 2011;106:946–954.

81. Verna EC, Hwang C, Stevens PD, et al. Pancreatic cancer screening in a prospective cohort of high-risk patients: A comprehensive strategy of imaging and genetics. *Clin Cancer Res*. 2010;16:5028–5037.

82. Langer P, Kann PH, Fendrich V, et al. Five years of prospective screening of high-risk individuals from families with familial pancreatic cancer. *Gut*. 2009;58:1410–1418.

83. Goggins M. Markers of pancreatic cancer: Working toward early detection. *Clin Cancer Res*. 2011;17:635–637.

12 Genetic Testing by Cancer Site

Stomach

Nicki Chun and James M. Ford

G astric cancer encompasses a heterogeneous collection of etiologic and histologic subtypes associated with a variety of known and unknown environmental and genetic factors. It is a global public health concern, accounting for 700,000 annual deaths worldwide and currently ranking as the fourth leading cause of cancer mortality, with a 5-year survival of only 20%. The incidence and prevalence of gastric cancer vary widely with Asian/Pacific regions bearing the highest rates of disease.

Recent and rapid advances in molecular genetics have provided an understanding of the cause for many inherited cancer syndromes, offering possibilities for individual genetic testing, family counseling, and preventive approaches. For most cancer syndromes, however, not every individual tested is found to have inherited a germline mutation in a candidate gene, suggesting additional uncharacterized alterations in other genes that result in similar outcomes. Nevertheless, the ability to genetically define many individuals and families with inherited cancer syndromes allows for a multidisciplinary approach to their management, often including consideration of surgical and medical preventive measures. Without question, such complex management and decision making should be centered in the high-risk cancer genetics clinic, where physicians, genetic counselors, and other health professionals jointly consider optimal management for patients and families at high risk for developing cancer.

Approximately 3% to 5% of gastric cancers are associated with a hereditary predisposition, including a variety of Mendelian genetic conditions and complex genetic traits. Identifying those gastric cancers associated with an inherited cancer risk syndrome is the purview of cancer genetics clinics. The keystone to any cancer genetics evaluation is a complete, three-generation family history. Pedigree analyses suggesting an inherited gastric cancer risk include familiar features such as multiple affected relatives tracking along one branch of the family in an autosomal dominant pattern, young ages at onset, and additional associated malignancies related to an identified syndrome. It is imperative to document the histology of the gastric tumors and other familial cancers as this is the initial node in the decision tree of an inherited gastric cancer syndrome differential. Finally, there are clinical criteria for recognized gastric cancer syndromes published by

167

expert consensus panels that assist genetic practitioners in assessing both the likelihood of identifying an underlying germline DNA mutation and guide management in the absence of a molecular confirmation. Herein, we review the literature regarding incidence, recurrence risks, and defined gastric cancer genetic syndromes to assist in providing genetic counseling for families affected by gastric cancer.

HISTOLOGIC DEFINITIONS AND DESCRIPTIONS

Gastric cancer has traditionally been subtyped pathologically according to Lauren's[1] classification published in 1965 and revised by Carneiro et al.[2] in 1995. The four histologic categories include (1) glandular/intestinal, (2) border foveal hyperplasia, (3) mixed intestinal/diffuse, and (4) solid/undifferentiated.

More clinically relevant, the majority of gastric cancers can be subdivided into intestinal type or diffuse type. Diffuse tumors exhibit isolated cells, typically developing below the mucosal lining, often spreading and thickening until the stomach appears hardened into the morphologic designation called "linitis plastica." Diffuse gastric tumors frequently feature "signet ring cells," named for the marginalization of the nucleus to the cell periphery due to high mucin content. Intestinal-type gastric tumors more often present as solid masses with atrophic gastritis and intestinal metaplasia at the periphery. The intestinal subtype is seen more commonly in older patients, whereas the diffuse type affects younger patients and has a more aggressive clinical course. The relative proportions of gastric cancer subtypes worldwide are 74% intestinal versus 16% diffuse and 10% other,[3] although diffuse gastric cancer is becoming relatively more common in the Western countries. The importance of distinguishing these two main histopathologic types of gastric cancer is highlighted by finding specific genetic changes associated with the different types. For the purposes of genetic counseling, E-cadherin (CDH1) mutations are found exclusively in the diffuse type.[4–8] Whereas intestinal-type hereditary gastric cancer families have been identified clinically, no genetic associations have yet been discovered.

As individual molecular profiling of solid tumors becomes more common in the future, we expect classification systems will evolve based on tumor biology more than histology. Advances in deciphering the mechanisms of gene alterations that lead to gastric cancer include gene mutation, amplification, deletion, and epigenetic methylation.[9] For example, two recent studies have performed whole-exome sequencing of human gastric tumors and identified a number of known (e.g., p53, PTEN, PIK3CA), but also previously unreported somatic gene mutations and pathway alterations. Both found ARID1A inactivating gene mutations in the majority of microsatellite-instable tumors, a member of the SWI-SNF chromatin remodeling family.[10,11] However, whether any of these somatic gene alterations are found to confer cancer risk when mutated in the germline remains to be determined.

ETIOLOGY

Analogous to other common cancers, a host of factors are implicated as causes of gastric cancer. Widely diverse geographical disparities suggest both environmental and genetic contributions. Furthermore, a strong association with endemic *Helicobacter pylori* carrier rates implicates infection as a major risk factor. There are likely to be a host of factors contributing to the development of most gastric cancers.

Environmental Risk Factors

Geographic variations in gastric cancer rates have prompted investigations of shared diet and lifestyle variables. Gastric cancer is correlated with the chronic ingestion of pickled vegetables, salted fish, excessive dietary salt, and smoked meats and with smoking.[12–16] Fruits and vegetables may have a protective effect. The influence of environmental factors as causes of gastric cancer is highlighted by declining rates of intestinal gastric cancer among immigrants from high-incident countries to low-incident countries.

Infectious Risk Factors

H. pylori infection is endemic in the Asian-Pacific basin.[17] Transmission routinely occurs through family contacts in childhood and leads to atrophic gastritis.[18,19] As evidenced by high indigenous infection rates, *H. pylori* is insufficient to singularly cause gastric cancer, suggesting complex interactions between virus and host genetic backgrounds. However, *H. pylori* species are consistently implicated as a major risk factor primarily associated with intestinal-type gastric cancer. Studies in a variety of high- and low-risk populations have found odds ratios ranging from 2.56 to 6 for noncardia gastric cancer.[20]

Epstein-Barr virus has recently been implicated in about 10% of gastric carcinoma worldwide or an estimated 80,000 cases annually. Epstein-Barr virus–associated gastric cancer shows some distinct clinicopathologic characteristics, such as male predominance, predisposition to the proximal stomach, and a high proportion in diffuse-type gastric carcinomas. Mechanistically, Epstein–Barr virus gastric tumors display epigenetic promoter methylation of many cancer-related genes, causing downregulation of their expression.[21]

Genetics

Five to ten percent of gastric cancer is associated with strong familial clustering and attributable to genetic factors. Shared environmental factors account for the majority of familial clustering of the intestinal type; however, approximately 5% of the total gastric cancer burden is thought to be due to germline mutations in genes causing highly penetrant, autosomal dominant gastric cancer risk of both intestinal and diffuse subtypes. We review the definitions of hereditary gastric cancer families and recognize genetic syndromes associated with increased gastric cancer risk.

EPIDEMIOLOGY OF GASTRIC CANCER

Gastric cancer is now the fourth most common malignancy worldwide, with rates having fallen steadily since 1975 when global statistics were first compared. The incidence and prevalence of gastric cancer vary widely among world populations. High-risk countries (reported incidence × 100,000 per year) include Korea (41.4), China (41.3), Japan (31.1), Portugal (34.4), and Colombia (20.3). Intermediate-risk countries include Malaysia, Singapore, and Taiwan (11 to 19), whereas low-risk areas include Thailand (8), Northern Europe (5.6), Australia (5.4), India (5.3), and North America (4.3). More than 70% of cases occur in developing countries, and men have roughly twice the risk of women.[22] In 2008, estimates of gastric cancer burden in the United States were 21,500 cases (13,190 men and 8,310 women) and 10,880 deaths.[23] The median age at diagnosis for gastric cancer is 71 years, and 5-year survival is approximately 25%.[24] Only 24% of stomach cancers are localized at the time of diagnosis, 30% have lymph node involvement, and another 30% have metastatic disease. Survival rates are predictably higher for those with localized disease, with corresponding 5-year survival rates of 60%.

The worldwide decline in the incidence of gastric cancer has been attributed to modifications in diet, improved food storage and preservation, and decreased *H. pylori* infection. Fresh fruit and vegetable consumption, refrigeration, decreased urban crowding, and improved living conditions have reduced *H. pylori* exposure and carrier rates. By contrast, the incidence of diffuse-type gastric cancer is stable, and in North America, it may even be increasing.[16,25–27]

FAMILIAL GASTRIC CANCER

Shared environmental factors, such as diet and *H. pylori* infection, account for the majority of familial clustering of the intestinal type of gastric cancer, with no known causative germline variants. However, few nongenetic risks for diffuse gastric cancer have been identified, supporting a larger role for hereditary factors. Approximately 5% of the total gastric cancer burden is thought to be due to germline mutations in genes causing a highly penetrant, autosomal dominant predisposition. The International Gastric Cancer Linkage Consortium (IGCLC) has redefined genetic classification of familial intestinal gastric cancer to reflect the background incidence rate in a population (Table 12.1).

Thus, countries with high incidence of intestinal-type gastric cancer (China, Korea, Japan, Portugal) use criteria analogous to the Amsterdam criteria invoked for Lynch syndrome:

(1) At least three relatives with intestinal gastric cancer, one a first-degree relative of the other two,
(2) at least two successive generations affected, and
(3) gastric cancer diagnosed before the age of 50 years in at least one individual.

In countries with a low incidence of intestinal-type gastric cancer (United States, United Kingdom):

(1) At least two first-/second-degree relatives affected by intestinal gastric cancer, one diagnosed before the age of 50 years; or
(2) three or more relatives with intestinal gastric cancer at any age.

TABLE 12.1	Clinical Criteria for CDH1 Testing Defined by IGCLC 2010

1. Two gastric cancer cases in the family: One confirmed diffuse type, one diagnosed at the age of <50 y
2. Three confirmed diffuse gastric cancers in first- or second-degree relatives independent of age
3. Diffuse gastric cancer diagnosed at age <40 y (no additional family history needed)
4. Personal or family history (first- or second-degree) of diffuse gastric cancer and lobular breast cancer, one diagnosed at age <50 y

From: Fitzgerald RC, Hardwick R, Huntsman D, et al. Hereditary diffuse gastric cancer: Updated consensus guidelines for clinical management and directions for future research. *J Med Genet.* 2010;47:436–444.

Familial intestinal gastric cancer families are similarly prevalent as familial diffuse gastric cancer families, yet a germline genetic defect underlying the disease remains yet to be identified.[28] Hemminki et al.[29] reported Swedish data on all available types of cancer in first-degree relatives by both parent and sibling probands. The relative risks (RRs) for gastric cancer were greater than 3 for siblings with any relative with gastric cancer and greater than 5 when a sibling was younger than 50 years. Shin et al.[30] assessed 428 gastric cancer subjects and 368 controls in Korea for the risk of gastric cancer in first-degree relatives and found an RR of 2.85 with one first-degree relative and greater than 5 in a first-degree relative with *H. pylori* and a positive family history. Therefore, in the high-incident countries of Japan and Taiwan, population screening for gastric cancer has greatly enhanced early detection, leading to 5-year survival rates of greater than 90%.[31]

HEREDITARY DIFFUSE GASTRIC CANCER

In 1999, the first IGCLC defined hereditary diffuse gastric cancer (HDGC) as families with (1) two cases diffuse gastric cancer in first-/second-degree relatives with one younger than 50 years, and (2) three cases diffuse gastric cancer at any age.[32] The first clear evidence for a gastric cancer susceptibility genetic locus was the identification in 1998 of a germline inactivating mutation in the gene encoding for E-cadherin (*CDH1*), in a large, five-generation Maori family from New Zealand with 25 kindred with early-onset diffuse gastric cancer.[33] The age at diagnosis of gastric cancer ranged upward from 14 years, with the majority occurring in individuals younger than 40 years. The pattern of inheritance of gastric cancer was consistent with an autosomal dominant susceptibility gene with incomplete penetrance. Similar reports of *CDH1* mutations in widely diverse HDGC cohorts from Asia, Europe, and North

America followed soon thereafter.[34–39] Germline *CDH1* mutations have been found to be associated with approximately 30% of families with HDGC, with a lifetime risk for gastric cancer of greater than 80%, and up to 60% risk for female carriers developing lobular breast cancer.[40] To date, *CDH1* is the only gene implicated in HDGC. Worldwide, about 100 *CDH1* mutation–positive families have been reported.[41]

E-CADHERIN MUTATIONS AND GASTRIC CANCER

The E-cadherin gene coding sequence gives rise to a mature protein consisting of three major domains, a large extracellular domain (exons 4 to 13) and smaller transmembrane (exons 13 to 14) and cytoplasmic domains (exons 14 to 16). As in other autosomal dominant cancer predisposing genes, only one *CDH1* allele is mutated in the germline, and the majority of genetic changes lead to truncation of the protein, with mutations distributed throughout the gene's 2.6 kb of coding sequence and 16 exons without any apparent hotspots. Somatic *CDH1* mutations have been identified in about half of sporadic diffuse gastric cancers, but occur rarely in intestinal gastric cancer. CDH1 encodes the calcium-dependent cell-adhesion glycoprotein E-cadherin. E-cadherin is a transmembrane protein that connects to the actin cytoskeleton through a complex with catenin proteins.[5,42] Functionally, E-cadherin impacts maintenance of normal tissue morphology and cellular differentiation. With regard to HDGC, it is believed that *CDH1* acts as a tumor suppressor gene, with mutation of *CDH1* leading to loss of cell adhesion, proliferation, invasion, and metastasis.[43]

GENETIC TESTING FOR HDGC

At the second meeting of the IGCLC in 2010, HDGC guidelines[44] were extended to recommend *CDH1* genetic testing to families with

(1) two cases of gastric cancer in which one case is histopathologically confirmed as diffuse and younger than 50 years,
(2) families with both lobular breast cancer and diffuse gastric cancer, with one diagnosed younger than 50 years, and
(3) probands diagnosed with diffuse gastric cancer younger than 40 years, with no family history of gastric cancer.

Using the initial IGCLC criteria for HDGC, *CDH1* mutation testing yielded a detection rate of 30% to 50%.[45] Interestingly, a pattern began to emerge of lower *CDH1* mutation rates among HDGC families in high gastric cancer incidence populations and higher rates in low-incident countries.[46,47] Other reports suggest that the rate of *CDH1* mutations in isolated cases of diffuse gastric cancer younger than 35 years is similar in both low- and high-risk countries hovering at around 20%.[48]

Approximately 50% to 70% of clinically diagnosed HDGC families have no identifiable genetic mutation. Multiple candidate loci have been investigated without identifying causative mutations that would account for the large number of non-CDH1 HDGC families.[49–51] Huntsman's group has published a report of multiplex ligation-dependant probe amplification-based exon duplication/deletion studies performed on 93 non-CDH1 families and found 6.5% carried large genomic deletions bringing the detection rate up to 45.6% in their cohort of 160 families.[52]

As *CDH1* mutation families were identified, data on these families provided the foundation for genetic counseling information. Initially, the cumulative risk of gastric cancer by the age of 80 years in HDGC families was initially estimated as 67% for men and 83% for women. The age at onset shows marked variation between and within families. The median age at onset in the 30 Maori *CDH1* mutation carriers who developed gastric cancer was 32 years, significantly younger than the median age of 43 years in individuals with gastric cancer from other ethnicities.[53] More recent reports of the lifetime risks of diffuse gastric cancer suggest greater than 80% in both men and women by the age of 80 years.[48,54]

The lifetime risk for lobular breast cancer among female *CDH1* carriers, originally estimated to be in the range of 20% to 40%, now approaches 60% with an average age of 53 years at the time of diagnosis.[36,54,55] Of note, *CDH1* mutations have been seen in up to 50% of sporadic lobular breast cancer. Pathologic similarities between diffuse gastric and lobular breast carcinomas such as high mucin content with associated signet ring features and loss of E-cadherin on immunohistochemistry hint at a common molecular mechanism.[56,57] To evaluate the *CDH1* carrier rate in women with lobular breast cancer without a family history of diffuse gastric cancer, a multicenter study of 318 women with lobular-type breast cancer diagnosed before the age of 45 years and known to be BRCA1/2-negative were sequenced for *CDH1* mutations. Only four possibly pathogenic mutations were identified for a rate of 1.3%, suggesting CDH1 is a rare cause of early lobular cancer without associated gastric cancer family history.[58]

Signet ring colon cancer has been reported in two families with germline CDH1, but no screening guidelines have been suggested.[45,59] Nonsyndromic cleft lip and/or palate was reported in seven individuals from three families in the Netherlands and in four individuals from two families in France. There is speculation that defects in the cell-adhesion role of E-cadherin may contribute to this developmental anomaly, although no association can be drawn from these scant case reports.[40,60]

Like other familial cancer syndromes with an autosomal dominant inheritance pattern, high penetrance for heterozygotes, and significant mortality unless diagnosed early, genetic counseling and testing should occur early, and a comprehensive screening plan developed, as well as consideration of prophylactic surgery. Pretest and posttest genetic counseling should be provided to individuals from HDGC kindred who are undergoing genetic testing for germline *CDH1* mutations. Since cases of gastric cancer in HDGC families have been reported in individuals as young as 14 years, HDGC may be considered one of the sets of hereditary cancer syndromes, such as MEN 2 associated medullary thyroid cancer, Li–Fraumeni syndrome (LFS), and familial adenomatous polyposis (FAP), in which genetic testing is potentially clinically useful in children.

SCREENING AND MANAGEMENT OF CANCER RISK IN HDGC

Diagnosing gastric cancer in its early stages provides the best chance for curative resection but is a difficult task. Symptoms due to gastric cancer do not appear until the disease is more advanced and are generally nonspecific. The survival of early gastric cancer (e.g., not beyond the mucosa or submucosa) is much better than advanced lesions, so identifying these lesions at the earliest of stages is imperative for optimal survival. Endoscopy is generally considered to be the best method to screen for gastric cancer, but diagnosing diffuse gastric carcinoma is most difficult, as these lesions tend not to form a grossly visible exophytic mass, but rather spread submucosally as single cells or clustered islands of cells. Improved chromoendoscopic-aided methods for directed biopsies to diagnose these early diffuse lesions may prove beneficial, but so far all approaches at screening, including computed tomography and positron emission tomography imaging, have proven disappointing.[61]

Given the inadequacy of clinical screening in HDGC, prophylactic total gastrectomy is offered to carriers of germline *CDH1* mutations.[62,63] In every published series of this approach, nearly all specimens contain multiple foci of intramucosal diffuse signet ring cell cancer. Currently, there is information available from 96 total gastrectomies in the setting of HDGC,[44] approximately three quarters of which were performed in asymptomatic *CDH1* carriers following negative screening endoscopy and biopsies. Only three cases did not show evidence for early invasive carcinoma, and in two of these, tiny foci of in situ signet ring cell carcinoma were observed.[44] Although malignant foci are generally localized to the proximal one-third of the stomach,[64] lesions may be distributed throughout the entire stomach, necessitating a total gastrectomy for comprehensive prevention. The optimal timing of prophylactic gastrectomy is unknown but is generally recommended when the unaffected carrier is 5 years younger than the youngest family member who has developed clinical symptoms of HDGC. Clinical management and screening strategies remain uncertain for families who meet criteria for HDGC but are negative for *CDH1* mutations or variants of unknown significance, although screening endoscopy is often suggested.

The impact and long-term outcomes of prophylactic gastrectomy on carriers' lifestyle and health are significant, particularly because 20% to 30% of carriers may never develop invasive gastric cancer. Certainly, all patients experience some level of morbidity, including diarrhea, weight loss, and difficulty eating. Mortality due to this indication for a gastrectomy has not been reported. Early evidence suggests that women can successfully carry healthy pregnancies after gastrectomy.[65] Most importantly, to date, there have been no reports of gastric cancer recurrence in a member of a HDGC family after prophylactic total gastrectomy.

Women with HDGC also exhibit up to 60% lifetime risk for developing breast cancer, primarily of the lobular type, and as more women are prevented from developing diffuse gastric cancer, breast cancer screening is of great relevance. The correct approach to screening for lobular breast cancer in women with HDGC is not known, but based on approaches used in other hereditary breast cancer susceptibility syndromes. Although prophylactic mastectomy has been shown to effectively prevent the development of breast cancer and to result in improved long-term survival in *BRCA1/2* mutation carriers, such an approach remains completely investigational for women in HDGC families. The prognosis of lobular cancers that develop in HDGC patients is currently unknown, and given the relatively late onset compared with breast cancers in *BRCA1/2* carriers, prophylactic mastectomies may not be appropriate. Standard screening recommendations therefore include annual breast magnetic resonance imaging and mammogram starting at the age of 35 years.[66,67] An open question is whether chemoprevention with tamoxifen may benefit women with HDGC, given its role in reducing breast cancer risk in half in women at elevated risk because of age, family history, or history of biopsy-proven lobular carcinoma in situ.[68]

In summary, individuals from HDGC families with inherited germline mutations in the *CDH1* gene face up to an 80% likelihood of developing gastric cancer and for women an additional 60% chance of developing lobular breast cancer during their lifetime, with significant risk beginning at relatively young ages. Such levels of overall cancer risk are similar to that of developing breast or colon cancer for carriers of *BRCA1* or 2 gene mutations, or mismatch repair gene mutations, respectively. Therefore, rigorous surveillance and consideration of prophylactic surgery are important for the management of these individuals. At the very least, regular endoscopic examination with random biopsy of the stomach should be performed every 6 to 12 months, probably starting 10 years earlier than the youngest affected patient in the family, or by the age of 25 years. Since mucosal abnormalities tend to occur late in diffuse gastric cancer and delay the endoscopic diagnosis, prophylactic gastrectomy should be seriously considered as a means of preventing gastric carcinoma, although it clearly comes with high morbidity. It is somewhat less clear as to the correct approach for screening and prevention of lobular breast cancer in women with HDGC. Adherence to standard recommendations for screening mammography for breast cancer should be followed. Consideration of investigative approaches to screening with magnetic resonance imaging and chemoprevention with tamoxifen or other agents are appropriate. The decision to perform prophylactic gastrectomy should be balanced with age-based risk, based on age-specific penetrance data, as well as many other personal factors. Therefore, it is essential that patients carrying the gene have the opportunity for extensive counseling, discussion, and reflection with knowledgeable clinicians, geneticists, and counselors before making the decision to proceed.

OTHER HEREDITARY CANCER SUSCEPTIBILITY SYNDROMES WITH INCREASED GASTRIC CANCER RISK

Lynch Syndrome

The seminal report of a family with dominantly inherited colon and gastrointestinal (GI) cancers in 1979 by Lynch and Lynch[69] began decades of defining and refining this hereditary syndrome. Lynch syndrome is caused by a germline mutation in a mismatch DNA repair gene (*MLH1*, *MSH2*, *MSH6*, *PMS2*, or *EPCAM*) and is thus associated with tumors exhibiting microsatellite instability (MSI). It is estimated that 2% to 4% of all diagnosed colorectal cancers[70] and 2% to 5% of all diagnosed endometrial cancers[71] are due to Lynch syndrome. With a frequency estimated at 1/440 in the United States,[72] it is similar to the BRCA carriage rate. The lifetime risks for Lynch syndrome associated cancers are highest for colorectal cancer at 52% to 82% (mean age at diagnosis 44 to 61 years), followed by an endometrial cancer risk of 25% to 60% in women (mean age at diagnosis 48 to 62 years), a 6% to 13% risk for gastric cancer (mean age at diagnosis 56 years), and 4% to 12% for ovarian cancer (mean age at diagnosis 42.5 years).[70–78]

Lynch-associated gastric cancers show predominantly intestinal histology (more than 90% of the cases). This correlation echoes the strong association between MSI tumor phenotype and intestinal gastric cancer. The International Collaborative Group on HNPCC developed the original Amsterdam Criteria in 1991. Revisions followed with Bethesda criteria outlined in 1997 and revised in 2004 with the inclusion of extra-colonic tumor risks including gastric cancer.[79,80]

MSI screening by molecular and/or immunohistochemistry for the four common Lynch protein products (MSH2, MSH6, MLH1, and PMS2) should be considered in families who meet the Bethesda criteria. As 15% of all gastric tumors exhibit MSI histology, the majority of these have acquired this mutator phenotype through sporadic mutations, and further germline testing of individuals with MSI-positive tumors is necessary to confirm a molecular diagnosis of Lynch syndrome.

Hereditary Breast/Ovarian Cancer Syndrome

Hereditary breast and ovarian cancer due to germline *BRCA1* and *BRCA2* mutations is perhaps the most well-defined and recognized inherited cancer syndrome. With a prevalence of 1/300 to 1/400 in most populations and up to 1/40 in selected groups with founder mutations, most notably those with Ashkenazi Jewish ancestry, it represents the most common of the hereditary disorders due to high-risk mutations. Carriers face a 5- to 6-fold increased risk of generally early-onset breast cancer and 10- to 20-fold increased risk for ovarian, fallopian, and primary peritoneal malignancies. Male carriers have a recognized increased risk for prostate cancer and male breast cancer. *BRCA1* and *BRCA2* have been implicated in multiple cellular functions but serve primary roles as tumor suppressor genes recruited to maintain genomic stability through DNA double-strand break repair. Following the cloning of the *BRCA1* and *BRCA2* genes in 1994 and 1995,[81,82] the Breast Cancer Linkage Consortium convened to pool data and generate a body clinical information to assist in counseling and management of BRCA carriers, resulting in a seminal publication outlining the spectrum of *BRCA* mutation–associated cancer risks. In 173 breast–ovarian cancer families with *BRCA2* mutations from 20 centers in Europe and North America, the RR of gastric cancer was 2.59 (95% confidence interval [CI], 1.46 to 4.61).[83] Carriers of the 6174 delT *BRCA2* Ashkenazi Jewish founder mutation in Israel found gastric cancer to be the most common malignancy after breast and ovarian. Conversely, 5.7% of patients with gastric cancer in Israel were found to carry this *BRCA2* mutation[84]; 20.7% of a Polish cohort of families with both gastric and breast malignancies were attributable to mutations in *BRCA2*. A *BRCA2* mutation was also found in 23.5% of women with ovarian cancer and a family history of stomach cancer in this population.[85,86]

Several studies have implicated *BRCA1* mutations as a risk factor for gastric cancer. A large Swedish population-based study published in 1999 involving 150 malignant tumors from 1,145 relatives in *BRCA1* found an RR = 5.86 (95% CI, 1.60 to 15.01) and observed that gastric cancer diagnosed before the age of 70 years was twice as common in carrier families compared with the general population. They did not observe the same risk with *BRCA2*.[87,88]

Brose et al.[89] observed the highest RR for gastric cancer (6.9) in 147 families with *BRCA1* mutations in Pennsylvania. Risch et al.[90] also observed an RR = 6.2 in first-degree relatives of 39 *BRCA1* mutation carrier families and to a lesser extent in 21 *BRCA2* families in Ontario, Canada.

More recently, a meta-analysis of more than 30 studies of tumor risk in *BRCA1* and *BRCA2* carriers found an RR of 1.69 (95% CI, 1.21 to 2.38) for gastric cancer, the highest risk after breast, ovarian, and prostate, followed closely by pancreatic cancer, with RR = 1.62 (1.31 to 2.00).[91] No pathology details were included in these studies, and it is unknown if one of the histologic subtypes of gastric cancer predominates in BRCA-associated tumors.

Familial Adenomatous Polyposis

FAP is a rare colon cancer syndrome associated with the striking presentation of early-onset multiple colonic adenomas and, in classic form, a near-complete certainty of early colon cancer without prophylactic surgical intervention. Incidence estimates for FAP range from 1/10,000 to 1/20,000, and almost one-third of those diagnosed carry a de novo mutation, making family history unreliable for ascertainment of many cases. Extracolonic findings include upper GI adenomas, fundic gland polyps, and desmoids tumors. A wide spectrum of extracolonic tumors can occur including relatively rare cancers such as hepatoblastomas, duodenal adenocarcinomas, and adrenal, pancreatic, thyroid, biliary tract, and brain tumors. Additional diagnostic aids can include the finding of congenital hypertrophy of the retinal pigment epithelium, supernumerary teeth, osteomas, cutaneous lipomas, and cysts.

It is estimated that the lifetime risk for upper GI cancer in FAP is approximately 4% to 12%, of which only 0.5% to 2% are gastric cancers, although this risk has been reported as sevenfold to 10-fold higher in Asia.[75,92,93] Approximately 50% of individuals with FAP have gastric fundus polyps, and 10% have adenomas of the stomach. Although gastric fundus polyps are unlikely to have malignant potential, gastric adenomas can occasionally develop into invasive disease.[94] Prophylactic gastrectomy is even discussed for diffuse fundic gland polyps showing high-grade dysplasia or large polyps.[95] Attenuated FAP is a muted form of classic FAP characterized by fewer than 100 colonic adenoma, a later median age and lower overall risk of colon cancer, and a high proportion of fundic gland polyps, suggesting a measurable risk for gastric cancer.[96–99]

Li–Fraumeni Syndrome

LFS is a devastating cancer syndrome with an extremely high risk for a multitude of tumor types. The most common malignancies are early-onset breast cancers and sarcomas followed by brain tumors, leukemia, and lung and then gastric cancer.[100] Four families were originally described by Drs. Li and Fraumeni[101] in 1969. The risk of an initial primary cancer is 50% by the age of 30 years and 90% by the age of 70 years,[102] with sex-specific differences in lifetime cancer risk of 73% in males and close to 100% in females primarily accounted for by an excess high breast cancer risk.[103] There are high risks for multiple primary cancers, with 60% of carriers developing a second tumor and 4% a third malignancy.[104] Previously thought to be extraordinarily rare with an incidence of 1/50,000 to 1/100,000, recently relaxed testing criteria suggest the actual carrier rate may be several times higher. Seventy percent of individuals who meet classic LFS clinical criteria are found to carry a *TP53* germline mutation. The de novo mutation rate is now estimated at 7% to 20%.[105] A negative family history can no longer exclude consideration of LFS, and clinical criteria have been updated to recommend P53 testing for single cases of adrenal cortical carcinoma, choroid plexus carcinoma, and breast cancer under the age of 30 years.

Although not one of the hallmark tumors of LFS, the International Agency for Research on Cancer database reports that gastric cancer frequency is up to 2.8% of LFS families.[106] Somatic TP53 alterations are associated with both the intestinal and diffuse forms of gastric cancer in equal frequency. However, *TP53* constitutional mutations are very rarely documented in the overall gastric cancer mutational spectrum. Among 62 TP53 mutant LFS families seen at the Dana-Farber Cancer Institute in Boston and the National Cancer Institute, gastric cancer was diagnosed in 4.9% of affected members.[107] The mean and median ages at gastric cancer diagnosis were 43 and 36 years, respectively (range, 24 to 74 years), compared with the median age of 71 years in the general population based on Surveillance Epidemiology and End Results data. Five families (8.1%) reported two or more cases of gastric cancer. Pathology review of the available tumors revealed both intestinal and diffuse histologies. A study of 180 families with LFS in the Netherlands found a concordant rate of gastric cancer among carriers with an RR = 2.6 (95% CI, 0.5 to 7.7).[108]

Peutz–Jeghers Syndrome

Peutz–Jeghers syndrome (PJS) is a rare inherited disorder of GI hamartomas, polyposis, and, most strikingly, early development of pigmented lesions on the lips, oral mucosa, and fingers. Incidence rates are estimated in the range of 1/25,000 to 1/250,000. Initially described by Peutz[109] in 1921 and subsequently by Jeghers et al.[110] in 1949, PJS is characterized by both hamartomatous and adenomatous polyposis throughout the GI tract and high predisposition to GI malignancies. The clinic diagnosis of PJS is made on the basis of histologically confirmed hamartomatous polyps and two of the following: Positive family history, hyperpigmentation of the digits and mucosa of the external genitalia, and small bowel polyposis.[111] The mucocutaneous hyperpigmentation characteristically occurs on the buccal mucosa or near the eyes, nose, mouth, axilla, or fingertips. Typically noticeable by the age of 5 years, they frequently fade by puberty. Classic pigmented lesions in a first-degree relative of a diagnosed individual are sufficient to meet criteria for PJS.

Chronic GI bleeds, anemia, and recurrent obstruction due to intussusception are frequent complications and often require surgical intervention. Among GI cancers, gastric cancer was found to be the third most frequent tumor in PJS, after small intestine and colorectal carcinoma. The cumulative cancer risk is 47% at the age of 65 years.[112] RRs reported for colon, stomach, and small intestine neoplasms have been as high as 84, 213, and over 500, respectively.[113] Increased risk is also present for other GI cancers (pancreatic, esophageal), as well as neoplasms outside the GI tract (lung, breast, ovarian, and endometrial). Other tumors associated with PJS are benign ovarian tumors called sex cord tumors with annular tubules, calcifying Sertoli tumors of the testes, and adenoma malignum of the cervix.

A Dutch team reviewed 20 PJS cohort studies, and one meta-analysis published between 1975 and 2007 with a total of 1,644 patients.[114,115] They found the cumulative lifetime risks of GI cancers of 38% to 66%, and for all cancers, a lifetime risk range of 37% to 93%. Specifically, the gastric cancer risks were 29%, the third most common malignancy after colorectal and breast. Understandably, this prompted a call for screening upper endoscopy every 2 to 5 years starting at the age of 20 years, whereas others suggest initiating endoscopy at the age of 8 years with addition of colonoscopy at the age of 20 years and breast screening at the age of 25 years.

STK11/LKB1 is the only gene identified to cause PJS, and mutations are found in 70% of those who meet clinical criteria.[116] Fifty percent of affected individuals have a family history of PJS, and 50% may represent de novo mutations, although the penetrance of PJS has yet to be confirmed. The absence of a mutation in *STK11* does not preclude a diagnosis of PJS in individuals meeting the clinical diagnostic criteria.

Juvenile Polyposis Syndrome

Juvenile polyposis syndrome (JPS) is another very rare, hereditary cancer syndrome with a broadly defined incidence rate between 1 in 16,000 and 1 in 100,000.[117–120] The diagnosis is based on the presence of multiple hamartomatous polyps with a distinct morphology termed "juvenile," although not restricted to development in childhood. Solitary juvenile polyps occur in 1% to 2% of the general population.

The diagnosis of JPS requires more than five juvenile polyps in the colorectum, multiple juvenile polyps throughout the GI tract, or a number of juvenile polyps in an individual with a known family history of juvenile polyps. There is wide interfamilial and intrafamilial variability in number and distribution of polyps. Juvenile polyps are commonly benign, but the risk of malignant transformation is present. Larger polyps have been noted to contain adenomatous regions resulting in a high lifetime risk of colorectal cancer approaching 20% by the age of 35 years and 68% by the age of 60 years. Gastric cancer has been found in 21% of JPS patients affected with gastric polyps, and increased incidence of pancreatic and small bowel cancers has also been reported (Table 12.2).[121]

TABLE 12.2	Inherited Cancer Syndromes with Associated Gastric Cancer (GC) Risks			
Cancer Syndrome	**Gene(s)**	**Frequency**	**Gastric Cancer Risk (%)**	**Reference**
HDGC	CDH1	Vary rare	>80	Fitzgerald et al.[44]
Hereditary breast/ ovarian cancer	BRCA1/2	1/40–1/400	2.6–5.5	Brose et al.[89]
Lynch syndrome	MLH1, MSH2, MSH6, PMS2, Epcam	1/440	6–13	Chen et al.,[72] Watson et al.[77]
Li–Fraumeni syndrome	P53	1/5,000	2.8	Gonzalez et al.[105]
FAP	APC	1/10–20,000	0.5–2.0	Garrean et al.[92]
Juvenile polyposis	SMAD4, BMPR1A	1/16–100,000	21	Howe et al.[121]
PJS	STK11	1/25–250,000	29	Giardiello et al.,[113] van Lier et al.[114]

Approximately 75% of JPS cases are familial, and 25% of JPS cases appear to be de novo. Two genes have been implicated as the cause of JPS in 40% of affected individuals: SMAD4 (or MADH4) and BMPR1A, with an approximate equal frequency.[121,122] The majority of JPS is due to as yet unidentified gene(s). Mutations in SMAD4 are also associated with hereditary hemorrhagic telangiectasia (HHT), also known as Osler–Weber–Rendu syndrome. HHT is associated with visceral bleeding, telangiectasias, or arteriovenous malformations. Currently, 15% to 22% of SMAD4 mutation carriers are suspected of having combined JPS/HHT.[123]

Surveillance recommendations for screening individuals with JPS include monitoring for rectal bleeding, anemia, and GI symptoms from infancy and additional complete blood count, upper endoscopy, and colonoscopy at the age of 15 years, or when symptoms are present. Endoscopy is repeated every 1 to 3 years, depending on polyp load. In families with SMAD4 mutations, HHT surveillance begins in early childhood.

CONCLUSIONS

Hereditary gastric cancer is a relatively unusual disease. Given the very poor prognosis for most gastric cancer patients once diagnosed, every effort should be made to identify lesions early when they are still curable. Genetic testing for gastric cancer susceptibility allows for identification of families with elevated risk for this and other tumors and development of rational surveillance strategies for early detection. Unfortunately, reliable screening tools for gastric cancer are not available, and prophylactic surgical gastrectomy has proven beneficial in certain autosomal dominant, high-penetrance genetic syndromes, including HDGC caused by germline *CDH1* mutations. Genetic testing for other gastric cancer risk genes may also be warranted as reviewed here. Major goals for clinical cancer genetics include identifying additional risk alleles to explain cancer susceptibility in families without known germline variants and to develop more robust tools for clinical screening for gastric cancer in high-risk individuals. Finally, the advent of whole genome sequencing of germline DNA and tumor genomes will lead to the rapid identification of novel variants and risk alleles of various penetrance. A challenge for the next generation of cancer genetics professionals will be the interpretation of multiple rare variants found in personal genomes and integration with schemes for prevention and early detection of gastric cancer.

REFERENCES

1. Lauren P. The two histological main types of gastric carcinoma: Diffuse and so-called intestinal-type carcinoma. An attempt at a histo-clinical classification. *Acta Pathol Microbiol Scand.* 1965;64: 31–49.
2. Carneiro F, Seixas M, Sobrinho-Simoes M. New elements for an updated classification of the carcinomas of the stomach. *Pathol Res Pract.* 1995;191:571–584.
3. Wu H, Rusiecki JA, Zhu K, et al. Stomach carcinoma incidence patterns in the United States by histologic type and anatomic site. *Cancer Epidemiol Biomarkers Prev.* 2009;18:1945–1952.
4. Machado JC, Soares P, Carneiro F, et al. E-cadherin gene mutations provide a genetic basis for the phenotypic divergence of mixed gastric carcinomas. *Lab Invest.* 1999;79:459–465.
5. Becker KF, Atkinson MJ, Reich U, et al. E-cadherin gene mutations provide clues to diffuse type gastric carcinomas. *Cancer Res.* 1994;54:3845–3852.
6. Tamura G, Sakata K, Nishizuka S, et al. Inactivation of the E-cadherin gene in primary gastric carcinomas and gastric carcinoma cell lines. *Jpn J Cancer Res.* 1996;87:1153–1159.
7. Muta H, Noguchi M, Kanai Y, et al. E-cadherin gene mutations in signet ring cell carcinoma of the stomach. *Jpn J Cancer Res.* 1996;87:843–848.
8. Carneiro F, Santos L, David L, et al. T (Thomsen-Friedenreich) antigen and other simple mucin-type carbohydrate antigens in precursor lesions of gastric carcinoma. *Histopathology.* 1994;24:105–113.
9. Jang BG, Kim WH. Molecular pathology of gastric carcinoma. *Pathobiology.* 2011;78:302–310.
10. Wang K, Kan J, Yuen ST, et al. Exome sequencing identifies frequent mutation of ARID1A in molecular subtypes of gastric cancer. *Nat Genet.* 2011;43:1219–1223.
11. Zang ZJ, Cutcutache I, Poon SL, et al. Exome sequencing of gastric adenocarcinoma identifies recurrent somatic mutations in cell adhesion and chromatin remodeling genes. *Nat Genet.* 2012;44:570–574.
12. Pedrazzani C, Corso G, Velho S, et al. Evidence of tumor microsatellite instability in gastric cancer with familial aggregation. *Fam Cancer.* 2009;8:215–220.
13. Palli D, Russo A, Ottini L, et al. Red meat, family history, and increased risk of gastric cancer with microsatellite instability. *Cancer Res.* 2001;61:5415–5419.
14. Buermeyer AB, Deschenes SM, Baker SM, et al. Mammalian DNA mismatch repair. *Annu Rev Genet.* 1999;33:533–564.
15. La Torre G, Chiaradia G, Gianfagna F, et al. Smoking status and gastric cancer risk: An updated meta-analysis of case-control studies published in the past ten years. *Tumori.* 2009;95:13–22.

16. McMichael AJ, McCall MG, Hartshorne JM, et al. Patterns of gastro-intestinal cancer in European migrants to Australia: The role of dietary change. *Int J Cancer.* 1980;25:431–437.

17. Nomura A, Stemmermann GN, Chyou PH, et al. Helicobacter pylori infection and gastric carcinoma among Japanese Americans in Hawaii. *N Engl J Med.* 1991;325:1132–1136.

18. Parsonnet J, Friedman GD, Vandersteen DP, et al. Helicobacter pylori infection and the risk of gastric carcinoma. *N Engl J Med.* 1991;325:1127–1131.

19. Helicobacter and Cancer Collaborative Group. Gastric cancer and Helicobacter pylori: A combined analysis of 12 case control studies nested within prospective cohorts. *Gut.* 2001;49:347–353.

20. Cavaleiro-Pinto M, Peleteiro B, Lunet N, et al. Helicobacter pylori infection and gastric cardia cancer: Systematic review and meta-analysis. *Cancer Causes Control.* 2011;22:375–387.

21. Chen JN, He D, Tang F, et al. Epstein-Barr virus–associated gastric carcinoma: A newly defined entity. *J Clin Gastroenterol.* 2010;46:262–271.

22. Ferlay J, Shin HR, Bray F, et al. Estimates of worldwide burden of cancer in 2008: GLOBOCAN 2008. *Int J Cancer.* 2008;127:2893–2917.

23. Jemal A, Siegel R, Ward E, et al. Cancer statistics, 2008. *CA Cancer J Clin.* 2008;58:71–96.

24. Correa P. Is gastric cancer preventable? *Gut.* 2004;53:1217–1219.

25. Henson DE, Dittus C, Younes M, et al. Differential trends in the intestinal and diffuse types of gastric carcinoma in the United States, 1973–2000: Increase in the signet ring cell type. *Arch Pathol Lab Med.* 2004;128:765–770.

26. Roosendaal R, Kuipers EJ, Buitenwerf J, et al. Helicobacter pylori and the birth cohort effect: Evidence of a continuous decrease of infection rates in childhood. *Am J Gastroenterol.* 1997;92:1480–1482.

27. Borch K, Jonsson B, Tarpila E, et al. Changing pattern of histological type, location, stage and outcome of surgical treatment of gastric carcinoma. *Br J Surg.* 2000;87:618–626.

28. Oliveira C, Seruca R, Carneiro F. Genetics, pathology, and clinics of familial gastric cancer. *Int J Surg Pathol.* 2006;14:21–33.

29. Hemminki K, Li X, Czene K. Swedish empiric risks: Familial risk of cancer: Data for clinical counseling and cancer genetics. *Int J Cancer.* 2004;108:109–114.

30. Shin CM, Kim N, Yang HJ, et al. Stomach cancer risk in gastric cancer relatives: Interaction between Helicobacter pylori infection and family history of gastric cancer for the risk of stomach cancer. *J Clin Gastroenterol.* 2010;44:e34–e39.

31. Yokota T, Kunii Y, Teshima S, et al. Significant prognostic factors in patients with early gastric cancer. *Int Surg.* 2000;85:286–290.

32. Caldas C, Carneiro F, Lynch HT, et al. Familial gastric cancer: Overview and guidelines for management. *J Med Genet.* 1999;36:873–880.

33. Guilford P, Hopkins J, Harraway J, et al. E-cadherin germline mutations in familial gastric cancer. *Nature.* 1998;392:402–405.

34. Gayther SA, Gorringe KL, Ramus SJ, et al. Identification of germ-line E-cadherin mutations in gastric cancer families of European origin. *Cancer Res.* 1998;58:4086–4089.

35. Guilford PJ, Hopkins JB, Grady WM, et al. E-cadherin germline mutations define an inherited cancer syndrome dominated by diffuse gastric cancer. *Hum Mutat.* 1999;14:249–255.

36. Keller G, Vogelsang H, Becker I, et al. Diffuse type gastric and lobular breast carcinoma in a familial gastric cancer patient with an E-cadherin germline mutation. *Am J Pathol.* 1999;155:337–342.

37. Richards FM, McKee SA, Rajpar MH, et al. Germline E-cadherin gene (CDH1) mutations predispose to familial gastric cancer and colorectal cancer. *Hum Mol Genet.* 1999;8:607–610.

38. Shinmura K, Kohno T, Takahashi M, et al. Familial gastric cancer: Clinicopathological characteristics, RER phenotype and germline p53 and E-cadherin mutations. *Carcinogenesis.* 1999;20:1127–1131.

39. Yoon KA, Ku JL, Yang HK, et al. Germline mutations of E-cadherin gene in Korean familial gastric cancer patients. *J Hum Genet.* 1999; 44:177–180.

40. Kluijt I, Siemerink EJ, Ausems MG, et al. CDH1-related hereditary diffuse gastric cancer syndrome: Clinical variations and implications for counseling. *Int J Cancer.* 2012;131:367–376. doi: 10.1002/ijc.26398.

41. Guilford P, Humar B, Blair V. Hereditary diffuse gastric cancer: Translation of CDH1 germline mutations into clinical practice. *Gastric Cancer.* 2010;13:1–10.

42. Grunwald GB. The structural and functional analysis of cadherin calcium-dependent cell adhesion molecules. *Curr Opin Cell Biol.* 1993;5:797–805.

43. Birchmeier W. E-cadherin as a tumor (invasion) suppressor gene. *Bioessays.* 1995;17:97–99.

44. Fitzgerald RC, Hardwick R, Huntsman D, et al. Hereditary diffuse gastric cancer: Updated consensus guidelines for clinical management and directions for future research. *J Med Genet.* 2010;47:436–444.

45. Brooks-Wilson AR, Kaurah P, Suriano G, et al. Germline E-cadherin mutations in hereditary diffuse gastric cancer: Assessment of 42 new families and review of genetic screening criteria. *J Med Genet.* 2004;41:508–517.

46. Oliveira C, de Bruin J, Nabais S, et al. Intragenic deletion of CDH1 as the inactivating mechanism of the wild-type allele in an HDGC tumour. *Oncogene.* 2004;23:2236–2240.

47. Suriano G, Yew S, Ferreira P, et al. Characterization of a recurrent germ line mutation of the E-cadherin gene: Implications for genetic testing and clinical management. *Clin Cancer Res.* 2005;11:5401–5409.

48. Oliveira C, Sousa S, Pinheiro H, et al. Quantification of epigenetic and genetic 2nd hits in CDH1 during hereditary diffuse gastric cancer syndrome progression. *Gastroenterology.* 2009;136:2137–2148.

49. Keller G, Vogelsang H, Becker I, et al. Germline mutations of the E-cadherin (CDH1) and TP53 genes, rather than of RUNX3 and HPP1, contribute to genetic predisposition in German gastric cancer patients. *J Med Genet.* 2004;41:e89.

50. Kim IJ, Park JH, Kang HC, et al. A novel germline mutation in the MET extracellular domain in a Korean patient with the diffuse type of familial gastric cancer. *J Med Genet.* 2003;40:e97.

51. Oliveira C, Ferreira P, Nabais S, et al. E-cadherin (CDH1) and p53 rather than SMAD4 and caspase-10 germline mutations contribute to genetic predisposition in Portuguese gastric cancer patients. *Eur J Cancer.* 2004;40:1897–1903.

52. Oliveira C, Senz J, Kaurah P, et al. Germline CDH1 deletions in hereditary diffuse gastric cancer families. *Hum Mol Genet.* 2009;18:1545–1555.

53. Pharoah PD, Guilford P, Caldas C. Incidence of gastric cancer and breast cancer in CDH1 (E-cadherin) mutation carriers from hereditary diffuse gastric cancer families. *Gastroenterology.* 2001;121:1348–1353.

54. Kaurah P, MacMillan A, Boyd N, et al. Founder and recurrent CDH1 mutations in families with hereditary diffuse gastric cancer. *JAMA.* 2007;297:2360–2372.

55. Schrader KA, Masciari S, Boyd N, et al. Hereditary diffuse gastric cancer: Association with lobular breast cancer. *Fam Cancer.* 2008;7:73–82.

56. Berx G, Becker KF, Hofler H, et al. Mutations of the human E-cadherin (CDH1) gene. *Hum Mutat.* 1998;12:226–237.

57. Berx G, Cleton-Jansen AM, Strumane K, et al. E-cadherin is inactivated in a majority of invasive human lobular breast cancers by truncation mutations throughout its extracellular domain. *Oncogene.* 1996;13:1919–1925.

58. Schrader KA, Masciari S, Boyd N, et al. Germline mutations in CDH1 are infrequent in women with early-onset or familial lobular breast cancers. *J Med Genet.* 2011;48:64–68.

59. Oliveira C, Bordin MC, Grehan N, et al. Screening E-cadherin in gastric cancer families reveals germline mutations only in hereditary diffuse gastric cancer kindred. *Hum Mutat.* 2002;19:510–517.

60. Frebourg T, Oliveira C, Hochain P, et al. Cleft lip/palate and CDH1/E-cadherin mutations in families with hereditary diffuse gastric cancer. *J Med Genet.* 2006;43:138–142.

61. Cisco RM, Ford JM, Norton JA. Hereditary diffuse gastric cancer: Implications of genetic testing for screening and prophylactic surgery. *Cancer.* 2008;113:1850–1856.

62. Huntsman DG, Carneiro F, Lewis FR, et al. Early gastric cancer in young, asymptomatic carriers of germ-line E-cadherin mutations. *N Engl J Med.* 2001;344:1904–1909.

63. Norton J, Ham C, Van Dam J, et al. CDH1 truncating mutations in the E-cadherin gene: An indication for total gastrectomy to treat hereditary diffuse gastric cancer. *Ann Surg.* 2007;45:873–879.

64. Rogers W, Dobo E, Norton J, et al. Risk-reducing total gastrectomy for germline mutations in E-cadherin (CDH1): Pathologic findings with clinical implications. *Am J Surg Pathol.* 2008;32:799–809.

65. Kaurah P, Fitzgerald R, Dwerryhouse S, et al. Pregnancy after prophylactic total gastrectomy. *Fam Cancer.* 2010;9:331–334.

66. Saslow D, Boetes C, Burke W, et al. American Cancer Society guidelines for breast screening with MRI as an adjunct to mammography. *CA Cancer J Clin.* 2007;57:75–89.

67. Daly M, Axilbund J, Buys S, et al. Genetic/familial high-risk assessment: Breast and ovarian. *J Natl Compr Cancer Netw.* 2010;8:562–594.

68. Wolmark N, Dunn BK. The role of tamoxifen in breast cancer prevention: Issues sparked by the NSABP Breast Cancer Prevention Trial (P-1). *Ann N Y Acad Sci.* 2001;949:99–108.

69. Lynch HT, Lynch PM. The cancer-family syndrome: A pragmatic basis for syndrome identification. *Dis Colon Rectum.* 1979;22:106–110.

70. Palomaki GE, McClain MR, Melillo S, et al. EGAPP supplementary evidence review: DNA testing strategies aimed at reducing morbidity and mortality from Lynch syndrome. *Genet Med.* 2009;11: 42–65.

71. Meyer LA, Broaddus RR, Lu KH. Endometrial cancer and Lynch syndrome: Clinical and pathologic considerations. *Cancer Control.* 2009;16:14–22.

72. Chen S, Wang W, Lee S, et al. Prediction of germline mutations and cancer risk in the Lynch syndrome. *JAMA.* 2006;296:1479–1487.

73. Aarnio M, Salovaara R, Aaltonen LA, et al. Features of gastric cancer in hereditary non-polyposis colorectal cancer syndrome. *Int J Cancer.* 1997;74:551–555.

74. Aarnio M, Sankila R, Pukkala E, et al. Cancer risk in mutation carriers of DNA-mismatch-repair genes. *Int J Cancer.* 1999;81:214–218.

75. Park YJ, Shin KH, Park JG. Risk of gastric cancer in hereditary nonpolyposis colorectal cancer in Korea. *Clin Cancer Res.* 2000;6:2994–2998.

76. Vasen HF, Wijnen JT, Menko FH, et al. Cancer risk in families with hereditary nonpolyposis colorectal cancer diagnosed by mutation analysis. *Gastroenterology.* 1996;110:1020–1027.

77. Watson P, Vasen HF, Mecklin JP, et al. The risk of extra-colonic, extra-endometrial cancer in the Lynch syndrome. *Int J Cancer.* 2008;123:444–449.

78. Gylling A, Abdel-Rahman WM, Juhola M, et al. Is gastric cancer part of the tumour spectrum of hereditary non-polyposis colorectal cancer? A molecular genetic study. *Gut.* 2007;56:926–933.

79. Rodriguez-Bigas MA, Boland CR, Hamilton SR, et al. A National Cancer Institute Workshop on Hereditary Nonpolyposis Colorectal Cancer Syndrome: Meeting highlights and Bethesda guidelines. *J Natl Cancer Inst.* 1997;89:1758–1762.

80. Umar A, Boland CR, Terdiman JP, et al. Revised Bethesda guidelines for hereditary nonpolyposis colorectal cancer (Lynch syndrome) and microsatellite instability. *J Natl Cancer Inst.* 2004;96: 261–268.

81. Miki Y, Swensen J, Shattuck-Eidens D, et al. A strong candidate for the breast and ovarian cancer susceptibility gene BRCA1. *Science.* 1994; 266:66–71.

82. Wooster R, Bignell G, Lancaster J, et al. Identification of the breast cancer susceptibility gene BRCA2. *Nature.* 1995;378:789–792.

83. The Breast Cancer Linkage Consortium. Cancer risks in BRCA2 mutation carriers. *J Natl Cancer Inst.* 1999;91:1310–1316.

84. Figer A, Irmin L, Geva R, et al. The rate of the 6174delT founder Jewish mutation in BRCA2 in patients with non-colonic gastrointestinal tract tumours in Israel. *Br J Cancer.* 2001;84:478–481.

85. Jakubowska A, Nej K, Huzarski T, et al. BRCA2 gene mutations in families with aggregations of breast and stomach cancers. *Br J Cancer.* 2002;87:888–891.

86. Jakubowska A, Scott R, Menkiszak J, et al. A high frequency of BRCA2 gene mutations in Polish families with ovarian and stomach cancer. *Eur J Hum Genet.* 2003;11:955–958.

87. Johannsson O, Loman N, Moller T, et al. Incidence of malignant tumours in relatives of BRCA1 and BRCA2 germline mutation carriers. *Eur J Cancer.* 1999;35:1248–1257.

88. Lorenzo B, Hemminki K. Risk of cancer at sites other than the breast in Swedish families eligible for BRCA1 or BRCA2 mutation testing. *Ann Oncol.* 2004;15:1834–1841.

89. Brose MS, Rebbeck TR, Calzone KA, et al. Cancer risk estimates for BRCA1 mutation carriers identified in a risk evaluation program. *J Natl Cancer Inst.* 2002;94:1365–1372.

90. Risch H, McLaughlin J, Cole D, et al. Prevalence and penetrance of germline BRCA1 and BRCA2 mutations in a population series of 649 women with ovarian cancer. *Am J Hum Genet.* 2001;68:700–710.

91. Friedenson B. BRCA1 and BRCA2 pathways and the risk of cancers other than breast or ovarian. *MedGenMed.* 2005;7:60.

92. Garrean S, Hering J, Saied A, et al. Gastric adenocarcinoma arising from fundic gland polyps in a patient with familial adenomatous polyposis syndrome. *Am Surg.* 2008;74:79–83.

93. Offerhaus GJ, Giardiello FM, Krush AJ, et al. The risk of upper gastrointestinal cancer in familial adenomatous polyposis. *Gastroenterology.* 1992;102:1980–1982.

94. Burt RW. Gastric fundic gland polyps. *Gastroenterology.* 2003;125:1462–1469.

95. Lynch HT, Snyder C, Davies JM, et al. FAP, gastric cancer, and genetic counseling featuring children and young adults: A family study and review. *Fam Cancer.* 2010;9:581–588.

96. Lynch HT, Smyrk T, McGinn T, et al. Attenuated familial adenomatous polyposis (AFAP). A phenotypically and genotypically distinctive variant of FAP. *Cancer.* 1995;76:2427–2433.

97. Abraham SC, Nobukawa B, Giardiello FM, et al. Fundic gland polyps in familial adenomatous polyposis: Neoplasms with frequent somatic adenomatous polyposis coli gene alterations. *Am J Pathol.* 2000;157:747–754.

98. Bianchi LK, Burke CA, Bennett AE, et al. Fundic gland polyp dysplasia is common in familial adenomatous polyposis. *Clin Gastroenterol Hepatol.* 2008;6:180–185.

99. Dunn K, Chey W, Gibbs J. Total gastrectomy for gastric dysplasia in a patient with attenuated familial adenomatous polyposis syndrome. *J Clin Oncol.* 2008;26:3641–3642.

100. Olivier M, Goldgar DE, Sodha N, et al. Li-Fraumeni and related syndromes: Correlation between tumor type, family structure, and TP53 genotype. *Cancer Res.* 2003;63:6643–6650.

101. Li F, Fraumeni JJ. Soft-tissue sarcomas, breast cancer, and other neoplasms. A familial syndrome? *Ann Intern Med.* 1969;71:747–752.

102. Malkin D, Li F, Strong L, et al. Germ line p53 mutations in a familial syndrome of breast cancer, sarcomas, and other neoplasms. *Science.* 1990;250:1233–1238.

103. Wu CC, Shete S, Amos CI, et al. Joint effects of germ-line p53 mutation and sex on cancer risk in Li-Fraumeni syndrome. *Cancer Res.* 2006;66:8287–8292.

104. Hisada M, Garber J, Fung C, et al. Multiple primary cancers in families with Li-Fraumeni syndrome. *J Natl Cancer Inst.* 1998;90:606–611.

105. Gonzalez K, Buzin C, Noltner K, et al. High frequency of de novo mutations in Li-Fraumeni syndrome. *J Med Genet.* 2009;46:689–693.

106. Corso G, Pedrazzani C, Marrelli D, et al. Familial gastric cancer and Li-Fraumeni syndrome. *Eur J Cancer Care (Engl).* 2010;19:377–381.

107. Masciari S, Dewanwala A, Stoffel EM, et al. Gastric cancer in individuals with Li-Fraumeni syndrome. *Genet Med.* 2011;13:651–657.

108. Ruijs MW, Verhoef S, Rookus MA, et al. TP53 germline mutation testing in 180 families suspected of Li-Fraumeni syndrome: Mutation detection rate and relative frequency of cancers in different familial phenotypes. *J Med Genet.* 2010;47:421–428.

109. Peutz J. Very remarkable case of familial polyposis of mucous membrane of intestinal tract and nasopharynx accompanied by peculiar pigmentations of skin and mucous membrane. *Nederl Maandschr Geneesk.* 1921;10:134–146.

110. Jeghers H, Mc KV, Katz KH. Generalized intestinal polyposis and melanin spots of the oral mucosa, lips and digits; a syndrome of diagnostic significance. *N Engl J Med.* 1949;241:1031–1036.

111. Giardiello FM, Welsh SB, Hamilton SR, et al. Increased risk of cancer in the Peutz-Jeghers syndrome. *N Engl J Med.* 1987;316:1511–1514.

112. Lim W, Olschwang S, Keller JJ, et al. Relative frequency and morphology of cancers in STK11 mutation carriers. *Gastroenterology.* 2004;126:1788–1794.

113. Giardiello F, Brensinger J, Tersmette A, et al. Very high risk of cancer in familial Peutz-Jeghers syndrome. *Gastroenterology.* 2000;119:1447–1453.

114. van Lier MG, Wagner A, Mathus-Vliegen EM, et al. High cancer risk in Peutz-Jeghers syndrome: A systematic review and surveillance recommendations. *Am J Gastroenterol.* 2010;105:1258–1264.

115. van Lier MG, Westerman AM, Wagner A, et al. High cancer risk and increased mortality in patients with Peutz-Jeghers syndrome. *Gut.* 2011;60:141–147.
116. Gruber SB, Entius MM, Petersen GM, et al. Pathogenesis of adenocarcinoma in Peutz-Jeghers syndrome. *Cancer Res.* 1998;58:5267–5270.
117. Allen BA, Terdiman JP. Hereditary polyposis syndromes and hereditary non-polyposis colorectal cancer. *Best Pract Res Clin Gastroenterol.* 2003;17:237–258.
118. Finan MC, Ray MK. Gastrointestinal polyposis syndromes. *Dermatol Clin.* 1989;7:419–434.
119. Lindor NM, Greene MH. The concise handbook of family cancer syndromes. Mayo Familial Cancer Program. *J Natl Cancer Inst.* 1998;90:1039–1071.
120. Utsunomiya J, Gocho H, Miyanaga T, et al. Peutz-Jeghers syndrome: Its natural course and management. *Johns Hopkins Med J.* 1975;136:71–82.
121. Howe JR, Sayed MG, Ahmed AF, et al. The prevalence of MADH4 and BMPR1A mutations in juvenile polyposis and absence of BMPR2, BMPR1B, and ACVR1 mutations. *J Med Genet.* 2004;41:484–491.
122. Sayed MG, Ahmed AF, Ringold JR, et al. Germline SMAD4 or BMPR1A mutations and phenotype of juvenile polyposis. *Ann Surg Oncol.* 2002;9:901–906.
123. Gallione C, Richards J, Letteboer T, et al. SMAD4 mutations found in unselected HHT patients. *J Med Genet.* 2006;43:793–797.

Robert Pilarski and Rebecca Nagy

13 Genetic Testing by Cancer Site
Endocrine System

A number of hereditary syndromes, caused by mutations in an even larger number of tumor suppressor genes and oncogenes, can cause tumors in organs of the endocrine system. Table 13.1 summarizes the major syndromes, genes, and endocrine organs affected.

MULTIPLE ENDOCRINE NEOPLASIA TYPE 1
Syndrome Description

Multiple endocrine neoplasia type 1 (MEN 1) is an autosomal dominant syndrome with an estimated incidence in the general population on the order of 1/100,000 to 10/100,000.[1,2] The major endocrine features of MEN 1 are parathyroid adenomas, enteropancreatic endocrine tumors, and pituitary tumors. A diagnosis of MEN 1 is made in a person with two of the three major endocrine tumors, or in an individual with at least one of these tumors if another relative has a diagnosis of MEN 1.[3–5] The age-related penetrance of MEN 1 is 45% at the age of 30 years, 82% at the age of 50 years, and 96% at the age of 70 years.[5–7]

The most common feature of MEN 1 is parathyroid adenoma, which results in primary hyperparathyroidism (PHPT). In approximately 50% to 85% of patients with MEN 1, PHPT will be the presenting manifestation. These tumors occur in 80% to 95% of patients by the age of 50 years,[5,8–10] and are typically multiglandular and often hyperplastic.[1] The average age at onset of PHPT in MEN 1 is 20 to 25 years, in contrast to that in the general population, which is in the 50s. Parathyroid carcinoma in MEN 1 is rare but has been described.[11–13]

Pancreatic endocrine tumors are the second most common endocrine manifestation in MEN 1, occurring in up to 30% to 80% of patients.[5,8] Gastrinomas and insulinomas are most common, followed by VIPomas (vasoactive intestinal peptide), glucagonomas, and somatostatinomas. These tumors are usually multicentric and can arise in the pancreas or more commonly as small (<0.5 cm) foci throughout

187

| TABLE 13.1 | Major Endocrine System Tumors and Associated Hereditary Syndromes |

| | Gene (Syndrome) | | | | |
Tumor Site/Type	MEN1 (MEN 1)	RET (MEN 2)	PTEN (CS/PHTS)	SDHX (HPCC/PGL)	VHL (VHL)
Adrenal (PC)		X		X	X
Carcinoid	X				X
Neuroendocrine	X			X	
Pancreas (islet cell)	X				X
Parathyroid	X	X			
Paraganglioma				X	X
Pituitary	X				
Thyroid		MTC	PTC, FTC		

PHTS, *PTEN* hamartoma tumor syndrome; HPCC/PGL, hereditary pheochromocytoma/paraganglioma syndrome.

the duodenum.[14] Gastrinomas represent 50% of the gastrointestinal neuroendocrine tumors in MEN 1 and are the major cause of morbidity and mortality in MEN 1 patients.[5,15] Most result in peptic ulcer disease (Zollinger–Ellison syndrome), and half are malignant at the time of diagnosis.[14–16] Nonfunctional tumors of the enteropancreas, some of which produce pancreatic polypeptide, are seen in 20% of patients.[17–19]

Approximately 15% to 50% of MEN 1 patients will develop a pituitary tumor.[5,8] Two-thirds are microadenomas (<1 cm in diameter), and the majority are prolactin secreting.[20] Other manifestations of MEN 1 include carcinoids of the foregut (typically bronchial or thymic), skin lipomas, facial angiomas, and collagenomas and adrenal cortical lesions, including cortical adenomas, diffuse or nodular hyperplasia, or rarely carcinoma.[7,21] Thyroid adenomas, pheochromocytoma (PC) (usually unilateral), spinal ependymoma, and leiomyoma have also been reported.[22]

Genetic Testing

MEN 1 is caused by mutations in the *MEN1* gene, which is located on chromosome 11q13. It is inherited in an autosomal dominant manner. Germline mutations are typically found in 80% to 95% of families with two or more affected members and in up to 65% of simplex cases (single case of MEN 1 with no family history).[4,23] Menin, the protein encoded by the *MEN1* gene, functions as a tumor suppressor gene and is involved in multiple cellular functions including transcription regulation, genomic stability, cell division, and cell cycle control (reviewed in[24]).

More than 1,100 mutations have been identified in the *MEN1* gene to date, and these are scattered across the entire coding region.[24] The majority of these are nonsense or frameshift mutations, and the remainder are missense or in-frame deletions that lead to expression of an altered protein. Splice-site mutations have also been described. There is currently no evidence of genotype–phenotype correlations, and interfamilial and intrafamilial variability is the rule.[25,26]

Whereas the *MEN1* mutation detection rate is quite high in simplex and familial cases, the greater diagnostic challenge for the clinician is when to order genetic testing in an individual who does not meet diagnostic criteria, but has one of the three component tumors. The prevalence of MEN 1 among patients with apparently sporadic component tumors varies widely by tumor type. Approximately one-third of patients with Zollinger–Ellison syndrome will carry an *MEN1* mutation.[27,28] In individuals with apparently isolated hyperparathyroidism (HPT) or pituitary adenomas, the mutation prevalence is lower, on the order of 2% to 5% for each,[20,29,30] but the prevalence is higher in individuals diagnosed with these tumors at younger ages (<30 years old). In a small series of patients with isolated foregut/midgut carcinoids, none of 68 were found to carry an *MEN1* mutation. Some authors suggest *MEN1* testing in those not meeting diagnostic criteria if one of the following is present: Gastrinoma at any age, multifocal pancreatic islet cell tumors at any age, parathyroid adenomas before the age of 30 years, multiglandular parathyroid adenomas, or recurrent HPT, or in individuals with one of the three main MEN 1 tumors plus one of the less common tumors/findings.[31]

Management

Screening and surveillance for MEN 1 should use a combination of biochemical screening and imaging as follows[3]:

- Annual serum prolactin and insulin-like growth factor 1 starting at the age of 5 years
- Annual fasting total serum calcium and/or ionized calcium and PTH starting at the age of 8 years
- Annual fasting serum gastrin starting at the age of 20 years; consider chromogranin A, glucagon, and proinsulin for other enteropancreatic tumors
- Annual fasting glucose starting at the age of 5 years
- Brain magnetic resonance imaging (MRI) at the age of 5 years, repeat every 3 to 5 years based on biochemical test results
- Abdominal computed tomography or MRI starting at the age of 20 years, repeat every 3 to 5 years based on biochemical test results

Surgical management of MEN 1 is complex and controversial given the multifocal and multiglandular nature of the disease and the high risk of tumor recurrence even after surgery. A full review of surgical options is outside the scope of this review, but this topic has been reviewed elsewhere.[32,33] Establishing the diagnosis of MEN 1 before making surgical decisions and referring affected individuals to a surgeon with experience in treating MEN 1 can be critical in preventing unnecessary surgeries or inappropriate surgical approaches.

MULTIPLE ENDOCRINE NEOPLASIA TYPE 2
Syndrome Description

Multiple endocrine neoplasia type 2 (MEN 2), caused by germline mutations in the *RET* proto-oncogene, is an autosomal dominant syndrome characterized by medullary thyroid cancer (MTC), PC, and/or HPT. Historically, families were classified into one of the three clinical subtypes, MEN 2A, MEN 2B, and familial medullary thyroid carcinoma (FMTC) based on the presence or absence of certain endocrine tumors and other phenotypic features. However, there is debate about whether FMTC represents a separate entity or is a variation of MEN 2A in which there is a lower lifetime risk and delay in the onset of the extrathyroidal manifestations.[34] Incorrect classification of families with MEN 2A as having FMTC may result in delayed diagnosis of PC, a disease with significant morbidity and mortality. For this reason, current management recommendations include screening for all three tumors in individuals carrying a germline *RET* mutation, with the exception of parathyroid screening in MEN 2B cases[35] (see section on management).

The endocrine tumors in MEN 2 are often multifocal and bilateral/multiglandular and present at an early age. MTC is present in up to 95% of mutation carriers, and the age at presentation varies, somewhat depending on the specific mutation. Early diagnosis of MTC is critical, given the poor overall survival for individuals diagnosed with distant metastases.[36–38] PCs are present in up to 50% of carriers, and the lifetime risk is also dependent on genotype. Although the PCs in MEN 2 rarely metastasize, they can be clinically significant because of intractable hypertension or anesthesia-induced hypertensive crises. Parathyroid abnormalities are the least common finding, occurring in up to 30% of patients. The parathyroid disease in MEN 2 can include benign parathyroid adenomas or multiglandular hyperplasia, but is typically asymptomatic or associated with only mild elevations in calcium.[39,40]

MEN 2A is diagnosed clinically by the occurrence of two or more of the specific endocrine tumors in a single individual or in close relatives. MEN 2A may also be suspected when MTC occurs at an early age (<50 years) or is bilateral or multifocal even in the absence of family history. Several large series indicate a mutation frequency of 1% to 7% in isolated cases of MTC.[40,41] Based on these data, it is widely recommended that *RET* gene mutation testing be performed for all cases of MTC, regardless of age at diagnosis and family history.[3,35,42]

MEN 2B, which makes up 5% of MEN 2 cases, is characterized by the early development of an aggressive form of MTC in all patients.[43] Patients with MEN 2B who do not undergo thyroidectomy at an early age (~1 year) are likely to develop metastatic MTC at an early age. PCs occur in about 50% of MEN 2B cases, and clinically significant parathyroid disease is very uncommon.[44] Individuals with MEN 2B can also have distinctive facies with enlarged lips, mucosal neuromas of the lips and tongue, medullated corneal nerve fibers, and an asthenic Marfanoid body habitus.[44] About 40% of patients have diffuse ganglioneuromatosis of the gastro-intestinal tract.[45]

Genetic Testing

MEN 2 is the result of germline mutations in the *RET* gene, located on chromosome region 10q11.2.[46,47] The *RET* gene is a proto-oncogene encoding a receptor tyrosine kinase with extracellular, transmembrane, and intracellular domains. *RET* mutations causing MEN 2 are activating mutations, resulting in a constitutively activated tyrosine kinase receptor.[48]

Genetic testing in MEN 2 is considered an important part of the management of at-risk family members. Since MTC and other tumors can develop in childhood, testing of children who have no symptoms is considered beneficial.[35] Timing of *RET* testing depends largely on the mutation present in the family. Several groups have developed mutation stratification systems to guide clinicians with regard to the appropriate timing of *RET* testing, prophylactic thyroidectomy, and biochemical screening.[3,35] These are based mainly on age at onset, aggressiveness of thyroid disease, and clinical phenotype, but have not been validated as clinical decision-making tools. The original stratification system was developed by the International RET Consortium.[3] A newer classification system by the American Thyroid Association[35] was published in 2009 (Table 13.2).

Approximately 95% of patients with MEN 2A or MEN 2B will have an identifiable germline *RET* mutation.[43] As mentioned previously, 1% to 7% of apparently sporadic cases of MTC will carry a germline *RET* mutation, underscoring the importance of testing all cases of MTC.[3,35,42] A targeted exon approach is most commonly used in families with MEN 2A. If the clinical suspicion is MEN 2B, a targeted mutation analysis can be used. If targeted testing in a family with a high clinical suspicion for MEN 2 is normal, sequencing of the remaining exons can then be performed. For families that do not have a detectable mutation, management recommendations can be based on the clinical features in the affected individual and in the family.

Management

Management of *RET* mutation carriers includes prophylactic thyroidectomy, as well as biochemical screening for PC and HPT.[3,35] The timing of these interventions has been largely based on genotype, but this remains controversial. Prophylactic thyroidectomy and parathyroidectomy with reimplantation of one or more parathyroid glands into the neck or forearm are a preventive option for all subtypes of MEN 2. For those with mutations associated with early-onset aggressive MTC, genetic testing alone is used to determine timing of surgery.[3,35] For individuals carrying lower- or intermediate-risk mutations (Table 13.2), some centers allow surgery to be delayed until biochemical screening becomes abnormal and/or the individual reaches a particular age.[35] This is still somewhat controversial; however, given the great intra-familial variability and the fact that MTC can be present even in the absence of an elevated basal or stimulated calcitonin.

TABLE 13.2	MEN 2 Mutation Classification System and Management Guidelines of the American Thyroid Association (ATA)			
ATA Risk Level	Mutated Codon(s)	Age at RET Testing	Age at Prophylactic Thyroidectomy	Timing and Frequency of Other Surveillance
A	768, 790, 791, 804, 891	<age 3–5 y	May delay surgery after age 5 y if criteria are met[a]	Age 20 y, repeat periodically
B	609, 611, 618, 620, 630, compound heterozygote: V804M + V778I	<age 3–5 y	Consider surgery before age 5 y; may delay surgery after age 5 y if criteria are met[a]	Age 8 y for codon 630; age 20 y for all others; repeat periodically
C	634	<age 3–5 y	Before age 5 y	Age 8 y, annually
D	883 and 918 Compound heterozygotes V804M + S904C V804M + E805K V804M + Y806C	ASAP and within the first year of life	ASAP and within the first year of life	Age 8 y, annually for PC only

[a]Criteria include a normal annual basal and/or stimulated serum count, normal annual neck ultrasound, less aggressive MTC family history, and family preference.

From: Kloos RT, Eng C, Evans DB, et al. Medullary thyroid cancer: Management guidelines of the American Thyroid Association. *Thyroid.* 2009;19:565–612.

Biochemical screening for parathyroid disease and PC is recommended, and the timing and frequency depend on the genotype and, in some cases, presence/absence of these tumors in the family (Table 13.2). Annual screening for hyperparathyroidism should include albumin-corrected calcium or ionized serum calcium with or without intact PTH measurement (American Thyroid Association, 2009). Screening for PC with plasma-free metanephrines and/or urinary fractionated metanephrines is recommended, given that these provide a higher diagnostic sensitivity than urinary catecholamines.[49,50] When biochemical screening suggests PC, MRI or computed tomography can be performed.[51,52] Confirmation of the diagnosis can be made using various anatomical and functional modalities.[52–54] Several reviews provide a succinct summary of the biochemical diagnosis, localization, and management of PC.[52,55] If surgical removal is required, laparoscopic adrenalectomy is the recommended approach for the treatment of unilateral PC.[56] For individuals with bilateral PC, cortical-sparing adrenalectomy is an option to minimize the risk of adrenal insufficiency.[56,57]

PTEN
Clinical Features

Germline mutations in the *PTEN* (phosphatase and tensin homolog on chromosome 10) gene have been associated with a number of related clinical disorders, including Cowden syndrome (CS), Bannayan–Riley–Ruvalcaba syndrome, a Proteus-like syndrome, adult Lhermitte–Duclos disease, and autism-like disorders with macrocephaly. Although CS is the only one with a documented risk for endocrine (thyroid) cancer, it is possible that any person with a *PTEN* mutation is at increased risk.[58]

The prevalence of CS, an autosomal dominant disorder, has been estimated to be between 1/200,000 and 1/250,000.[59] Diagnostic criteria for CS were initially developed in 1996,[60] and subsequent modifications have been proposed.[61–63] A clinical diagnosis requires a requisite number of clinical features, which are divided into groups of "pathognomonic," "major," and "minor" criteria (Table 13.3).

Cancer rates in CS have historically been reported as 25% to 50% for breast cancer, 3% to 10% for thyroid cancer, and 5% to 10% for endometrial cancer, based on compilations of cases published in the early literature.[64–66] Thyroid cancer in CS is exclusively of follicular or papillary histology. More recently, an increased risk for colon cancer has been reported.[67] Although recent reports from two large cohorts found cancer rates similar to these,[67,68] a follow-up report on one of these cohorts projected lifetime cancer risks of 85% for breast cancer, 35% for thyroid cancer, 28% for endometrial cancer, 34% for kidney cancer, and 9% for colon cancer.[69] However, these high risks are subject to significant selection bias and should be considered with caution, given their discrepancy with clinical experience with CS patients.

Benign lesions are also seen in CS and include mucocutaneous lesions (trichilemmomas, acral keratoses, and papillomatous papules, seen in most patients), thyroid abnormalities (goiter, adenoma in 50% to 67%), benign breast lesions (fibroadenomas, fibrocystic disease in 40% to 75% of females), gastrointestinal polyps (≥80%), macrocephaly (≥80%), and uterine fibroids (25% to 44% of females).[68,69]

Genetic Testing

The *PTEN* tumor suppressor gene is a dual-specificity phosphatase with multiple and as yet incompletely understood roles in cellular regulation. It is known to signal down the PI3K/Akt pathway to cause G1 cell cycle arrest and apoptosis, and has also been shown to regulate cell-survival pathways, such as the mitogen-activated kinase pathway.[70] Although it is generally reported that germline *PTEN* mutations are found in 80% of CS patients, based on initial reports in 1997,[71–73] more recent data suggest that it is much lower,[67–69] and there is reason to consider revising the diagnostic criteria.[68] A small number of studies suggest that gene deletions or rearrangements are rare in CS.[74,75] Approximately 2% of all CS patients in one study had a variant in the *PTEN* promoter.[74] Although not definitive, protein expression studies suggested that these variants could be deleterious. The new mutation rate for *PTEN* is unknown. Testing criteria for CS have been developed and are updated annually by the National

TABLE
13.3 **CS Diagnostic Criteria**

Pathognomonic criteria
- Lhermitte–Duclos disease (LDD)—adult
- Mucocutaneous lesions
     Trichilemmomas, facial
     Acral keratoses
     Papillomatous lesions

Major criteria
- Breast cancer
- Thyroid cancer (papillary or follicular)
- Macrocephaly (≥97th percentile)
- Endometrial cancer

Minor criteria
- Other structural thyroid lesions (e.g., adenoma, multinodular goiter)
- Mental retardation (i.e., IQ ≤75)
- Gastrointestinal hamartomas
- Fibrocystic disease of the breast
- Lipomas
- Fibromas
- Genitourinary tumors (e.g., uterine fibroids, renal cell carcinoma) or
- Genitourinary structural malformations
- Uterine fibroids

Operational diagnosis in an individual (any of the following):
(1) Mucocutaneous lesions alone, if
     (a) There are ≥6 facial papules, of which ≥3 must be trichilemmoma, or
     (b) Cutaneous facial papules and oral mucosal papillomatosis, or
     (c) Oral mucosal papillomatosis and acral keratoses, or
     (d) Palmoplantar keratoses, ≥6
(2) ≥2 major criteria, but one must include macrocephaly or LDD; or
(3) One major and three minor criteria; or
(4) Four minor criteria

Operational diagnosis in a family where one individual is diagnostic for CS:
(1) One pathognomonic criterion; or
(2) Any one major criterion with or without minor criteria; or
(3) Two minor criteria; or
(4) History of Bannayan–Riley–Ruvalcaba syndrome[58]

Comprehensive Cancer Network.[76] Clinical *PTEN* testing is available in a number of national laboratories.

Germline genetic variants were found in the *SDHB* and *SDHD* genes in one report in a cohort of patients with CS- or a CS-like phenotype.[77] None of the patients with genetic variants met current CS diagnostic criteria, however, and the clinical significance of these variants has been questioned, given that most had previously been identified as benign polymorphisms.[78] More recently, germline methylation of the *KILLIN* gene has been suggested to be related to CS as well.[79]

Management

Management guidelines for individuals with CS have been adopted by the National Comprehensive Cancer Network[76] and include annual physical examinations, monthly breast self-examinations, and a baseline thyroid ultrasound (with consideration of repeating annually), starting at the age of 18 years; clinical breast examinations every 6 months, starting at the age of 25 years; annual mammography and breast MRI screening starting at the age of 30 to 35 years; consideration of colonoscopy every 5 to 10 years, starting at the age of 35 years; consideration of an annual dermatologic examination; and consideration of participation in clinical trials for endometrial cell cancer screening.

SDHX/TMEM127/MAX
Clinical Features

Mutations in four genes of the succinate dehydrogenase (SDH) complex, *SDHA*, *SDHB*, *SDHC*, and *SDHD* (collectively referred to as *SDHX*), and several interacting genes have been shown to cause the autosomal dominant hereditary paraganglioma–pheochromocytoma (PGL/PCC) syndrome. The SDH complex is part of both the mitochondrial–respiratory chain (complex II) and the Krebs cycle.[80] The specific clinical phenotype varies, somewhat depending on the gene involved, as discussed below.

Individuals with *SDHB* mutations tend to present with sympathetic PGLs and less commonly PCC and parasympathetic PGL. There is a higher rate of malignancy and mortality with *SDHB* mutations compared with other SDH genes.[80] An analysis of 378 published cases with *SDHB* mutations found that 78% had PGL (71% sympathetic), and 25% had PCC (all unilateral), with a mean age at presentation of 33 years.[81] Up to 31% had malignant tumors. In one study of 32 metastatic PCC/PGL patients whose tumor was diagnosed before age 20 years, 23 (72%) had *SDHB* mutations.[82] The penetrance of *SDHB* mutations has been estimated to be 77% by the age of 50 years.[83] The risks for renal cell carcinoma and oncocytoma also appear to be increased.[84,85]

SDHD mutations most commonly cause multifocal parasympathetic PGL. A review of the clinical features of 289 patients with *SDHD* mutations found that 92%

had PGL (56% multiple), 24% had PCC (all unilateral), and only 4% had malignant disease.[81] The mean age at presentation is 35 years,[86] and the penetrance is estimated to be 86% by the age of 50 years.[83] *SDHD* mutations appear to be maternally imprinted such that tumors develop only when a mutation is inherited from the father.[87] However, several rare cases of maternal transmission have been reported.[88,89]

SDHC mutations are rare in patients with PCC/PGL. They mainly cause nonmalignant parasympathetic PGL (and rarely PCC) and were found in 4% of such patients in one study.[90] The average age at presentation is 43 years.[81]

More recently, mutations in the *SDHAF2* (also called *SDH5*), *SDHA*, *TMEM127*, and *MAX* genes have also been found in hereditary PGL/PCC. Given their rarity, and their recent discoveries, less is known about their clinical presentation. Mutations in *SDHAF2/SDH5* have been described in a number of families with head and neck PGL, but to date no cases with PCC have been reported.[91,92] It appears that there is genetic imprinting, with paternal transmission required for tumor development.[91,92] Biallelic SDHA mutations have been known to cause inherited juvenile encephalopathy/Leigh syndrome,[93] but it was only recently that heterozygous mutations have been found in a few individuals with PCC or PGL.[94,95] Mutations in *TMEM127* were first identified[96] in 2010 and were initially felt to be associated exclusively with PC.[97] However, several cases with extra-adrenal tumors have been reported.[98] *TMEM127* mutations are relatively rare causes of PCC and PGL—mutations were found in only 6 (1%) of 559 PCC cases and none of 72 PGL cases who did not carry mutations in *SDHB*, *SDHD*, *RET*, or *VHL*.[99] In addition, the age at diagnosis of PCC is not significantly earlier than average (41.5 years), and malignancy is infrequent.[96,97] Exome sequencing was used to identify *MAX* gene mutations in 12 individuals with hereditary PCC in one study.[100] Most cases (67%) were bilateral, and an association with malignancy was suggested, as was the possibility that paternal transmission was required for tumor development.

Genetic Testing

Although approximately 10% of PCC patients have a clinically apparent hereditary syndrome, studies have shown that up to 25% of "sporadic" cases also have germline mutations in either *SDHB*, *SDHD*, *RET*, or *VHL*.[101] Similarly, analysis of 445 patients with PGL found mutations in *SDHB*, *SDHC*, or *SDHD* in 220 (50%).[102] Whereas some have called for genetic testing for all PCC/PGL, others have called for a targeted approach. A number of algorithms have been proposed whereby testing decisions are based on a variety of factors including presence of clinical features, early age at diagnosis, location and laterality of tumor(s), positive family history, and presence of malignancy.[81,103] Clinical testing is available in the United States for all of these genes except *MAX*.

Management

The management of PCC and PGL is primarily surgical, and it is critical that patients undergo preoperative catecholamine and metanephrine screening to detect functional disease, which could precipitate anesthesia-induced hypertensive crisis during surgery. For at-risk patients with known mutations, there are no consensus guidelines as to the appropriate screening protocols. Although it is generally felt that MRI and/or functional imaging and measurement of blood/urine metanephrines be performed on a regular basis, the specifics vary among centers.[104]

VON HIPPEL–LINDAU AND PHEOCHROMOCYTOMA

von Hippel–Lindau (VHL) disease is not often characterized as an endocrine-related disorder. However, the presence of PC and, rarely, pancreatic neuroendocrine tumors in VHL warrants a brief discussion in this section. Herein, we will also briefly review the genetic approach to the patient presenting with sporadic PC, as this is not an uncommon reason for referral for genetic counseling and risk assessment, and a significant proportion of these individuals will have an underlying hereditary condition. Additional information about other VHL and other VHL-related tumors (i.e., renal cell carcinoma) can be found in the section on urinary tract cancers.

VHL is an inherited multisystem disease predisposing to retinal and central nervous system hemangioblastomas, renal cell carcinoma, PC, pancreatic islet cell tumors, and endolymphatic sac tumors. It has an estimated birth incidence of 1 in 36,000 per year,[105] and is inherited in an autosomal dominant manner with a high degree of interfamilial and intrafamilial variability.[106] The penetrance is age dependent, but reaches ~95% by the age of 65 years.[105,107] Four subtypes have been described on the basis of genotype–phenotype correlations.[107] PC is the main endocrine-related tumor associated with VHL. As in other hereditary syndromes, VHL-associated PCs are typically multifocal and/or bilateral and present at an earlier age than sporadic tumors and rarely metastatic.[107]

PC can be seen in several different hereditary conditions in addition to VHL, including neurofibromatosis type 1 (NF1), MEN 2, and the hereditary paraganglioma/PC syndromes.[108] One study of 271 patients with apparently sporadic PC analyzed the *NF1* (diagnosis made on the basis of clinical features, not genetic testing), *RET*, *VHL*, *SDHB*, and *SDHD* genes.[109] Upon further scrutiny, 166 (25.9%) of the 271 had a positive family history, and in these 166 families, germline mutations were detected in *RET* (*n* = 31), *VHL* (*n* = 56), *NF1* (*n* = 14), *SDHB* (*n* = 34), or *SDHD* (*n* = 31). Interestingly, 12.7% of those with no other syndromic features and/or family history (after rigorous clinical evaluation) also carried mutations.

These data indicate that a significant proportion of individuals presenting with apparently sporadic PC are carriers of germline genetic mutations. Referral to a genetic specialist may be warranted in all cases of apparently isolated PC, but is certainly appropriate in those diagnosed at or younger than 35 years and those with metastatic disease or multifocal and/or bilateral disease. Several clinical and genetic screening algorithms have been proposed to assist clinicians in deciding which genes to test and in which order,[52,109,110] as testing for mutations in five different genes in every patient may not be feasible or cost-effective.

REFERENCES

1. Chandrasekharappa S, Teh B. Clinical and molecular aspects of multiple endocrine neoplasia type 1. In: Dahia PLM, Eng C, eds. *Genetic Disorders of Endocrine Neoplasia, Vol. 28. Front Horm Res.* Basel, Switzerland: Karger; 2001:50–80.

2. Kouvaraki MA, Lee JE, Shapiro SE, et al. Genotype-phenotype analysis in multiple endocrine neoplasia type 1. *Arch Surg.* 2002;137:641–647.

3. Brandi M, Gagel R, Angeli A, et al. Consensus guidelines for diagnosis and therapy of MEN type 1 and type 2. *J Clin Endocrinol Metab.* 2001;86:5658–5671.

4. Chandrasekharappa SC, Guru SC, Manickam P, et al. Positional cloning of the gene for multiple endocrine neoplasia type 1 (MEN 1) gene. *Science.* 1997;276:404–407.

5. Trump D, Farren B, Wooding C, et al. Clinical studies of multiple endocrine neoplasia type 1 (MEN1). *QJM.* 1996;89:653–669.

6. Carty SE, Helm AK, Amico JA, et al. The variable penetrance and spectrum of manifestations of multiple endocrine neoplasia type 1. *Surgery.* 1998;124:1106–1114.

7. Machens A, Schaaf L, Karges W, et al. Age-related penetrance of endocrine tumours in multiple endocrine neoplasia type 1 (MEN1): A multicentre study of 258 gene carriers. *Clin Endocrinol (Oxf).* 2007;67:613–622.

8. Thakker RV. Multiple endocrine neoplasia type 1 (MEN1). In: DeGroot LJ, Besser GK, Burger HG, et al., eds. *Endocrinology.* Philadelphia, PA: WB Saunders; 1995.

9. Brandi ML, Marx SJ, Aurbach GD, et al. Familial multiple endocrine neoplasia type 1. A new look at pathophysiology. *Endocrinol Rev.* 1987;8:391–405.

10. Benson L, Ljunghall S, Akerstrom G, et al. Hyperparathyroidism presenting as the first lesion in multiple endocrine neoplasia type 1. *Am J Med.* 1987;82:731–737.

11. Agha A, Carpenter R, Bhattacharya S, et al. Parathyroid carcinoma in multiple endocrine neoplasia type 1 (MEN1) syndrome: Two case reports of an unrecognised entity. *J Endocrinol Invest.* 2007;30:145–149.

12. Shih RY, Fackler S, Maturo S, et al. Parathyroid carcinoma in multiple endocrine neoplasia type 1 with a classic germline mutation. *Endocr Pract.* 2009;15:567–572.

13. Sato M, Miyauchi A, Namihira H, et al. A newly recognized germline mutation of MEN1 gene identified in a patient with parathyroid adenoma and carcinoma. *Endocrine.* 2000;12:223–226.

14. Pipeleers-Marichal M, Somers G, Willems G, et al. Gastrinomas in the duodenums of patients with multiple endocrine neoplasia type 1 and the Zollinger–Ellison syndrome. *N Engl J Med.* 1990;322:723–727.

15. Norton JA, Fraker DL, Alexander HR, et al. Surgery to cure the Zollinger–Ellison syndrome. *N Engl J Med.* 1999;341:635–644.

16. Weber H, Venzon D, Lin J, et al. Determinants of metastatic rate and survival in patients with Zollinger–Ellison syndrome: A prospective long-term study. *Gastroenterology.* 1995;108:1637–1649.

17. Skosgeid B, Rastad J, Öberg K. Multiple endocrine neoplasia type 1. Clinical features and screening. *Endocrinol Metab Clin N Am.* 1994;23:1–18.

18. Marx SJ. Multiple endocrine neoplasia type 1. In: Vogelstein B, Kinzler KW, eds. *The Genetic Basis of Human Cancer.* New York City: McGraw Hill; 2002:475–499.

19. Thomas-Marques L, Murat A, Delemer B, et al. Prospective endoscopic ultrasonographic evaluation of the frequency of nonfunctioning pancreaticoduodenal endocrine tumors in patients with multiple endocrine neoplasia type 1. *Am J Gastroenterol.* 2006;101:266–273.

20. Corbetta S, Pizzocaro A, Peracchi M, et al. Multiple endocrine neoplasia type 1 in patients with recognized pituitary tumours of different types. *Clin Endocrinol (Oxf).* 1997;47:507–512.

21. Pieterman CR, Schreinemakers JM, Koppeschaar HP, et al. Multiple endocrine neoplasia type 1 (MEN1): Its manifestations and effect of genetic screening on clinical outcome. *Clin Endocrinol (Oxf).* 2009;70:575–581.

22. Gibril F, Schumann M, Pace A, et al. Multiple endocrine neoplasia type 1 and Zollinger–Ellison syndrome: A prospective study of 107 cases and comparison with 1009 cases from the literature. *Medicine (Baltimore).* 2004;83:43–83.

23. Larsson C, Skosgeid B, Öberg K, et al. Multiple endocrine neoplasia type 1 gene maps to chromosome 11 and is lost in insulinoma. *Nature.* 1988;332:85–87.

24. Lemos MC, Thakker RV. Multiple endocrine neoplasia type 1 (MEN1): Analysis of 1336 mutations reported in the first decade following identification of the gene. *Hum Mutat.* 2008;29:22–32.

25. Giraud S, Zhang CX, Serova-Sinilnikova OM, et al. Germ-line mutation analysis in patients with multiple endocrine neoplasia type 1 and related disorders. *Am J Hum Genet.* 1998;63: 455–467.

26. Wautot V, Vercherat C, Lespinasse J, et al. Germline mutation profile of MEN1 in multiple endocrine neoplasia type 1: Search for correlation between phenotype and the functional domains of the MEN1 protein. *Hum Mutat.* 2002;20:35–47.

27. Roy PK, Venzon DJ, Shojamanesh H, et al. Zollinger-Ellison syndrome. Clinical presentation in 261 patients. *Medicine (Baltimore).* 2000;79:379–411.

28. Bardram L, Stage JG. Frequency of endocrine disorders in patients with the Zollinger-Ellison syndrome. *Scand J Gastroenterology.* 1985;20:233–238.

29. Uchino S, Noguchi S, Sato M, et al. Screening of the MEN1 gene and discovery of germ-line and somatic mutations in apparently sporadic parathyroid tumors. *Cancer Res.* 2000;60:5553–5557.

30. Scheithauer BW, Laws ERJ, Kovacs K, et al. Pituitary adenomas of the multiple endocrine neoplasia type 1 syndrome. *Semin Diagn Pathol.* 1987;4:205–211.

31. Newey PJ, Thakker RV. Role of multiple endocrine neoplasia type 1 mutational analysis in clinical practice. *Endocr Pract.* 2011;17(suppl 3):8–17.

32. Pieterman CR, van Hulsteijn LT, den Heijer M, et al. Primary hyperparathyroidism in MEN1 patients: A cohort study with longterm follow-up on preferred surgical procedure and the relation with genotype. *Ann Surg.* 2012;255:1171–1178.

33. Pieterman CR, Vriens MR, Dreijerink KM, et al. Care for patients with multiple endocrine neoplasia type 1: The current evidence base. *Fam Cancer.* 2010;10:157–171.

34. Pacini F, Castagna MG, Cipri C, et al. Medullary thyroid carcinoma. *Clin Oncol (R Coll Radiol).* 2010;22:475–485.

35. Kloos RT, Eng C, Evans DB, et al. Medullary thyroid cancer: Management guidelines of the American Thyroid Association. *Thyroid.* 2009;19:565–612.

36. Fuchshuber PR, Loree TR, Hicks WL Jr, et al. Medullary carcinoma of the thyroid: Prognostic factors and treatment recommendations. *Ann Surg Oncol.* 1998;5:81–86.

37. Dottorini ME, Assi A, Sironi M, et al. Multivariate analysis of patients with medullary thyroid carcinoma. Prognostic significance and impact on treatment of clinical and pathologic variables. *Cancer.* 1996;77:1556–1565.

38. Kebebew E, Ituarte PH, Siperstein AE, et al. Medullary thyroid carcinoma: Clinical characteristics, treatment, prognostic factors, and a comparison of staging systems. *Cancer.* 2000;88:1139–1148.

39. Kraimps JL, Denizot A, Carnaille B, et al. Primary hyperparathyroidism in multiple endocrine neoplasia type IIA: Retrospective French multicentric study. Groupe d'Etude des Tumeurs a Calcitonine (GETC, French Calcitonin Tumors Study Group), French Association of Endocrine Surgeons. *World J Surg.* 1996;20:808–812; discussion 812–813.

40. Eng C, Mulligan LM, Smith DP, et al. Low frequency of germline mutations in the RET proto-oncogene in patients with apparently sporadic medullary thyroid carcinoma. *Clin Endocrinol (Oxf).* 1995;43:123–127.

41. Wohllk N, Cote GJ, Bugalho MM, et al. Relevance of RET proto-oncogene mutations in sporadic medullary thyroid carcinoma. *J Clin Endocrinol Metab.* 1996;81:3740–3745.

42. National Comprehensive Cancer Network. The NCCN Clinical Practice Guidelines in Oncology: Thyroid Cancer (Version 2.2012). NCCN Clinical Practice Guidelines in Oncology (NCCN Guidelines), Vol. 2012. 2012.

43. Eng C, Clayton D, Schuffenecker I, et al. The relationship between specific RET proto-oncogene mutations and disease phenotype in multiple endocrine neoplasia type 2. International RET mutation consortium analysis. *JAMA.* 1996;2776:1575–1579.

44. Morrison PJ, Nevin NC. Multiple endocrine neoplasia type 2B (mucosal neuroma syndrome, Wagenmann-Froboese syndrome). *J Med Genet.* 1996;33:779–782.

45. Brauckhoff M, Gimm O, Weiss CL, et al. Multiple endocrine neoplasia 2B syndrome due to codon 918 mutation: Clinical manifestation and course in early and late onset disease. *World J Surg.* 2004;28:1305–1311.

46. Mole SE, Mulligan LM, Healey CS, et al. Localisation of the gene for multiple endocrine neoplasia type 2A to a 480 kb region in chromosome band 10q11.2. *Hum Mol Genet.* 1993;2:247–252.

47. Gardner E, Papi L, Easton DF, et al. Genetic linkage studies map the multiple endocrine neoplasia type 2 loci to a small interval on chromosome 10q11.2. *Hum Mol Genet.* 1993;2:241–246.

48. Takahashi M, Asai N, Iwashita T, et al. Molecular mechanisms of development of multiple endocrine neoplasia 2 by RET mutations. *J Intern Med.* 1998;243:509–513.

49. Lenders JW, Pacak K, Walther MM, et al. Biochemical diagnosis of pheochromocytoma: Which test is best? *JAMA.* 2002;287:1427–1434.

50. Boyle JG, Davidson DF, Perry CG, et al. Comparison of diagnostic accuracy of urinary free metanephrines, vanillyl mandelic acid, and catecholamines and plasma catecholamines for diagnosis of pheochromocytoma. *J Clin Endocrinol Metab.* 2007;92:4602–4608.

51. Pacak K. Preoperative management of the pheochromocytoma patient. *J Clin Endocrinol Metab.* 2007;92:4069–4079.

52. Pacak K, Eisenhofer G, Ahlman H, et al. Pheochromocytoma: recommendations for clinical practice from the First International Symposium. October 2005. *Nat Clin Pract Endocrinol Metab.* 2007;3: 92–102.

53. van der Harst E, de Herder WW, Bruining HA, et al. [(123)I]metaiodobenzylguanidine and [(111) In]octreotide uptake in benign and malignant pheochromocytomas. *J Clin Endocrinol Metab.* 2001;86:685–693.

54. Timmers HJ, Taieb D, Pacak K. Current and future anatomical and functional imaging approaches to pheochromocytoma and paraganglioma. *Horm Metab Res.* 2012;44:367–372.

55. Reisch N, Peczkowska M, Januszewicz A, et al. Pheochromocytoma: Presentation, diagnosis and treatment. *J Hypertens.* 2006;24:2331–2339.

56. Yip L, Lee JE, Shapiro SE, et al. Surgical management of hereditary pheochromocytoma. *J Am Coll Surg.* 2004;198:525–534; discussion 525–534.

57. Asari R, Scheuba C, Kaczirek K, et al. Estimated risk of pheochromocytoma recurrence after adrenal-sparing surgery in patients with multiple endocrine neoplasia type 2A. *Arch Surg.* 2006;141:1199–1205; discussion 1205.

58. Pilarski R. Cowden syndrome: A critical review of the clinical literature. *J Genet Couns.* 2009;18:13–27.

59. Nelen MR, Kremer H, Konings IB, et al. Novel PTEN mutations in patients with Cowden disease: Absence of clear genotype–phenotype correlations. *Eur J Hum Genet.* 1999;7:267–273.

60. Nelen MR, Padberg GW, Peeters EAJ, et al. Localization of the gene for Cowden disease to 10q22-23. *Nat Genet.* 1996;13:114–116.

61. Eng C. Will the real Cowden syndrome please stand up: Revised diagnostic criteria. *J Med Genet.* 2000;37:828–830.

62. Pilarski R, Eng C. Will the real Cowden syndrome please stand up (again)? Expanding mutational and clinical spectra of the PTEN hamartoma tumour syndrome. *J Med Genet.* 2004;41:323–326.

63. Zbuk KM, Stein, JL, Eng C. PTEN Hamartoma Tumor Syndrome (PHTS). GeneReviews at GeneTests: Medical Genetics Information Resource [database online]. 2006. Available at http://www.genetests.org.

64. Starink TM, van der Veen JPW, Arwert F, et al. The Cowden syndrome: A clinical and genetic study in 21 patients. *Clin Genet.* 1986;29:222–233.

65. Starink TM. Cowden's disease: Analysis of fourteen new cases. *J Am Acad Dermatol.* 1984;11:1127–1141.

66. Salem OS, Steck WD. Cowden's disease (multiple hamartoma and neoplasia syndrome). A case report and review of the English literature. *J Am Acad Dermatol.* 1983;8:686–696.

67. Heald B, Mester J, Rybicki L, et al. Frequent gastrointestinal polyps and colorectal adenocarcinomas in a prospective series of PTEN mutation carriers. *Gastroenterology.* 2010;139:1927–1933.

68. Pilarski R, Stephens JA, Noss R, et al. Predicting PTEN mutations: An evaluation of Cowden syndrome and Bannayan–Riley–Ruvalcaba syndrome clinical features. *J Med Genet.* 2011;48:505–512.

69. Tan MH, Mester JL, Ngeow J, et al. Lifetime cancer risks in individuals with germline PTEN mutations. *Clin Cancer Res.* 2012;18:400–407.

70. Tamguney T, Stokoe D. New insights into PTEN. *J Cell Sci.* 2007;120:4071–4079.

71. Nelen MR, van Staveren CG, Peeters EAJ, et al. Germline mutations in the PTEN/MMAC1 gene in patients with Cowden disease. *Hum Mol Genet.* 1997;6:1383–1387.

72. Liaw D, Marsh DJ, Li J, et al. Germline mutations of the PTEN gene in Cowden disease, an inherited breast and thyroid cancer syndrome. *Nat Genet.* 1997;16:64–67.

73. Marsh DJ, Coulon V, Lunetta KL, et al. Mutation spectrum and genotype–phenotype analyses in Cowden disease and Bannayan–Zonana syndrome, two hamartoma syndromes with germline PTEN mutation. *Hum Mol Genet.* 1998;7:507–515.

74. Zhou XP, Waite KA, Pilarski R, et al. Germline PTEN promoter mutations and deletions in Cowden/Bannayan–Riley–Ruvalcaba syndrome result in aberrant PTEN protein and dysregulation of the phosphoinositol-3-kinase/Akt pathway. *Am J Hum Genet.* 2003;73:404–411.

75. Chibon F, Primois C, Bressieux JM, et al. Contribution of PTEN large rearrangements in Cowden disease: A MAPH screening approach. *J Med Genet.* 2008;45:657–665.

76. National Comprehensive Cancer Network. The NCCN Genetic Familial High-Risk Assessment: Breast and Ovarian. (Version 1.2011). NCCN Clinical Practice Guidelines in Oncology, Vol. 2011. 2011.

77. Ni Y, Zbuk KM, Sadler T, et al. Germline mutations and variants in the succinate dehydrogenase genes in Cowden and Cowden-like syndromes. *Am J Hum Genet.* 2008;83:261–268.

78. Bayley JP. Succinate dehydrogenase gene variants and their role in Cowden syndrome. *Am J Hum Genet.* 2011;88:674–675; author reply 676.

79. Bennett KL, Mester J, Eng C. Germline epigenetic regulation of KILLIN in Cowden and Cowden-like syndrome. *JAMA.* 2011;304:2724–2731.

80. Gimenez-Roqueplo AP, Favier J, Rustin P, et al. Mutations in the SDHB gene are associated with extra-adrenal and/or malignant phaeochromocytomas. *Cancer Res.* 2003;63:5615–5621.

81. Welander J, Soderkvist P, Gimm O. Genetics and clinical characteristics of hereditary pheochromocytomas and paragangliomas. *Endocr Relat Cancer.* 2011;18:R253–R276.

82. King KS, Prodanov T, Kantorovich V, et al. Metastatic pheochromocytoma/paraganglioma related to primary tumor development in childhood or adolescence: Significant link to SDHB mutations. *J Clin Oncol.* 2011;29:4137–4142.

83. Neumann HP, Pawlu C, Peczkowska M, et al. Distinct clinical features of paraganglioma syndromes associated with SDHB and SDHD gene mutations. *JAMA.* 2004;292:943–951.

84. Ricketts C, Woodward ER, Killick P, et al. Germline SDHB mutations and familial renal cell carcinoma. *J Natl Cancer Inst.* 2008;100:1260–1262.

85. Henderson A, Douglas F, Perros P, et al. SDHB-associated renal oncocytoma suggests a broadening of the renal phenotype in hereditary paragangliomatosis. *Fam Cancer.* 2009;8:257–260.

86. Ricketts CJ, Forman JR, Rattenberry E, et al. Tumor risks and genotype–phenotype–proteotype analysis in 358 patients with germline mutations in SDHB and SDHD. *Hum Mutat.* 2010;31:41–51.

87. van der Mey AG, Maaswinkel-Mooy PD, Cornelisse CJ, et al. Genomic imprinting in hereditary glomus tumours: Evidence for new genetic theory. *Lancet.* 1989;2:1291–1294.

88. Pigny P, Vincent A, Cardot Bauters C, et al. Paraganglioma after maternal transmission of a succinate dehydrogenase gene mutation. *J Clin Endocrinol Metab.* 2008;93:1609–1615.

89. Yeap PM, Tobias ES, Mavraki E, et al. Molecular analysis of pheochromocytoma after maternal transmission of SDHD mutation elucidates mechanism of parent-of-origin effect. *J Clin Endocrinol Metab.* 2011;96:E2009–E2013.

90. Schiavi F, Boedeker CC, Bausch B, et al. Predictors and prevalence of paraganglioma syndrome associated with mutations of the SDHC gene. *JAMA.* 2005;294:2057–2063.

91. Hao HX, Khalimonchuk O, Schraders M, et al. SDH5, a gene required for flavination of succinate dehydrogenase, is mutated in paraganglioma. *Science.* 2009;325:1139–1142.

92. Bayley JP, Kunst HP, Cascon A, et al. SDHAF2 mutations in familial and sporadic paraganglioma and phaeochromocytoma. *Lancet Oncol.* 2010;11:366–372.

93. Horvath R, Abicht A, Holinski-Feder E, et al. Leigh syndrome caused by mutations in the flavoprotein (Fp) subunit of succinate dehydrogenase (SDHA). *J Neurol Neurosurg Psychiatry.* 2006;77:74–76.

94. Burnichon N, Briere JJ, Libe R, et al. SDHA is a tumor suppressor gene causing paraganglioma. *Hum Mol Genet.* 2010;19:3011–3020.

95. Korpershoek E, Favier J, Gaal J, et al. SDHA immunohistochemistry detects germline SDHA gene mutations in apparently sporadic paragangliomas and pheochromocytomas. *J Clin Endocrinol Metab.* 2011;96:E1472–E1476.

96. Qin Y, Yao L, King EE, et al. Germline mutations in TMEM127 confer susceptibility to pheochromocytoma. *Nat Genet.* 2010;42:229–233.

97. Yao L, Schiavi F, Cascon A, et al. Spectrum and prevalence of FP/TMEM127 gene mutations in pheochromocytomas and paragangliomas. *JAMA.* 2010;304:2611–2619.

98. Neumann HP, Sullivan M, Winter A, et al. Germline mutations of the TMEM127 gene in patients with paraganglioma of head and neck and extraadrenal abdominal sites. *J Clin Endocrinol Metab.* 2011;96:E1279–E1282.

99. Abermil N, Guillaud-Bataille M, Burnichon N, et al. TMEM127 screening in a large cohort of patients with pheochromocytoma and/or paraganglioma. *J Clin Endocrinol Metab.* 2012;97:E805–E809.

100. Comino-Mendez I, Gracia-Aznarez FJ, Schiavi F, et al. Exome sequencing identifies MAX mutations as a cause of hereditary pheochromocytoma. *Nat Genet.* 2011;43:663–667.

101. Neumann HP, Bausch B, McWhinney SR, et al. Germ-line mutations in nonsyndromic pheochromocytoma. *N Engl J Med.* 2002;346:1459–1466.

102. Burnichon N, Rohmer V, Amar L, et al. The succinate dehydrogenase genetic testing in a large prospective series of patients with paragangliomas. *J Clin Endocrinol Metab.* 2009;94:2817–2827.

103. Jafri M, Maher ER. The genetics of phaeochromocytoma: Using clinical features to guide genetic testing. *Eur J Endocrinol.* 2012;166:151–158.

104. Rubinstein WS. Endocrine cancer predisposition syndromes: Hereditary paraganglioma, multiple endocrine neoplasia type 1, multiple endocrine neoplasia type 2, and hereditary thyroid cancer. *Hematol Oncol Clin North Am.* 2010;24:907–937.

105. Maher ER, Iselius L, Yates JRW, et al. von Hippel-Lindau disease: A genetic study. *J Med Genet.* 1991;28:443–447.

106. Neumann HPH, Wiestler OD. Clustering of features of von Hippel–Lindau syndrome: Evidence for a complex genetic locus. *Lancet.* 1991;337:1052–1054.

107. Maher ER, Neumann HP, Richard S. von Hippel–Lindau disease: A clinical and scientific review. *Eur J Hum Genet.* 2011;19:617–623.

108. Maher ER, Eng C. The pressure rises: Update on the genetics of phaeochromocytoma. *Hum Mol Genet.* 2002;11:2347–2354.

109. Gimenez-Roqueplo AP, Lehnert H, Mannelli M, et al. Phaeochromocytoma, new genes and screening strategies. *Clin Endocrinol (Oxf).* 2006;65:699–705.

110. Erlic Z, Rybicki L, Peczkowska M, et al. Clinical predictors and algorithm for the genetic diagnosis of pheochromocytoma patients. *Clin Cancer Res.* 2009;15:6378–6385.

14 Genetic Testing by Cancer Site

Skin

Michele Gabree and Meredith Seidel

Many hereditary cancer predisposition syndromes are associated with cutaneous findings. Identification of unique dermatologic features provides an opportunity to distinguish hereditary cancer syndromes with similar associated internal malignancies. Although skin findings are an important diagnostic tool for a number of cancer syndromes, including Cowden syndrome, Birt–Hogg–Dubé, hereditary leiomyomatosis renal cell carcinoma, and others (Table 14.1), this section will focus on skin cancer as well as tumor syndromes with cutaneous findings that are not included elsewhere in this book, including hereditary melanoma, basal cell nevus syndrome (BCNS), and neurofibromatosis type 1 (NF1) and neurofibromatosis type 2 (NF2).

The identification of dermatologic abnormalities and their association with internal malignancies often require thorough observation from clinicians. A consultation with a dermatologist may be helpful to identify specific dermatologic abnormalities. In some cases, biopsy and pathology may be necessary for a diagnosis.

GENETIC COUNSELING

Genetic counseling for hereditary skin diseases is similar to the process for other cancer predisposition syndromes. The genetic counseling process generally includes a detailed family and medical history, risk assessment, discussion of benefits, and limitations of available genetic testing, including possible test results, discussion of medical management, and implications for family members.[19] Dermatologic evaluation and review of pathology records pertaining to the cutaneous findings may provide clarification on specific dermatologic observations. Consultation with a dermatologist and/or other specialist who is knowledgeable about hereditary syndromes is often essential to a clinical evaluation. When possible, reviewing the medical records of family members is also helpful to confirm dermatologic diagnoses, as reports of some skin findings in family members may contain some inaccuracies.[20]

TABLE

14.1

Summary of Hereditary Cancer Syndromes with Cutaneous Features

	Cutaneous Features	Internal Tumor Site
Benign cutaneous features prominent		
Cowden syndrome[1,2]	Trichilemmoma, palmoplantar keratoses, oral mucosal papillomas, cutaneous facial papules, lipomas, macular pigmentation of the glans penis	Breast, thyroid, uterus
Birt–Hogg–Dubé[3]	Fibrofolliculomas, trichodiscomas, angiofibromas, perifollicular fibromas, acrochordons	Kidney
Childhood cancer syndrome (homozygous Lynch syndrome)[4]	Neurofibromas, CALMs	Hematologic, neural system, colon, small intestine, urinary tract
Hereditary leiomyomatosis renal cell carcinoma[5]	Cutaneous leiomyomas	Kidney, uterus
Multiple endocrine neoplasia, type 2B[6]	Mucosal neuromas of the lips/ tongue	Thyroid, adrenal gland, gastrointestinal tract
NF1[7,8]	Neurofibromas (cutaneous and subcutaneous), CALMs, freckling (inguinal, axillary), hypopigmented macules, cutaneous angiomas xanthogranulomas, glomus tumors, hyperpigmentation	Brain, spine, peripheral nervous system, optic pathway, small intestine, neuroendocrine, breast
NF2[7,9]	CALMs (usually 1–3), plaque lesions, intradermal schwannomas, subcutaneous schwannomas, cutaneous neurofibromas (uncommon)	Brain, spine, peripheral nervous system, optic pathway
Peutz–Jeghers syndrome[10]	Mucocutaneous pigmentation	Breast, stomach, small intestine, colon, pancreas, ovary, testicle

(*Continued*)

	Cutaneous Features	Internal Tumor Site
Tuberous sclerosis complex[11]	Hypomelanotic macules, facial angiofibromas, shagreen patches, fibrous facial plaques, ungual fibromas	Brain, kidney, heart, neuroendocrine
Benign cutaneous features sometimes present		
Multiple endocrine neoplasia type 1[12]	Facial angiofibromas, collagenomas, lipomas	Pituitary, pancreas, parathyroid, gastroenteropancreatic tract
Familial adenomatous polyposis[13]	Lipomas, fibromas, and epidermal cysts	Colon, thyroid, small intestine, liver, brain, pancreas, ampulla of Vater
Skin cancer prominent		
BCNS[14]	Basal cell carcinoma	Brain, ovary, heart
Hereditary melanoma[15]	Melanoma, dysplastic nevi	Pancreas
Xeroderma pigmentosum[16]	Melanoma, basal cell and squamous cell carcinoma, severe sunburn, lentigos, xerosis, erythema, actinic keratoses, poikiloderma	Oral cavity
Skin cancer sometimes present		
Hereditary breast and ovarian cancer syndrome[17]	Melanoma	Breast, ovary, prostate, pancreas
Lynch syndrome[18]	Sebaceous neoplasms, keratoacanthomas	Colon, uterus, stomach, ovary, hepatobiliary tract, urinary tract, small intestine, brain

HEREDITARY SKIN CANCER AND THE NEUROFIBROMATOSES

In addition to a few known single-gene disorders associated with skin cancers, confounding environmental factors, including solar ultraviolet radiation, as well as other genetic factors also are known to be associated with a varying degree of skin cancer risk. Separately, other hereditary tumor and cancer predisposition syndromes, such as NF1 and NF2, contain benign cutaneous features as common and sometimes predominant findings. General characteristics of a hereditary cancer predisposition syndrome include multiple tumors or cutaneous features in one individual, multiple affected family members, and individuals or families with related tumors, cancers, or unique physical characteristics. In some cases, young age at onset may also suggest a higher likelihood of a hereditary syndrome.

Hereditary Melanoma

Approximately 10% of melanoma cases are attributed to hereditary predisposition. Hereditary melanoma has been associated with mutations in two genes, cyclin-dependent kinase inhibitor 2A (*CDKN2A*) and cyclin-dependent kinase 4 (*CDK4*). Mutations in *CDK4* are rare and have been identified in only a few hereditary melanoma families.[21] Of families with hereditary melanoma, defined as three or more diagnoses of melanoma in one family, approximately 20% to 40% will have a detectable mutation in *CDKN2A*.[22]

CDKN2A and *CDK4* both function as tumor suppressors. *CDKN2A* encodes two transcripts: p16 and p14ARF through alternate reading frames. The majority of *CDKN2A* mutation-carrying families have been found to have mutations that affect the p16 protein. Mutations affecting the function of p14ARF are reportedly rare in cutaneous melanoma families.[23]

Phenotype

Hereditary melanoma has also been referred to as familial atypical mole melanoma syndrome.[24] Although the presence of atypical moles has been associated with an increased risk for melanoma, it has not been identified as a strong predictor of *CDKN2A* mutation status.[25,26]

The penetrance of *CDKN2A* mutations has been observed to be dependent on geography. This is likely due to varying environmental and other genetic factors across geographic regions. A study of *CDKN2A* carriers selected based on positive personal and family history of melanoma observed the melanoma risk for *CDKN2A* mutation carriers to be 58% in Europe, 76% in the United States, and 91% in Australia.[27] In a population-based study of patients with melanoma, the penetrance of *CDNK2A* mutations was observed to be lower (28% risk for melanoma by the age of 80 years).[28] Variants in the melanocortin 1 receptor (*MC1R*) gene have been associated with increased *CDKN2A* penetrance.[29] The prevalence of *MC1R* has been observed to differ with ethnic background and is one example of a genetic factor influencing melanoma risk that varies by geographical region.[30]

In addition to melanoma, other cancers have also been observed in increased frequency in *CDKN2A* mutation carriers. Most notably, an increased risk for pancreatic cancer has been reported in some *CDKN2A* mutation–carrying families.[31] Less commonly, an increased risk for other cancers, including neural system tumors, non-melanoma skin cancers, uveal melanoma, and head and neck cancers, has also been reported in individuals with *CDKN2A* mutations.[31,32]

TABLE 14.2	**Referral Criteria for Hereditary Melanoma Genetic Counseling**

Three or more relatives on the same side of the family with melanoma

Three or more primary melanomas in one individual

Pancreatic cancer and melanoma on the same side of the family

From: Leachman SA, Carucci J, Kohlmann W, et al. Selection criteria for genetic assessment of patients with familial melanoma. *J Am Acad Dermatol*. 2009;61:677e1–677e14.

In the United States, which is an area of moderate to high melanoma incidence, genetic counseling for hereditary melanoma has been generally recommended in families in which (1) three or more relatives are affected with melanoma; (2) one individual has three or more primary melanomas; or (3) both pancreatic cancer and melanoma are present in one family (Table 14.2).[15] Early age at onset in the absence of a family history of melanoma is not highly suggestive of a *CDKN2A* mutation.[33,34]

Genetic Testing

Clinical testing for *CDKN2A* and *CDK4* is available in the United States at several commercial laboratories. However, some of the laboratories offering hereditary melanoma testing perform analysis of only *CDKN2A*, given the relatively low-frequency *CDK4* mutations reported.

The utility of genetic testing for *CDKN2A* mutations remains a source of debate. This is partly due to the relatively low frequency of *CDKN2A* mutations in families with melanoma. In addition, many individuals with a personal and/or family history of melanoma are under close surveillance and aware of risk-reduction recommendations; therefore, genetic test results would not alter clinical management.[25] Also, the role of pancreatic cancer surveillance in *CDKN2A* carriers remains under investigation. Some studies have suggested that knowledge of *CDKN2A* mutation status improves short-term compliance to risk-reducing behaviors.[35,36] However, information regarding the long-term impact of *CDKN2A* testing is limited at this time. The possible genetic test results for an individual undergoing *CDKN2A* genetic testing are shown in Table 14.3.

Individuals with a *CDKN2A* mutation have a 50% of passing the mutation on to their children.

Medical Management

CDKN2A mutation carriers, or individuals at 50% risk to be a carrier, should be monitored carefully for melanoma through clinical and self-examinations

TABLE 14.3	*CDKN2A* Genetic Testing Results and Medical Management Recommendations

Test Result	Medical Management
CDKN2A mutation positive	Melanoma surveillance • Clinical skin examination with dermatologist every 4–6 mo • Biopsy should be performed on suspected lesions • Avoid prolonged direct sunlight and use sun-protective clothing and sunscreen • Monthly self-skin examinations • Inform at-risk relatives Pancreatic cancer surveillance[a] • Recommended for individuals with a family history of pancreatic cancer and may be considered in other cases • Refer to gastroenterologist for discussion of pancreatic screening options • Inform at-risk relatives
CDKN2A variation of unknown significance	Etiology of the melanoma remains unknown • Consider if genetic testing is indicated for other affected relatives • Proband and family remain at increased risk for melanoma • Screening recommendations should be based on personal and family history
CDKN2A mutation negative	No mutation previously identified in family: • Etiology of the melanoma remains unknown • Consider if genetic testing is indicated for other affected relatives • Proband and family remain at increased risk for melanoma • Screening recommendations should be based on personal and family history Mutation previously identified in family: • Proband and family remain at increased risk for melanoma, although the risk is lower than for relatives who carry a *CDKN2A* mutation • Screening recommendations should be based on personal and family history

[a]To date, pancreatic cancer surveillance has not been proven to be effective at improving pancreatic cancer outcome.

(Table 14.3). In addition, *CDKN2A* carriers are recommended to avoid prolonged direct sunlight and utilize sun-protective clothing and sunscreen.[25,37]

Individuals who test negative for a familial *CDKN2A* mutation may also have an increased risk for melanoma. However, this risk has been observed to be lower than the melanoma risk for *CDKN2A* mutation carriers.[28]

As noted in Table 14.3, *CDKN2A* mutation carriers, especially those with a family history of pancreatic cancer, are candidates for pancreatic cancer surveillance and should discuss the risks, benefits, and limitations of screening with a gastroenterology specialist.[38] However, to date, the effectiveness of pancreatic surveillance remains under investigation.[39]

Basal Cell Nevus Syndrome

BCNS, also known as Gorlin syndrome or nevoid basal cell carcinoma syndrome, is an autosomal dominant syndrome associated with cutaneous findings, including basal cell carcinoma, as well as skeletal system, nervous system, and ocular abnormalities.[40] Although BCNS has complete penetrance, the expression is variable.[41]

BCNS is thought to be relatively uncommon, and the incidence of BCNS has been estimated to be 1:30,827 to 1:57,000.[42] The variable expression may cause difficulty in diagnosing BCNS.

BCNS has been associated with mutations in the *patched gene 1 (PTCH1)* gene. *PTCH1* functions as a tumor suppressor in the sonic hedgehog (Shh) pathway, which is also involved in embryonic development.[43] Chromosomal abnormalities of 9q22.3 region, which includes *PTCH1*, have been reported in a few individuals with features of BCNS as well as other features, including short stature, developmental delay, and seizures.[44] Rarely, mutations in other genes, including *SUFU* and *PTCH2*, have also been reported in individuals with features of BCNS.[45,46]

Phenotype

The phenotype of BCNS is variable, and some characteristics are present at different life stages. Therefore, it is important to obtain a complete medical history, including physical examination and dermatologic, cardiac, and gynecologic examinations as well as radiologic studies to confirm a diagnosis of BCNS.

The clinical manifestations of BCNS include the following:

Skin

Basal Cell Carcinoma

Approximately 50% to 75% of individuals with BCNS will develop basal cell carcinomas.[47] Typically, basal cell carcinomas develop in the late teens through the 30s, but some published reports have indicated the detection of basal cell carcinomas in early childhood in individuals with BCNS. The presence of basal cell carcinomas is also dependent on other factors, including skin type and radiation exposure, including sun exposure.[40,41]

Noncancerous Cutaneous Features

The majority of individuals with BCNS will have multiple nevi present by adulthood.[40] In addition, BCNS is associated with an increased prevalence of facial milia, dermoid cysts, and skin tags. Palmar and plantar pits are also a common feature of BCNS and usually are evident by early adulthood.[40]

Skeletal

Skeletal abnormalities, including rib and spinal abnormalities, are reported with increased frequency in BCNS. The majority of individuals with BCNS are reported to have macrocephaly.[48]

Central Nervous System

Ectopic Calcification

Ectopic calcification, particularly of the falx celebri, has been reported as a common finding in individuals with BCNS.[48]

Brain Tumor

Although other types of brain tumors have been reported in individuals with BCNS, medulloblastoma, typically desmoplastic type, is the most common.[49] Approximately 5% of individuals with BCNS are diagnosed with medulloblastoma, usually around 2 years of age.

Other Features

Jaw Keratocysts

Approximately 75% of affected individuals with BCNS develop multiple jaw keratocysts.[50]

Characteristic Facial Features

Facial features characteristic of BCNS including macrocephaly, bossing of the forehead, coarse facial features, and facial milia have been observed in approximately 60% of BCNS cases.[14]

In addition to the above features, congenital malformations such as cleft lip/palate, polydactyly, and eye anomalies have also been reported as features of BCNS.[40]

Additional associated tumors including cardiac and ovarian fibromas have also been reported to occur with increased frequency in BCNS.[51,52]

Diagnosis and Genetic Testing

A diagnosis of BCNS was initially based on clinical criteria; however, the availability of molecular testing has identified mutations in individuals with a more variable phenotype. The First International Colloquium on BCNS concluded that the clinical criteria should be used to consider a suspected diagnosis of BCNS rather than as diagnostic criteria.[53] The colloquium recommends that a suspected diagnosis of BCNS be considered in individuals with an identified *PTCH1* mutation and one major clinical criterion, individuals who express two major criteria, and individuals with one major and two minor criteria (Table 14.4).

Genetic testing for the *PTCH1* gene is clinically available. Approximately 50% to 85% of individuals with clinical features of BCNS will have a detectable mutation in the *PTCH1* gene through gene sequencing analysis. Deletions and duplications of the *PTCH1* gene have also been reported.[54]

Approximately 20% to 30% of individuals with BCNS are de novo, meaning that neither parent carries the associated gene mutation.[14] Individuals affected with BCNS have a 50% chance of having an affected child. In cases where a mutation has been identified, testing is an option for at-risk family members. In addition, both preconception genetic diagnosis and prenatal testing are available for known *PTCH1* mutations.

Medical Management

Because of the many variable symptoms of BCNS, individuals with BCNS should be referred to an appropriate specialist depending on the symptoms.

TABLE 14.4	Clinical Criteria for Suspected Diagnosis of BCNS

Major criteria
- Early-onset/multiple basal cell carcinoma
- Odontogenic keratocyst of the jaw (<20 y of age)
- Palmaroplantar pitting
- Calcification of the falx cerebri
- Medulloblastoma (usually desmoplastic)
- First-degree relative with BCNS

Minor criteria
- Rib anomalies
- Skeletal malformations and radiologic changes
- Macrocephaly
- Cleft lip/palate
- Ovarian/cardiac fibroma
- Lymphomesenteric cysts
- Ocular abnormalities

From: Bree AF, Shah MR. Consensus statement from the first international colloquium on basal cell nevus syndrome (BCNS). *Am J Med Genet A.* 2011;155A:2091–2097.

Basal Cell Carcinoma

Early diagnosis is important for management and to limit cosmetic damage. Surgery, oral retinoids, topical therapies, and photodynamic therapy have all been utilized with varying degrees of success for individuals with BCNS.[47]

Medulloblastoma

Consideration of developmental assessment and physical examination every 6 months is an option for children during infancy and early childhood. Imaging for medulloblastoma surveillance is not currently recommended.[14]

Jaw Keratocysts

Clinical examinations and imaging are recommended for individuals with BCNS, starting during childhood. These tumors may sometimes be detected during routine dental examinations.[55]

Ovarian and Cardiac Fibromas

Affected individuals with cardiac fibromas should be referred to a cardiologist. Ovarian fibromas also warrant a specialty referral and may require surgery, ideally with the aim of preserving fertility.[56]

Radiation Exposure

Given the known increased risk for basal cell carcinoma, it is recommended that individuals with BCNS avoid sun exposure. In addition, it is recommended that other radiation exposure also be avoided if possible, including radiation as treatment for medulloblastoma.[49]

Neurofibromatosis Type 1

NF1 is one of the most common genetic disorders, affecting an estimated 1:2,500 to 1:3,000 individuals at birth.[7] Formerly known as von Recklinghausen disease or peripheral neurofibromatosis, manifestations of the disease affect multiple areas of the body, including, but not limited to, the central and peripheral nervous systems, skin, eyes, skeleton, gastrointestinal system, and the cardiovascular system. Historically, observations of patients with NF1 date back to the 13th century, but the disorder was first formally described in 1882 by Friedrich von Recklinghausen.[7,57,58]

NF1 is a completely penetrant autosomal dominant condition with widely variable expression, both within and between families.[59] No ethnic, racial, or sex predilection has been observed.[57] NF1 is caused by mutations in the NF1 gene on 17q11.2. The protein product of NF1 is neurofibromin, a GTPase activating protein that is expressed across many tissue types and in particularly high levels within neurocutaneous tissue. It acts as a negative regulator of intracellular Ras signaling pathways involved in cell growth and proliferation.[7,60,61] More recently, NF1 has also been linked to the development of skeletal muscle.[62]

Phenotype

In 1987, the National Institutes of Health developed clinical diagnostic criteria for NF1 (Table 14.5) on which diagnosis of the disease is most often based.[59] The disease usually presents in childhood, beginning with skin findings, which are often present by 1 year of age. In general, the clinical manifestations of NF1 are age-dependent: By the age of 6 years, approximately 90% of individuals with NF1 meet diagnostic criteria; by 8 years of age, 97% meet criteria, and virtually all meet the criteria by the time they are 20 years old.[59]

Skin

Among the numerous and variable clinical manifestations of NF1, cutaneous findings feature prominently and can even be the sole basis for a diagnosis of NF1. The following skin findings are hallmark features of NF1, and each is a component of the diagnostic criteria (Table 14.5).

Café-Au-Lait Macules (CALMs)

Café-au-lait macules (CALMs) are the most common and often the earliest presenting feature of NF1. CALMs may be congenital and are observed in almost all

TABLE 14.5	NIH Diagnostic Criteria: Neurofibromatosis Type 1

Clinical diagnosis of NF1 can be made for an individual exhibiting any two (or more) of the following:
Six or more café-au-lait macules:
- ≥5 mm prepubertal
- ≥15 mm postpubertal

Two or more neurofibromas of any type, or one or more plexiform neurofibromas
Freckling in the axillary or inguinal region
Optic glioma
Two or more Lisch nodules (iris hamartomas)
A distinctive osseous lesion such as sphenoid dysplasia or tibial pseudoarthrosis
A first-degree relative with NF1 as defined by the above criteria

From: Evans DG, Raymond FL, Barwell JG, et al. Genetic testing and screening of individuals at risk of NF2. *Clin Genet.* 2012;82:416–424. doi: 10.1111/j.1399-0004.2011.01816.x.

patients with NF1 within the first year of life. They often become larger and more numerous through adolescence and may fade as an adult.[57]

Intertriginous Freckling

Skinfold freckling, or Crowe sign, is a cardinal feature of NF1.[59] Freckling occurs most often in the axillary and inguinal regions of the body and is exhibited by up to 90% of patients, usually beginning in childhood. Freckling may also be found in other areas of the body including beneath the breasts in females, on the neck, above the eyelids, around the mouth, and on the trunk in adults.[58]

Neurofibromas

The hallmark feature of NF1, neurofibromas can develop in almost any part of the body, including on or just below the surface of the skin. Cutaneous neurofibromas vary in size (<1 mm to large/disfiguring) and number; they are soft and fleshy and may be raised or flat, ranging in color from blue/purple to brown to flesh colored. Subcutaneous neurofibromas are firm, tender nodules that are often visible beneath the skin. Cutaneous and/or subcutaneous neurofibromas usually manifest later than CALMs and freckling, either later in childhood or in early adolescence.[58,59]

Less common, nondiagnostic cutaneous features of NF1 include hyperpigmentation, which may be generalized or appearing in conjunction with affected body areas in segmental NF1, glomus tumors, hypopigmented macules (usually on the trunk), xanthogranulomas, cutaneous angiomas, and pruritus.[7,57,60]

Neurologic

Tumors of the central and peripheral nervous systems are prevalent among individuals with NF1. These include spinal neurofibromas, peripheral nerve sheath tumors, plexiform neurofibromas, and astrocytomas. In addition, optic pathway gliomas (OPGs) are slow-growing tumors occurring among 15% to 20% of patients, usually by the age of 6 years. OPGs are symptomatic in only 5% of individuals, in which case they are most often diagnosed by the age of 3 years.[7,57,60]

A variety of nontumor neurologic manifestations are reported among individuals with NF1. These include learning disabilities, which occur in 60% or more of children with NF1, decreased IQ (occasionally <70), attention-deficit/hyperactivity disorder, and other behavior difficulties. Unidentified bright objects, or UBOs, are a characteristic magnetic resonance imaging (MRI) finding in NF1. The clinical significance of UBOs is not known, but some evidence correlates UBO prevalence with severity of cognitive and behavioral difficulties.[58,59] Seizure disorders and multiple sclerosis also occur at a higher frequency in NF1, and Chiari type I malformation, aqueductal stenosis, and macrocephaly have all been reported.[7,59]

Eye

Lisch nodules, or melanocytic iris hamartomas, are asymptomatic eye findings present in most individuals with NF1, usually by the age of 5 to 10 years. Lisch nodules are pathognomonic for NF1 and are most reliably detected by an experienced ophthalmologist by slit-lamp examination.[7,8,60] Glaucoma, choroidal abnormalities, and ptosis are less common but have all been reported in patients with NF1.[7]

Skeletal

Bony growths and other abnormalities of the bone are key features of NF1. Diagnostic bone findings include thinning of the long-bone cortex (with or without pseudoarthrosis) and sphenoid wing dysplasia. In addition, there is an increased frequency of short stature, scoliosis, and, more recently noted, osteopenia and osteoporosis among individuals with NF1.[7,57,60]

Cardiovascular

Cardiovascular complications occur at a higher frequency among patients with NF1 and include congenital heart disease (pulmonary stenosis, coarctation of the aorta), hypertension, cerebrovascular disease, and renal artery stenosis.[7,63] Pulmonary stenosis is more prevalent among patients with classic NF1 but may also be found as part of a variant phenotype that combines features of NF1 and Noonan syndrome.[59]

Other Features

Respiratory Complications

Respiratory complications include restrictive lung disease caused by compression from neurofibroma and metastases from malignant peripheral nerve sheath tumors.[7]

NF1-associated Malignancies

The overall increased risk of cancer in NF1 patients is 2.7-fold, and the cumulative risk for patients older than 50 years is 20%.[61] Malignant peripheral nerve sheath tumors are the most common cancerous tumors in NF1. Other malignancies include chronic myelogenous leukemia, astrocytoma, rhabdomyosarcoma, gastrointestinal stromal tumors, carcinoid tumors (small intestine), pheochromocytomas (although usually not malignant), and breast carcinoma.[61] There are also a few reports of higher rates of melanoma seen in NF1; however, this association remains controversial.[57]

Diagnosis and Genetic Testing

Up to 50% of individuals with NF1 have no family history and represent de novo mutations. The *NF1* gene has one of the highest spontaneous mutations rates, about

1:10,000, and more than 500 pathogenic mutations have been identified.[61] The reason for the high mutation rate is not fully understood, but may be due in part to the large size of the gene.[59]

Although diagnosis of NF1 is almost always made on a clinical basis using the established criteria, genetic testing is available and can be useful, particularly in certain situations. Mutations are identifiable in 95% of individuals who meet the NF1 clinical diagnostic criteria.[64] In young children with no family history who do not yet meet the diagnostic criteria, genetic testing may aid in differentiating NF1 from other disorders with phenotypic overlap such as Legius syndrome, familial café-au-lait spots, and NF2. Genetic testing may also help identify rare variant forms of the disease that do not satisfy the National Institutes of Health criteria. In families with a previously identified mutation, prenatal diagnosis and prenatal testing are available. A common challenge in prenatal counseling and testing for NF1 arises from the variability and unpredictability of the disease presentation.[7,65]

Given the wide variability in expression of the disease even among members of the same family, it stands to reason that very few genotype–phenotype correlations have been described. It has been noted that individuals carrying a deletion of an entire NF1 allele (approximately 4% to 5% of cases) are likely to exhibit a more severe phenotype, including a greater number of cutaneous neurofibromas, often occurring at younger ages. Cognitive abnormalities are also more frequent and severe, and somatic overgrowth, large hands and feet, and dysmorphic facial features have been reported.[63] In addition, individuals with a 3-base-pair in-frame deletion of exon 17 of NF1 may exhibit the common nontumor cutaneous features of NF1, without cutaneous or surface plexiform neurofibromas.[63]

In addition to the high rate of spontaneous mutations, another challenge associated with genetic counseling for NF1 is the high rate of mosaicism. Approximately 40% to 50% of cases are segmental, or mosaic, representing postzygotic NF1 mutations. In these cases, recurrence risks can be difficult to predict; however, they are usually estimated to be less than 1% unless the germline is affected. Indeed, there are cases of individuals with segmental NF1 bearing children with constitutional disease.[63]

Medical Management

Management of NF1 requires multidisciplinary input and, ideally, should be overseen by practitioners experienced in caring for patients with neurofibromatosis.[58,60]

Recommended surveillance for children with NF1 may vary somewhat by center, but typically includes annual physical and ophthalmologic examination until the age of 8 years. Between the ages of 8 and 18 years, examinations every other year may be sufficient.[58,60,64] Blood pressure monitoring should take place at least annually because of the risk of pheochromocytoma and renal artery stenosis.[58,64] In addition, annual neurologic examinations are advisable, with consideration of neuroimaging in the presence of any abnormal findings.[58] In addition, ongoing developmental and neuropsychological evaluation is recommended to assess cognitive function and to identify learning disabilities.[8,57]

Screening by way of MRI, electroencephalogram, and/or x-ray may be dictated by symptoms, clinical findings, and/or personal and family history. For certain findings more frequent monitoring may be indicated and, in some cases, treatment may be available.

Plexiform Neurofibroma

Perform MRI every 6 to 12 months to monitor growing lesions. Depending on the location of the lesion, surgical debulking may be possible but is often incomplete, resulting in regrowth.[8,60,64]

Optic Pathway Gliomas

Once identified, MRI is used to monitor OPGs. Quarterly ophthalmologic evaluation is suggested for the first year, followed by annual examination of patients for at least 3 years or until the age of 8 years. Evaluation by endocrinology may be recommended. For symptomatic OPGs, chemotherapy treatment is available, but radiotherapy is not recommended.[8,57]

Malignant Peripheral Nerve Sheath Tumor

Monitor individuals with plexiform neurofibroma for increased size and pain, as well as changes in tumor texture; monitor unexplained neurologic changes. If possible, complete surgical resection is desired, but should be followed by radiation therapy if it is not complete.[8,64]

Cutaneous Neurofibromas

Surgical removal of neurofibromas may be possible when necessary for cosmetic or pain-related reasons.[8,57]

As necessary, referrals should be made to a variety of specialties, including cardiology, nephrology, plastic surgery, otolaryngology, and gastroenterology.

Neurofibromatosis Type 2

NF2 was first described by J. H. Wishart in 1822, at least 50 years prior to von Recklinghausen's description of NF1. Although there is relatively little overlap in the clinical phenotype of the two conditions, NF2 is much less common and was, until relatively recently, often mistaken as a variant form of NF1. It was not until 1987 when linkage studies attributed the conditions to two different genes on different chromosomes that the diseases were formally recognized as separate. Although more common than it was once thought to be, the estimated incidence of NF2 is approximately 1/10 of that of NF1, or 1:30,000 to 1:40,000.[66]

NF2 is inherited in an autosomal dominant manner and is virtually 100% penetrant by the age of 60 years.[9] It is caused by mutations in the NF2 gene on chromosome

22q12. The product of the *NF2* gene is the protein known as merlin (moesin–ezrin–radixin-like protein) or schwannomin, and it is thought to function in cell membrane protein organization, cellular adhesion, and negative regulation of cellular growth, proliferation, and motility.[60,64] The specific mechanism of the tumor suppressor function of merlin has not yet been fully elucidated and is an area of active investigation.[60]

A key difference between NF1 and NF2 relates to cutaneous findings, which, in NF2, may aid in diagnosis but are not diagnostic in and of themselves. The cardinal feature of NF2 is vestibular schwannoma, which arise bilaterally on the 8th cranial nerve in almost all cases of the disease.[7]

Phenotype

Contrary to the name of the disorder, schwannomas and meningiomas, not neurofibromas, are the most prominent tumor types found in NF2.[9,67] Individuals with NF2 most often present between 20 and 30 years of age with hearing loss (frequently unilateral) related to the presence of a vestibular schwannoma. Tinnitus, dizziness, and imbalance are also common adult symptoms at presentation.[9] Although children may also develop similar symptoms, they are more likely to present with less common features of NF2, making examination of other systems the key to accurate diagnosis. In these cases, neurologic examination, eye examination, and careful examination of the skin become crucial.[64] Several sets of NF2 diagnostic criteria exist, and the criteria may still be evolving[68]; however, currently, the most widely used criteria set is the Manchester Diagnostic Criteria, shown in Table 14.6.[60]

TABLE 14.6	**Diagnostic Criteria for NF2**

Manchester Diagnostic Criteria for NF2

- Bilateral vestibular schwannoma

or

- First-degree family member with NF2 and unilateral vestibular schwannoma, or any two of meningioma, glioma, neurofibroma, schwannoma, posterior subcapsular lenticular opacities

or

- Unilateral vestibular schwannoma and any two of meningioma, glioma, neurofibroma, schwannoma, posterior subcapsular lenticular opacities

or

- Multiple meningiomas (≥2) and unilateral vestibular schwannoma or any two of glioma, neurofibroma, schwannoma, cataract

Skin

Although not hallmarks of the disease, the cutaneous manifestations of NF2 are prevalent and can be detected in up to 70% of cases.[7] As with NF1, skin findings include CALMs; however, when CALMs are present in NF2, it is generally fewer, about 1 to 3 per person. Individuals with NF2 may also exhibit plaque lesions on the surface of the skin, intradermal schwannomas, subcutaneous schwannomas, and, very rarely,[7,57,60] cutaneous neurofibromas.[7,9]

Neurologic

Tumors

Bilateral vestibular schwannomas occur in 90% to 95% of NF2 patients.[7] Although malignancy is rare, the location of growth is a common cause of increased morbidity, often causing progressive hearing loss and balance issues.[58] Schwannomas of other cranial nerves are not uncommon among NF2 patients[9]; in addition, spinal and peripheral nerve schwannomas often develop.[64] Meningiomas are the second most common tumor type, found in 58% to 75% of patients with NF2. Both cranial and spinal meningiomas can be found in NF2.[64] More rare, but also observed, are spinal and brainstem ependymomas, as well as spinal and cranial astrocytoma.[7]

Peripheral Neuropathy

The majority of patients with NF2 will develop peripheral neuropathy within their lifetime, often in childhood presenting as a hand or foot drop, or a palsy. Neuropathy is sometimes but not always related to tumor compression.[9]

Eye

Subcapsular lenticular opacities are a key diagnostic feature of NF2. They are found in 60% to 81% of patients and may develop into cataracts.[9,58] Additional ocular findings include epiretinal membranes, or thin translucent or semitranslucent sheets of fibrous tissue, which usually do not decrease visual acuity.[9] In addition, retinal hamartomas appear in 6% to 22% of NF2 patients and can cause a loss of visual acuity.[9]

Diagnosis and Genetic Testing

In patients with suspected NF2 and a positive family history (two or more family members affected), genetic testing reveals mutations in 90% or more. However, approximately 50% of individuals with NF2 represent de novo mutations in the *NF2* gene. In isolated cases of classic NF2 with no known family history, mutations are identified in approximately 60% to 72%. In families with an identified mutation, presymptomatic genetic testing of at-risk family members is important for management of the disease. Prenatal genetic testing and preimplantation genetic diagnosis are also available.[69]

Somatic mosaicism is observed in roughly 33% of individuals with de novo cases of NF2, and identification of these individuals often relies on confirming the presence of the same mutation in tissue from two distinct NF2-related lesions.[67] Finally, for some mutations, genotype–phenotype correlation data are available.[9]

Medical Management

In general, as with NF1, it is best if NF2 patients are able to be followed by experienced practitioners in a comprehensive clinic setting. Screening recommendations may include initiation of MRI screening for vestibular schwannomas at the age of 10 years, as symptoms of the tumors are rare in younger patients. When present, growth of vestibular schwannomas is best measured by tumor volume using MRI.[60] Head and spinal MRI is the primary screening tool and should be performed every 2 years for at-risk children younger than 20 years with no symptoms or tumors. After the age of 20 years, the tumors grow slower and screening can be decreased to every 3 to 5 years.[69] Annual ophthalmologic examination is recommended from infancy in at-risk or affected individuals. In addition, the following annual examinations, initiated in infancy, may be recommended: Neurologic examination and audiology with auditory brainstem evoked potentials.[9]

When it is possible, surgery is the primary mode of treatment for NF2 tumors, with the intent of improving quality of life and maintenance of function. Surgery is not always possible and, in some cases, radiation therapy may be used as an alternative. Overall, patients with NF2 have a shorter life expectancy.[60]

CONCLUSIONS

Dermatologic examinations, when combined with a thorough personal and family medical history, play an important role in the diagnosis of many cancer predisposition syndromes. Although some cutaneous features are strongly indicative of a specific diagnosis, others may be less common or less strongly associated with a particular syndrome; therefore, it remains important to consider these findings in the context of a patient's complete medical and family history. The current availability of molecular testing for many hereditary syndromes has significantly advanced the ability to distinguish and confirm a suspected clinical diagnosis. In addition to the syndromes listed above, it is important to note that other cancer predisposition syndromes may also have cutaneous components, and with the advancement of molecular testing, additional syndromes are likely to be identified in the future.

REFERENCES

1. Pilarski R. Cowden syndrome: A critical review of the clinical literature. *J Genet Couns.* 2009;18:13–27.
2. Hobert JA, Eng C. PTEN hamartoma tumor syndrome: An overview. *Genet Med.* 2009;11:687–694.

3. Menko FH, van Steensel MA, Giraud S, et al. Birt-Hogg-DubØ syndrome: Diagnosis and management. *Lancet Oncol.* 2009;10:1199–1206.

4. Kruger S, Kinzel M, Walldorf C, et al. Homozygous PMS2 germline mutations in two families with early-onset haematological malignancy, brain tumours, HNPCC-associated tumours, and signs of neurofibromatosis type 1. *Eur J Hum Genet.* 2008;16:62–72.

5. Badeloe S, Frank J. Clinical and molecular genetic aspects of hereditary multiple cutaneous leiomyomatosis. *Eur J Dermatol.* 2009;19:545–551.

6. Moline J, Eng C. Multiple endocrine neoplasia type 2: An overview. *Genet Med.* 2011;13:755–764.

7. Ferner RE. The neurofibromatoses. *Pract Neurol.* 2010;10:82–93.

8. Williams VC, Lucas J, Babcock MA, et al. Neurofibromatosis type 1 revisited. *Pediatrics.* 2009;123:124–133.

9. Asthagiri AR, Parry DM, Butman JA, et al. Neurofibromatosis type 2. *Lancet.* 2009;373:1974–1986.

10. Beggs AD, Latchford AR, Vasen HF, et al. Peutz-Jeghers syndrome: A systematic review and recommendations for management. *Gut.* 2010;59:975–986.

11. Borkowska J, Schwartz RA, Kotulska K, et al. Tuberous sclerosis complex: Tumors and tumorigenesis. *Int J Dermatol.* 2011;50:13–20.

12. Winship IM, Dudding TE. Lessons from the skin—cutaneous features of familial cancer. *Lancet Oncol.* 2008;9:462–472.

13. Burger B, Cattani N, Trueb S, et al. Prevalence of skin lesions in familial adenomatous polyposis: A marker for presymptomatic diagnosis? *Oncologist.* 2011;16:1698–1705.

14. Evans DG, Farndon PA. Nevoid basal cell carcinoma syndrome. In: Pagon RA, Bird TD, Dolan CR, Stephens K, Adam MP, eds. *GeneReviews™ [Internet].* Seattle, WA: University of Washington, Seattle; 1993.

15. Leachman SA, Carucci J, Kohlmann W, et al. Selection criteria for genetic assessment of patients with familial melanoma. *J Am Acad Dermatol.* 2009;61:677e1–677e14.

16. Kremer KH, DiGiovana JJ. Xeroderma pigmentosum. In: Pagon RA, Bird TD, Dolan CR, Stephens K, Adam MP, eds. *GeneReviews™ [Internet].* Seattle, WA: University of Washington, Seattle; 1993.

17. Cancer risks in BRCA2 mutation carriers. The Breast Cancer Linkage Consortium. *J Natl Cancer Inst.* 1999;91:1310–1316.

18. Dores GM, Curtis RE, Toro JR, et al. Incidence of cutaneous sebaceous carcinoma and risk of associated neoplasms: Insight into Muir-Torre syndrome. *Cancer.* 2008;113:3372–3381.

19. Robson ME, Storm CD, Weitzel J, et al. American Society of Clinical Oncology policy statement update: Genetic and genomic testing for cancer susceptibility. *J Clin Oncol.* 2010;28:893–901.

20. Hemminki K, Eng C. Clinical genetic counselling for familial cancers requires reliable data on familial cancer risks and general action plans. *J Med Genet.* 2004;41:801–807.

21. Goldstein AM, Chidambaram A, Halpern A, et al. Rarity of CDK4 germline mutations in familial melanoma. *Melanoma Res.* 2002;12:51–55.

22. Hayward NK. Genetics of melanoma predisposition. *Oncogene.* 2003;22:3053–3062.

23. Goldstein AM, Chan M, Harland M, et al. High-risk melanoma susceptibility genes and pancreatic cancer, neural system tumors, and uveal melanoma across GenoMEL. *Cancer Res.* 2006;66:9818–9828.

24. Newton Bishop JA, Bataille V, Pinney E, et al. Family studies in melanoma: Identification of the atypical mole syndrome (AMS) phenotype. *Melanoma Res.* 1994;4:199–206.

25. Newton Bishop JA, Gruis NA. Genetics: What advice for patients who present with a family history of melanoma? *Semin Oncol.* 2007;34:452–459.

26. Bishop JN, Harland M, Randerson-Moor J, et al. Management of familial melanoma. *Lancet Oncol.* 2007;8:46–54.

27. Bishop DT, Demenais F, Goldstein AM, et al. Geographical variation in the penetrance of CDKN2A mutations for melanoma. *J Natl Cancer Inst.* 2002;94:894–903.

28. Begg CB, Orlow I, Hummer AJ, et al. Lifetime risk of melanoma in CDKN2A mutation carriers in a population-based sample. *J Natl Cancer Inst.* 2005;97:1507–1515.

29. Demenais F, Mohamdi H, Chaudru V, et al. Association of MC1R variants and host phenotypes with melanoma risk in CDKN2A mutation carriers: A GenoMEL study. *J Natl Cancer Inst.* 2010;102:1568–1583.

30. Raimondi S, Sera F, Gandini S, et al. MC1R variants, melanoma and red hair color phenotype: A meta-analysis. *Int J Cancer.* 2008;122:2753–2760.

31. de Snoo FA, Bishop DT, Bergman W, et al. Increased risk of cancer other than melanoma in CDKN2A founder mutation (p16-Leiden)–positive melanoma families. *Clin Cancer Res.* 2008;14:7151–7157.

32. Randerson-Moor JA, Harland M, William S, et al. A germline deletion of p14(ARF) but not CDKN2A in a melanoma-neural system tumour syndrome family. *Hum Mol Genet.* 2001;10:55–62.

33. Tsao H, Zhang X, Kwitkiwski K, et al. Low prevalence of germline CDKN2A and CDK4 mutations in patients with early-onset melanoma. *Arch Dermatol.* 2000;136:1118–1122.

34. Berg P, Wennberg AM, Tuominen R, et al. Germline CDKN2A mutations are rare in child and adolescent cutaneous melanoma. *Melanoma Res.* 2004;14:251–255.

35. Aspinwall LG, Leaf SL, Kohlmann W, et al. Patterns of photoprotection following CDKN2A/p16 genetic test reporting and counseling. *J Am Acad Dermatol.* 2009;60:745–757.

36. Aspinwall LG, Leaf SL, Dola ER, et al. CDKN2A/p16 genetic test reporting improves early detection intentions and practices in high-risk melanoma families. *Cancer Epidemiol Biomarkers Prev.* 2008;17:1510–1519.

37. Eckerle Mize D, Bishop M, Reese E, et al. Familial atypical multiple mole melanoma syndrome. In: Riegert-Johnson DL, Boardman LA, Hefferon T, Roberts M, eds. *Cancer Syndromes [Internet].* Bethesda, MD: National Center for Biotechnology Information (US); 2009.

38. Bartsch DK, Sina-Frey M, Lang S, et al. CDKN2A germline mutations in familial pancreatic cancer. *Ann Surg.* 2002;236:730–737.

39. Verna EC, Hwang C, Stevens PD, et al. Pancreatic cancer screening in a prospective cohort of high-risk patients: A comprehensive strategy of imaging and genetics. *Clin Cancer Res.* 2010;16:5028–5037.

40. Lo Muzio L. Nevoid basal cell carcinoma syndrome (Gorlin syndrome). *Orphanet J Rare Dis.* 2008;3:32.

41. Tom WL, Hurley MY, Oliver DS, et al. Features of basal cell carcinomas in basal cell nevus syndrome. *Am J Med Genet A.* 2011;155A:2098–2104.

42. Evans DG, Howard E, Giblin C, et al. Birth incidence and prevalence of tumor-prone syndromes: Estimates from a UK family genetic register service. *Am J Med Genet A.* 2010;152A:327–332.

43. Lupi O. Correlations between the sonic hedgehog pathway and basal cell carcinoma. *Int J Dermatol.* 2007;46:1113–1117.

44. Yamamoto K, Yoshihashi H, Furuya N, et al. Further delineation of 9q22 deletion syndrome associated with basal cell nevus (Gorlin) syndrome: Report of two cases and review of the literature. *Congenit Anom (Kyoto).* 2009;49:8–14.

45. Pastorino L, Ghiorzo P, Nasti S, et al. Identification of a SUFU germline mutation in a family with Gorlin syndrome. *Am J Med Genet A.* 2009;149A:1539–1543.

46. Fan Z, Li J, Du J, et al. A missense mutation in PTCH2 underlies dominantly inherited NBCCS in a Chinese family. *J Med Genet.* 2008;45:303–308.

47. Go JW, Kim SH, Yi SY, et al. Basal cell nevus syndrome showing several histologic types of Basal cell carcinoma. *Ann Dermatol.* 2011;23(suppl 1):S36–S40.

48. Kimonis VE, Mehta SG, Digiovanna JJ, et al. Radiological features in 82 patients with nevoid basal cell carcinoma (NBCC or Gorlin) syndrome. *Genet Med.* 2004;6:495–502.

49. Amlashi SF, Riffaud L, Brassier G, et al. Nevoid basal cell carcinoma syndrome: Relation with desmoplastic medulloblastoma in infancy. A population-based study and review of the literature. *Cancer.* 2003;98:618–624.

50. Mohtasham N, Nemati S, Jamshidi S, et al. Odontogenic keratocysts in nevoid basal cell carcinoma syndrome: A case report. *Cases J.* 2009;2:9399.

51. Ball A, Wenning J, Van Eyk N. Ovarian fibromas in pediatric patients with basal cell nevus (Gorlin) syndrome. *J Pediatr Adolesc Gynecol.* 2011;24:e5–e7.

52. Bossert T, Walther T, Vondrys D, et al. Cardiac fibroma as an inherited manifestation of nevoid basal-cell carcinoma syndrome. *Tex Heart Inst J.* 2006;33:88–90.

53. Bree AF, Shah MR. Consensus statement from the first international colloquium on basal cell nevus syndrome (BCNS). *Am J Med Genet A.* 2011;155A:2091–2097.

54. Takahashi C, Kanazawa N, Yoshikawa Y, et al. Germline PTCH1 mutations in Japanese basal cell nevus syndrome patients. *J Hum Genet.* 2009;54:403–408.

55. Casaroto AR, Loures DC, Moreschi E, et al. Early diagnosis of Gorlin-Goltz syndrome: Case report. *Head Face Med.* 2011;7:2.

56. Morse CB, McLaren JF, Roy D, et al. Ovarian preservation in a young patient with Gorlin syndrome and multiple bilateral ovarian masses. *Fertil Steril.* 2011;96:e47–e50.

57. Boyd KP, Korf BR, Theos A. Neurofibromatosis type 1. *J Am Acad Dermatol.* 2009;61:1–14.

58. Yohay K. Neurofibromatosis types 1 and 2. *Neurologist.* 2006;12:86–93.

59. Radtke HB, Sebold CD, Allison C, et al. Neurofibromatosis type 1 in genetic counseling practice: Recommendations of the National Society of Genetic Counselors. *J Genet Couns.* 2007;16:387–407.

60. Ahmad S, ed. Neurodegenerative Diseases. Vol. 724. Landes Bioscience and Springer Science+Business Media; 2012.

61. Patil S, Chamberlain RS. Neoplasms associated with germline and somatic NF1 gene mutations. *Oncologist.* 2012;17:101–116.

62. Kossler N, Stricker S, Rödelsperger C, et al. Neurofibromin (Nf1) is required for skeletal muscle development. *Hum Mol Genet.* 2011;20:2697–2709.

63. Friedman J. Neurofibromatosis 1. June 2, 2009. Available at: http://www.ncbi.nlm.nih.gov/books/NBK1109/. Accessed March 6, 2012.

64. Ardern-Holmes SL, North KN. Therapeutics for childhood neurofibromatosis type 1 and type 2. *Curr Treat Options Neurol.* 2011;13:529–543.

65. Ponder MMF, Hallowell N, Statham H, et al. Genetic counseling, reproductive behavior and future reproductive intentions of people with neurofibromatosis type 1 (NF1). *J Genet Couns.* 1998;7:331–344.

66. Evans DG. Neurofibromatosis type 2 (NF2): A clinical and molecular review. *Orphanet J Rare Dis.* 2009;4:16.

67. Goutagny S, Kalamarides M. Meningiomas and neurofibromatosis. *J Neurooncol.* 2010;99:341–347.

68. Baser ME, Friedman JM, Joe H, et al. Empirical development of improved diagnostic criteria for neurofibromatosis 2. *Genet Med.* 2011;13:576–581.

69. Evans DG, Raymond FL, Barwell JG, et al. Genetic testing and screening of individuals at risk of NF2. *Clin Genet.* 2012;82:416–424. doi: 10.1111/j.1399-0004.2011.01816.x.

Gene Index

Gene	Page(s)	Cancer Site
APC	111	Colon (Polyposis Syndromes)
BMPR1A	111	Colon (Polyposis Syndromes)
	167	Stomach
BRCA1	71	Breast
	93	Ovary
	133	Uterus
	157	Pancreas
	167	Stomach
BRCA2	71	Breast
	93	Ovary
	133	Uterus
	157	Pancreas
	167	Stomach
CDH1	71	Breast
	167	Stomach
CDK4	203	Skin
CDKN2A	157	Pancreas
	203	Skin
CTFR	157	Pancreas
CTRC	157	Pancreas
EPCAM	93	Ovary
	133	Uterus
	167	Stomach
FH	133	Uterus
	143	Urinary Tract
FLCN	143	Urinary Tract
MEN1	187	Endocrine System
MEN2	187	Endocrine System
MLH1	93	Ovary
	125	Colon (Nonpolyposis Syndromes)
	133	Uterus
	143	Urinary Tract
	167	Stomach
MSH2	93	Ovary
	125	Colon (Nonpolyposis Syndromes)

Syndrome Index

Term Index